Introduction to Evidence-Based Practice

A PRACTICAL GUIDE FOR NURSING

DavisPlus...
Online Resource Center

DavisPlus is your online source for a wealth of learning resources and teaching tools, as well as electronic and mobile versions of our products.

STUDENTS

Unlimited FREE access.
No password.
No registration.
No fee.

INSTRUCTORS

Upon Adoption.
Password-protected library of title-specific, online course content.

Visit http://davisplus.fadavis.com

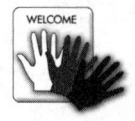 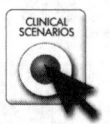  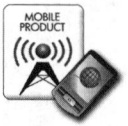  

Explore more online resources from F.A.Davis...

DAVIS'S DRUG GUIDE.com
powered by
Unbound Medicine®

www.drugguide.com
is Davis's Drug Guide Online, the complete Davis's Drug Guide for Nurses® database of over 1,100 monographs on the web.

Taber's Online
powered by
Unbound Medicine®

www.tabersonline.com
delivers the power of Taber's Cyclopedic Medical Dictionary on the web. Find more than 60,000 terms, 1,000 images, and more.

DAVIS'S Laboratory and Diagnostic Tests with Nursing Implications
powered by
Unbound Medicine®

www.LabDxTest.com
is the complete database for Davis's Comprehensive Handbook of Laboratory and Diagnostic Tests with Nursing Implications online. Access hundreds of detailed monographs.

www.FADavis.com

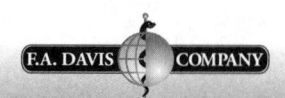

Introduction to Evidence-Based Practice

A PRACTICAL GUIDE FOR NURSING

Lisa Hopp, PhD, RN
Professor, Nursing and Director
Indiana Center for Evidence Based Nursing
Practice: A Collaborating Centre of the
Joanna Briggs Institute
Purdue University Calumet
Hammond, Indiana

Leslie Rittenmeyer, PsyD, RN, CNE
Professor, Nursing and Deputy Director
Indiana Center for Evidence Based Nursing
Practice: A Collaborating Centre of the
Joanna Briggs Institute
Purdue University Calumet
Hammond, Indiana

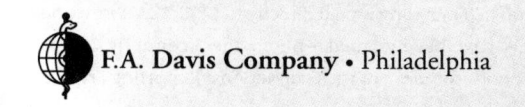
F.A. Davis Company • Philadelphia

F.A. Davis Company
1915 Arch Street
Philadelphia, PA 19103
www.fadavis.com

Printed in the United States of America

Last digit indicates print number: 10 9 8 7 6 5 4 3 2

Publisher, Nursing: Joanne Patzek DaCunha
Director of Content Development: Darlene D. Pedersen
Project Editor: Elizabeth Hart
Illustration and Design Manager: Carolyn O'Brien

As new scientific information becomes available through basic and clinical research, recommended treatments and drug therapies undergo changes. The author(s) and publisher have done everything possible to make this book accurate, up to date, and in accord with accepted standards at the time of publication. The author(s), editors, and publisher are not responsible for errors or omissions or for consequences from application of the book, and make no warranty, expressed or implied, in regard to the contents of the book. Any practice described in this book should be applied by the reader in accordance with professional standards of care used in regard to the unique circumstances that may apply in each situation. The reader is advised always to check product information (package inserts) for changes and new information regarding dose and contraindications before administering any drug. Caution is especially urged when using new or infrequently ordered drugs.

Library of Congress Cataloging-in-Publication Data
Hopp, Lisa, 1956-
 Introduction to evidence-based practice : a practical guide for nursing / Lisa Hopp, Leslie Rittenmeyer. — 1st ed.
       p. ; cm.
Includes bibliographical references and index.
ISBN 978-0-8036-2328-6 (pbk. : alk. paper)
I. Rittenmeyer, Leslie. II. Title.
[DNLM: 1. Evidence-Based Nursing. 2. Models, Nursing. 3. Nursing Process. WY 100.7]

610.73—dc23

                              2011043019

For my mate, Eric, who inspires me to think big; for my parents, who taught me to work hard; for my girls, who are my reason to be; and for patients, who are the reason we nurse.

-LH

This book is dedicated to my husband Dennis, who worries that I spend too much time on my computer; our family, who sustains me; and to nurses at the bedside, who are heroic in their everyday work.

-LR

FOREWORD

Pressure ulcers, catheter-acquired urinary tract infections, falls, safe medication administration, and many other health problems are universal. As I interact with nurses, physicians, physiotherapists, and other health-care providers across the world, I am struck by the commonness of our problems and our desire to improve outcomes. Our cultures, contexts, and worldviews certainly vary; remarkably, we can share the same body of evidence. The way we use the evidence and how patients respond and experience their health are unique.

In this book, you will learn how to use the evidence-based practice process to provide the best nursing care possible in your local context. You will find that evidence-based practice is not merely an interesting academic exercise that you just "get through" in your undergraduate studies. Rather, you will learn how evidence informs the practical, everyday actions that you take on behalf of your patients.

Drs. Hopp and Rittenmeyer have written the book in any easy-to-read and pragmatic way. You will quickly understand how to begin using evidence to make the best decisions for your nursing practice. The authors intend that any nurse or student can use the book to get started with evidence. I particularly like that each chapter begins with a clinical story that you will likely connect to your own practice. These stories illustrate how practical and fundamental it is to have the right knowledge for the right patient at the right time.

You are busy clinicians, thinking on your feet. This book is meant to help you think in action but use the best available evidence with your clinical expertise to make decisions incorporating your patients' preferences and values. The time has come for a book that allows clinicians and students to learn about evidence-based practice in a straightforward, clear, and uncluttered manner.

Alan Pearson RN, ONC, DipNEd, MSc, PhD, FRCNA, FCN, FAAG, FRCN
Executive Director
The Joanna Briggs Institute

We conceptualized this text around the belief that nurses want what is best for their patients. Through our work in the evidence-based practice movement, we have come to learn that this is not always a simple endeavor. The rapid explosion of information and its sources has contributed to the complexity of practicing in a way that yields desirable outcomes. In order to access, appraise, and utilize the available information, students and practicing nurses alike need to learn first about evidence-based practice. In this book, we present the elemental principles that demystify the process in a way that is easily accessible and excites passion for patient care. We are keenly aware that there is significant need for nurses to gain a global perspective in order to truly find and implement the best available evidence. We believe this book provides that perspective as well.

We intend that clinicians and students will find the book useful. Its aim is to present a comprehensive survey of evidence-based nursing practice that faculty can use throughout an undergraduate curriculum and clinical educators can use throughout a staff development program. Our goal is to provide information that is thorough yet concise and practical for clinicians, students, and faculty. Each chapter begins with a clinical story that serves as a real-world illustration of evidence-based practice in action.

We have designed the material to be flexible. Educators may use the book across a curriculum or program as learning about evidence-based practice unfolds. Alternatively, they may use it as the primary text for a course focused on evidence-based practice. We also believe this book could be valuable for any practicing nurses who want to learn the basic principles of evidence-based nursing practice.

In Unit I, we set the stage by addressing the basic questions of what evidence-based nursing practice is, how it makes a difference, and where evidence comes from. We present a global perspective in terms of both the history of evidence-based practice and appropriate sources of evidence. In Unit II, we address a sample of pragmatic models and framework of evidence-based practice. We emphasize that models help structure the process of making changes in practice. We have picked models that help individual nurses or systems transfer evidence into everyday nursing practice. Unit III deconstructs the evidence-based process from asking a question through evaluation. Using Hayes's "5As" structure, we align evidence-based practice and the nursing process. Finally, in Unit IV, we put it all together in examples of the entire evidence-based practice process in nursing specialty areas. Each chapter is structured in a parallel fashion to illustrate how evidence-based practice can address a nurse-sensitive outcome. These chapters integrate the evidence-based practice process from problem recognition to outcome evaluation and quality improvement.

It is our hope that we have constructed a book that has utility in the beginning, middle, and end of an undergraduate curriculum or staff development program. We intend that it will remain not on bookshelves but in the hands of students and nurses as a useful resource for basic information about evidence-based practice.

CONTRIBUTORS

Michelle Block, RN, MS, PhD(c)
Assistant Professor, Nursing
Purdue University Calumet
Hammond, Indiana

Marsha Ellett, PhD, RN
Professor, Department of Family
  Health
School of Nursing
Indiana University
Indianapolis, Indiana

Peggy Gerard, PhD, RN
Dean, School of Nursing
Purdue University Calumet
Hammond, Indiana

Dolores Huffman, RN, PhD
Associate Professor, Nursing
Purdue University Calumet
Hammond, Indiana

Ellen Moore, DNP, RN, FNP-BC
Professor, Nursing
Purdue University Calumet
Hammond, Indiana

Cheryl Moredich, RN, MS
Associate Professor, Nursing
Purdue University Calumet
Hammond, Indiana

**Alan Pearson, RN, ONC, DipNED,
MSc, PhD, FRCNA, FCN, FAAG,
FRCN**
Professor of Evidence-Based Health
  Care
University of Adelaide
Executive Director
Joanna Briggs Institute
Adelaide, South Australia

Beth Vottero, PhD, RN, CNE
Assistant Professor, Nursing
Purdue University Calumet
Hammond, Indiana

Jane Walker, PhD, RN
Associate Professor, Nursing
Purdue University Calumet
Hammond, Indiana

Kim Whalen, MLIS
Assistant Professor of Library Services
Valparaiso University
Valparaiso, Indiana

REVIEWERS

Sharon Abbate, EdD, MS, BSN, RN
Assistant Professor, College of Nursing
University of St. Francis
Joliet, Illinois

Sherry Abel, RN, BSN,MS
Assistant Professor
South University
Tampa, Florida

Faisal H. Aboul-Enein, DrPH, RN, MSN, MPH, NP, BC
Clinical Assistant Professor
Texas Woman's University,
College of Nursing
Houston Texas

Betty Abraham-Settles, RN, MSN
Nursing Instructor
University of South Carolina Aiken
Aiken, South Carolina

Judith Alexander, RN, DNS
Associate Professor
Armstrong Atlantic State University
Savannah, Georgia

Donna Bailey, PhD
Part-time, Adjunct Instructor
School of Nursing at Thomas Edison
  State College
Trenton, New Jersey

Karen S. Benjamin, RN, MSN
Assistant Lecturer
RN-BSN Distance Learning Degree
  Program
University of Wyoming,
Fay W. Whitney School of Nursing
Laramie, Wyoming

Sara Berger, MSN, RN-BC
Assistant Professor
Medcenter One College of Nursing
Bismarck, North Dakota

Tracy L. Brewer, DNP, RNC
Assistant Professor
Wright State University
Dayton, Ohio

Tammy Buchholz, MSN, RN
Assistant Professor
Medcenter One College of Nursing
Bismarck, North Dakota

Margaret Bultas, PhD, RN, CPNP-PC
Assistant Professor
Goldfarb School of Nursing at Barnes
  Jewish College
St. Louis, Missouri

Mary P. Curtis, PhD, RN, ANP-C
Associate Professor of Nursing
Goldfarb School of Nursing at Barnes
  Jewish College
St. Louis, Missouri

Laurie Doerner, RN, MSN
Assistant Professor/Nursing
Oral Roberts University,
Anna Vaughn College of Nursing
Tulsa, Oklahoma

Susan M. Eley, PhD, FNP-BC
Assistant Professor
Indiana State University
Terre Haute, Indiana

Roseanne Fairchild, PhD, RN
Assistant Professor of Nursing
Indiana State University
Terre Haute, Indiana

Dale B. Gressle, MSN, RN
Assistant Professor
Cabarrus College of Health Sciences
Concord, North Carolina

**Kristen Jones, BScN, RN,
MPH(N), PhD student**
Lecturer
Lakehead University
Thunder Bay, Ontario, Canada

**Jane M. Langemeier, RN, MSN,
PhD**
Assistant Professor
Clarkson College of Nursing
Omaha, Nebraska

**Barbara J. Lockwood, PhD,
RN, CNE**
Associate Professor and MSN
  Coordinator
Aurora University
Aurora, Illinois

**Violet Malinski, PhD, MA,
BSN, RN**
Associate Professor
Hunter College School of Nursing
New York, New York

Laura Mallett, MSN, RN
Assistant Lecturer
University of Wyoming
Laramie, Wyoming

Cindy Manning, RN, MSN
Professor
Blinn Collge
Bryan, Texas

Joan McCleish, RN, PhD
Dean of Institutional Research,
  Assessment, Distance Ed
Mercy College of Health Sciences
Des Moines, Iowa

Anne McNamara, RN, PhD
Dean and Professor
Grand Canyon University
Phoenix, Arizona

**Carmella M. Moran, PhD, MSN,
BSN, RN**
Director, School of Nursing
Aurora University
Aurora, Illinois

Gayle Preheim, EdD
Program Coordinator
University of Colorado, Denver
College of Nursing
Aurora, Colorado

Wanda Rose, PhD, RN, BC
Associate Professor
Medcenter One College of Nursing
Bismarck, North Dakota

Linda M. Schultz, PhD, CRRN
Assistant Professor
Maryville University
St. Louis, Missouri

**Margo L Thompson, RN, MA,
MSN, EdD, CNE**
Nursing Faculty Coordinator/Academic
  Advisor
Webster University
Kansas City, Missouri

**Patricia Vermeersch, PhD,
GNP-BC**
Associate Professor
Wright State University
Dayton, Ohio

Jennie Wagner, MS
Professor
University of North Carolina at
  Chapel Hill
Chapel Hill, North Carolina

Diane Wilhite, RN, MSN
Nursing Instructor
Wallace State Community College
Hanceville, Alabama

ACKNOWLEDGMENTS

Many people have supported us throughout the writing of this book. We have the good fortune to work with colleagues whom we look forward to seeing every day and who make our days at the university seem like working from home.

If we spend a bit too much time at work, it is because of the commitment and friendships we share with our fellow faculty at Purdue University Calumet. We are particularly thankful for Dean Peggy Gerard's support, whose leadership earns our school the highest respect of our university colleagues and whose friendship we treasure.

To our contributors, Jane Walker, Dee Huffman, Beth Vottero, Cheryl Moredich, Peggy Gerard, Michelle Block, Kim Whalen, Marsha Ellet, and Alan Pearson, we thank you for your willingness to contribute your stories, scholarly work, and collegiality. Your individual perspectives and unique talents added dimension and depth to the book.

At F.A. Davis, we would like to thank Jonathan Joyce for getting us started and keeping us focused on our audience. Our editors Joanne DaCunha, Beth LoGuidice, and Liz Hart have kept us moving forward with the persistent kindness and nudging of gentlewomen.

Finally, we acknowledge our global colleagues within the Joanna Briggs Collaboration and Institute for their commitment to improve the health of people in every nation through evidence-based practice.

CONTENTS

Background and Context
What Is Evidence-Based Practice and Who Cares?

This unit sets the stage for learning about evidence-based practice. In Chapter 1 you will learn the history of evidence-based practice worldwide and its progress in the United States. In Chapter 2, you will learn how to carefully define evidence-based practice by understanding each of its key elements and how it makes a difference in everyday clinical nursing practice. In Chapter 3, a global leader in evidence-based practice will discuss the importance of global thinking and use of international evidence. These chapters are fundamental to understanding how evidence-based practice fits in your clinical practice as well as nurses' practice worldwide. Each chapter begins with a clinical story, and the story unfolds throughout each chapter. This will help you connect new concepts with clinical practice.

CHAPTER 1

Professional Nursing and Evidence-Based Practice

Lisa Hopp

- Define *evidence-based practice* in the context professional nursing.
- Defend the importance of using evidence to make professional nursing decisions.
- Differentiate clinical decisions based on nursing traditions from those based on evidence.
- Describe how evidence-based practice evolved from research utilization.

Agency for Healthcare Research and Quality (AHRQ)
Bibliographic databases
Centers for Medicare and Medicaid Services (CMS)
Cochrane Collaboration
Conduct and Utilization of Research in Nursing (CURN) Project
Cumulative Index of Nursing and Allied Health Literature (CINAHL)
Evidence-based practice

Institute of Medicine (IOM)
Joanna Briggs Institute (JBI)
Medical Literature Analysis and Retrieval System (MEDLINE)
National Guideline Clearinghouse
Nursing traditions
Randomized controlled trial (RCT)
Research utilization
Western Interstate Commission on Higher Education (WICHE) Project

Clinical Story

It is 10:00 p.m. Maria is caring for a 50-year-old female patient who had abdominal surgery about 8 hours ago. Maria also has four other postsurgical patients assigned to her. She enters the room to assess the patient's vital signs and comfort level and to check her abdominal wound dressing. She sees that the patient has an IV catheter for fluid and medications and an indwelling urinary catheter. The patient tells Maria that her pain level is 5/10 and that she is reluctant to move around because "it hurts too much."

Maria knows that the patient's pain control is a priority and that abdominal surgery patients typically receive IV fluids until they are ready to drink fluids by mouth. The urinary catheter is a convenient and accurate way to measure urine output, and the patient does not have to get up to go to the bathroom as frequently when she has significant surgical pain. Conversely, Maria wonders if she should remove the urinary catheter because it poses a risk for infection. She decides to ask a more senior nurse about discontinuing the catheter.

The senior nurse tells Maria that in the past, they usually left the catheter in until the patient could get up to go to the bathroom easily. However, the surgical floor recently piloted a new evidence-based policy in which nurses discontinue the urinary catheter as soon as the patient is alert enough to urinate on her own or at midnight, whichever comes first. Maria asks the senior nurse if she thinks there are any risks to taking the catheter out now. The senior nurse says that she really has not given it much thought and that she is in the habit of leaving it in until the patient is up and about regularly.

When Maria returns to the room, she and the patient discuss the option of taking the catheter out to avoid the chance of infection, and Maria explains that the patient will need to get out of bed to void. The patient states that she would not want an infection and would ask for pain medication if she needed it. Weighing all of the information, Maria discontinues the catheter and requests that the patient ask for help the first time she needs to void. ■

Introduction

When nurses begin their day, they face many decisions. They decide when and how to assess their patients. They use what they learn from their assessment and the patient's desires to plan mutually determined goals. As expert nurses plan, they choose which interventions will most likely help them meet these goals. In other words, they use the nursing process to do what is best for their patients. Evidence-based practice is concerned with how to make these everyday decisions using the best available evidence from research, professional nursing expertise, and the patient's preferences.

What Is Evidence-Based Practice?

Evidence-based practice is about doing what works and doing it the right way to achieve the best possible patient outcomes (Muir-Gray, 1997, p. 18). More formally, it is "the conscientious, explicit, and judicious use of current best evidence in making decisions about the care of individual patients. . . . [It] means integrating individual clinical expertise with the best available external clinical evidence from systematic research" (Sackett, Rosenberg, Muir-Gray, et al., 1996, 71). Nursing leaders in evidence-based practice have adapted this definition to include four components that influence decisions: (1) the best available research evidence, (2) clinical expertise, (3) resources, and (4) patient preferences (DiCenso, Cullum, and Ciliska, 1998; Muir-Gray, 1997).

Each part of this definition is important. First, "conscientious, explicit and judicious" means that nurses think carefully, weigh their use of information, and are able to tell others why they use the information. "Current best evidence" implies that someone must first thoroughly search and then judge the quality of the information to determine if the evidence is indeed the best that is available. In other words, the definition indicates that nurses do not use any evidence that happens to be handy. Rather, they find and choose the highest quality information. When professional nurses make evidence-based decisions about individual patients, they also incorporate what they know from their clinical experience and past practices. However, clinical expertise means something different from **nursing traditions,** or, more simply, doing what you always do for no other reason than habit. Clinical expertise requires being able to tell others what you know, thinking about what you know, talking about what you know, and asking others to critique what you know; clinical expertise is practical know-how that someone else validates (Rycroft-Malone, Seers, Titchen, et al., 2004). Professional nurses incorporate patient preferences to morally and ethically provide care. Although much remains to be learned about how best to incorporate patient desires into clinical decisions, patient preferences include both what individuals prefer, and what groups within a community prefer (Rycroft-Malone, Seers, et al., 2004). Finally, the component "available resources" refers to the reality of limited health-care dollars, human resource challenges such as adequate nurse–patient ratios, and the availability of technology. Perhaps the most complex aspect of evidence-based decision making is how to weigh the benefit, harms, and costs of providing the best care.

In this chapter's clinical story, Maria did what many nurses do first—she asked someone whose opinion she valued. Maria discovered that although this nurse had many years of experience, she admitted that she had not given the issue much thought and that habit influenced her practice. Although Maria's colleague had certainly cared for many patients with a urinary catheter, her practical know-how would not hold up to scrutiny or critique if she can justify this particular practice only because "that's the way she has always done it." Maria was right to pursue the issue further by examining the policy for the evidence that supports the recommendation to discontinue the catheter. In addition, she included patient preference in the decision, having offered the patient information about best practice and risks.

As you learn more about evidence-based practice, remember that it is like a three-legged stool where the best available evidence from research, clinical expertise, and patient preferences support the best patient outcomes within a context of limited resources.

Why Is Evidence-Based Practice Important?

Rycroft-Malone, Buchnall, and Melnyk (2004) boldly stated, "One of the most prominent themes ever to characterize international health care is evidence-based practice" (p. 1). In the United States, many organizations, governments, regulators, and patients are calling for health-care providers to practice using evidence. Logic would indicate that the best, most current, information should inform nursing decisions. However, published studies about the effectiveness of using research in practice shows only modest improvements in patient outcomes. One study showed an overall 28% improvement in patient outcomes when nurses used research rather than standard interventions (Cheater, Becker, and Olson, 1988). Because this evidence is not current and the authors conducted the study before the evidence-based practice movement began, it is time to revisit the issue of the effectiveness of using evidence in practice. It is very clear that evidence-based practice is here to stay, and most experts believe that when nurses use evidence to inform their decisions, patient outcomes will be the best they can be (Box 1■1).

Nurse scientists have been producing research since nursing's earliest days. Although the number of research studies continues to grow, there are still relatively few studies about how best to use this research. The general public may believe that as soon as scientists discover something that improves patient outcomes, health-care providers quickly adopt this new information. Unfortunately, new knowledge does not transfer quickly or easily, and a great deal of geographic variation exists in the United States (Institute of Medicine of the National Academies [IOM], 2008). Furthermore, treatments that evidence shows are effective are still not consistently used. For example, the Dartmouth Atlas Project showed that, even among highly rated hospitals,

---

BOX 1■1   Significance of Evidence-Based Practice

- International importance
- Large, regional variations in use of evidence-based practices
- Rapid development of research but slow adoption of evidence-based practices
- Only about half of all patients in the United States receive recommended care
- There is a 28% improvement rate in patient outcomes when nurses use interventions based on research versus standard care
- "Pay-for-performance" requires that evidence-based practices are used
- "Know-do gap" keeps patients from receiving the best care

only 40% to 83% of patients had beta blockers (a highly effective medicine that helps protect the heart from another heart attack and decreases sudden death and other causes of mortality) prescribed at discharge after having a heart attack (Wennberg, 2002). Evidence-based practice aims to speed up the transfer of new knowledge into everyday practice.

A Brief History of Evidence-Based Practice

In some ways, evidence-based practice is nothing new. But since the 1990s, evidence-based practice has become a major movement in how nurses and all health professionals think about making clinical decisions. Florence Nightingale was one of the first nurses to advocate for health-care workers to create, interpret, and use research findings to give the best care. She understood the scientific method, statistics, and epidemiology, and she tried to influence health ministers to make better use of data they collected to improve health (McDonald, 2001). However, it was not until nurses were adequately educated and could fund research that findings were available to use.

In the 1970s, nursing leaders focused on a process called **research utilization.** Estabrooks (1999) defined *research utilization* as a "complex process in which knowledge, in this case in the form of research, is transformed from the findings of one or more studies into possible nursing interventions, the ultimate goal of which is use in practice" (p. 204). Today we consider evidence-based practice as an umbrella term that includes research utilization. Two big national projects in the United States were the **Conduct and Utilization of Research in Nursing (CURN) Project** and the **Western Interstate Commission on Higher Education (WICHE) Project.** Their goal was to increase the use of research by improving how nurses evaluated research. These projects helped nurses improve their appraisal skills and appropriate use of individual pieces of research. But these efforts predated our understanding that single studies rarely provide an adequate answer and the syntheses of many studies provide stronger evidence. The importance of patient preferences and clinical expertise are now stressed as part of the equation of best practice.

Some 80 years after Nightingale's frustration with how decision makers ignored the evidence, British epidemiologist and physician Archie Cochrane shocked the medical community when he publically complained that physicians did not pay attention to evidence when they made clinical decisions (Cochrane Collaboration, n.d.). Like Nightingale, he saw that many infant deaths could have been prevented if only physicians made decisions based on many large, rigorous studies. Although he died before his idea became a reality, in 1992 the **Cochrane Collaboration** established its first collection of research trials on the health of mothers and babies. Cochrane emphasized that a particular type of study, the **randomized controlled trial (RCT),** was the best way to test whether an intervention works. An RCT is an experiment using human beings in which the investigator randomly assigns participants in the trial to either a treatment or control (no treatment) group. It is now considered the gold standard of effectiveness in research because it balances other confounding influences between groups and allows the researcher to link cause (treatment or control) with the effect (clinical outcome). This idea still guides the work of the Cochrane Collaboration, and its library of reviews of international evidence is regarded as one of the premier primary sources of evidence about the effectiveness of interventions, particularly for medicine (Cochrane Collaboration, n.d.).

Although the Cochrane Library contains some evidence that is directly related to the effects of nursing interventions, another organization is aimed at evidence more directly related to nursing and nurse midwifery. In 1996, Alan Pearson and colleagues founded the **Joanna Briggs Institute (JBI)** in Adelaide, South Australia (Jordan, Donnelly, and Pittman, 2006). Like that of the Cochrane Collaboration, JBI's purpose is to develop a worldwide collaboration to address global health priorities through synthesis and dissemination of systematic reviews of evidence. The founders took a broader view of what constitutes legitimate evidence, including findings from many kinds of rigorous research, experience, and expertise. In addition, JBI focuses on all aspects of evidence-based practice, not only the summary of evidence. The collaboration now includes centers and members distributed throughout the world, representing diverse populations. The work of the institute and collaborating centers continues its strong focus on nursing and nurse midwifery but also embraces multiple health-care disciplines (Jordan et al., 2006).

In the United States, evidence-based practice efforts at the federal level have come from the **Agency for Healthcare Research and Quality (AHRQ),** which is considered the nerve center of evidence-based practice activity in the United States. In 1997, the AHRQ began awarding 5-year contracts to evidence-based practice centers in the United States and Canada for the production of technology assessment; health reports; and systematic reviews that have particular clinical, social, or economic importance. The agency also manages the **National Guideline Clearinghouse,** which is an online collection of guidelines for clinical practice. Many nurses rely on this resource for evidence-based guidelines, and it is particularly important when searching for practice guidelines. The user needs to be a good consumer of this and any information called evidence based. Many organizations may develop guidelines about the same health problem; therefore, you may find many guidelines about certain topics and no guidelines about others. Another important organization that has had a deep impact on evidence-based practice in the United States is the **Institute of Medicine (IOM).** The IOM is a nongovernmental organization within the National Academies of Science; its job is to study and advise about all scientific matters, including health. It is highly regarded because of the way it studies problems and holds open, public meetings during deliberations.

The IOM has published a series of reports about the safety of patients and the quality of health care in the United States. These reports have caused many in the United States to take notice of the imbalance between what it spent on health care, compared with the outcomes. In one report, authors estimated that only about 55% of Americans receive recommended care, that inadequate care resulted in 18,000 unnecessary deaths annually from heart attacks, and, on average, that 17 years pass before a new discovery becomes routine practice (IOM, 2003). Because of these reports, the IOM and other organizations have called for significant changes to accelerate the integration of evidence into practice.

Are U.S. Nurses Ready for Evidence-Based Practice?

Many agencies and groups are requiring nurses and other health-care professionals to use evidence to support their decisions. Accrediting groups, such as the Joint Commission, and payers such as the **Centers for Medicare and Medicaid Services (CMS),** the federal agency that administers Medicare and monitors Medicaid programs offered by states, require hospitals to demonstrate that evidence informs their policies. The focus on patient safety has shown a spotlight on evidence-based practice. In 2008, CMS denied payment for certain hospital-acquired conditions that could have been prevented if the health-care team used evidence-based practices (Centers for Medicare and Medicaid Services [CMS], 2009). Many of these conditions are highly sensitive to nursing care. For example, in the clinical story, Maria could insert, manage, and decide when to discontinue her patient's short-term urinary catheters. If a Medicare patient in a hospital acquires a urinary tract infection after the catheter is inserted, then the hospital will not receive any reimbursement related to the infection. Researchers have estimated the cost of this type of infection could range from $839 to $4693 (1997 U.S. dollars), depending on how severe the infection becomes (Karchmer, Giannetta, Muto, et al., 2000). More patients can die, and lengths of stay can be longer, adding to cost (Chant, Smith, Marshall, et al., 2011). This "Pay-for-performance" incentive and other pressures have motivated hospitals to increase capacity and to use evidence-based practice. Ultimately, these incentives may stimulate support for nurses to enable them to use evidence in their everyday practice.

The call for evidence-based practice is strong, but are nurses in the United States ready to respond? Schools of nursing are working hard to prepare their graduates to use evidence to make clinical decisions (Box 1■2). Prior to the 1990s, graduates of baccalaureate programs may have been somewhat prepared to use individual reports of research. More commonly, students learned practices steeped in traditions, learning the profession while in their clinical courses or through what they read in textbooks. In 2005, Pravikoff, Tanner, and Pierce found that nurses in the United States lacked many of the fundamental skills and resources needed for evidence-based practice (Pravikoff et al., 2005). For example, when nurses search for evidence, they need to know how to use **bibliographic databases** in which the health-care literature is indexed. Nearly 75% of respondents had never searched the **Cumulative Index of Nursing and Allied Health Literature (CINAHL),** the primary bibliographic database for nursing research, and nearly as many (58%) had never searched **Medical Literature Analysis and Retrieval System (MEDLINE),** the primary bibliographic database for medicine and other health professions. In addition, most did not seek the help of a librarian (83%) or the hospital's library (82%). Even if they did know how to use the databases, only about half of the respondents thought they had access to the Internet. The investigators also asked about barriers (other than time) that prevented them from using evidence. Many of the top individual barriers related to knowledge and skills in finding, understanding, and analyzing research, and some respondents lacked access to a computer or library. Top institutional barriers included higher priorities, staffing, budget, and training challenges, and the feeling that evidence-based practice was not possible "in the real world."

BOX 1■2   **Interdisciplinary Rounds**

Evidence-based practice is not unique to nursing. All health-related fields—medicine, physiotherapy, pharmacy, dentistry—are becoming evidence based. Evidence-based practice can provide a common language and path to pursue best practices with other disciplines.

Example:

When designing an evidence-based protocol to discontinue urinary catheters as soon as possible after surgery, nurses would consider evidence from the Centers for Disease Control and Prevention and international practice guidelines. They would need to collaborate with infectious disease specialists, urologists, surgeons, and other physicians to develop a policy that is acceptable to the local providers yet consistent with the best available evidence.

To negotiate the process successfully, the lead nurses would need to be able to find, evaluate, and interpret the best available evidence and to advocate for the integration of patient preferences.

These challenges may seem overwhelming, but the emphasis on evidence-based practice in all disciplines will surely bring progress to how we improve skills, provide resources, and bridge the "know-do" gap (Box 1■3). The rest of this book is aimed at demystifying evidence-based practice so that students and practicing nurses can do what works and what is right for patients.

■ Summary

Evidence-based practice is more than using research. Maria, the new nurse in the clinical story, made a decision to discontinue the patient's catheter; she used evidence

BOX 1■3   **Tools for Learning and Practice**

- Search the Internet for the Cochrane Collaboration and the Joanna Briggs Institute. Explore the sites and bookmark for future use.
- Search the Internet for the Agency for Healthcare Research and Quality (AHRQ); explore and bookmark. Search the site for the "patient safety handbook for nurses" and bookmark for future use.
- Use Google or another search engine to search for the phrase "evidence-based practice." Explore the sites and bookmark for later evaluation of their usefulness and genuineness.

from research and the patient's preferences, and reconsidered her unit's nursing traditions. In her conversation with the senior nurse, Maria discovered that even though this nurse had several years of experience, she admitted that she had not thought about this common, basic decision. By acting to prevent a complication, Maria also helped avoid costs that the hospital may not have recovered if the patient developed an infection because of the catheter. This scenario illustrates that the best practice can and should be a combination of the best available evidence (the evidence-based policy), the patient's desires, and a reexamination of traditions. The definition of evidence-based practice as a three-legged stool points to using particular types of information to guide practice, and acknowledges that expert knowledge gained from experience and from patients is important to making good clinical decisions.

The Cochrane Collaboration and the Joanna Briggs Institute have led international efforts to develop libraries of the best available evidence and tools for evidence implementation. Even though nurses in the United States may report that they do not possess some of the basic skills needed for using evidence in their practice, many governmental and nongovernmental agencies are calling for better safety and quality outcomes through the use of best available research evidence. Schools of nursing, students, and practicing nurses need to work together to meet the challenge of informing all aspects of patient care with evidence, not habit and tradition.

CHAPTER QUESTIONS

1. Define *evidence-based practice.*

2. What factors have contributed to making evidence-based practice a prominent theme in the United States and abroad?

3. What are the Cochrane Collaboration and the Joanna Briggs Institute?

4. What is the difference between using evidence to inform practice and using traditions to inform clinical decisions? Do you think that nursing traditions have a place in clinical decisions?

5. How do research utilization and evidence-based practice compare?

6. Explain what is meant by the "know-do" gap. Provide an example.

7. Think about a common nursing practice such as bathing. How do you think evidence-based practice might guide how we bathe patients in different situations? Is there a place for evidence-based practice in simple skills such as bathing patients? Why or why not?

References

Centers for Medicare and Medicaid Services (2009, April 15). Hospital acquired infections (present on admission indicator). Retrieved August 17, 2009, from http://www.cms.hhs.gov/HospitalAcqCond/.

Chant, C., Smith, O. M., Marshall, J. C., et al. (2011). Relationship of catheter-associated urinary tract infection to mortality and length of stay in critically ill patients: A systematic review and meta-analysis of observational studies. *Critical Care Medicine, 39,* 1167–1173. doi:10.1097/CCM.0b013e31820a8581

Cheater, B. S., Becker, A. M., & Olson, R. K. (1988). Nursing interventions and patient outcomes: A meta-analysis of studies. *Nursing Research, 37,* 303–307.

Cochrane Collaboration. (n.d.). Chronology of Cochrane Collaboration. Retrieved January 9, 2009, from http://www.cochrane.org/docs/cchronol.htm

DiCenso, A., Cullum, N., & Ciliska, D. (1998). Implementing evidence-based nursing: Some misconceptions. *Evidence-Based Nursing, 1,* 38–39.

Estabrooks, C. A. (1999). The conceptual structure of research utilization. *Research in Nursing and Health, 22,* 203–216.

Institute of Medicine of the National Academies. (2003). *Priority areas for national priority: Transforming health care quality.* Washington, DC: National Academies Press.

Institute of Medicine of the National Academies. (2008). *Knowing what works in health care: A roadmap for the nation.* Washington, DC: National Academies Press.

Jordan, Z., Donnelly, P., & Pittman, E. (2006). *A short history of a big idea: The Joanna Briggs Institute 1996–2006.* Melbourne: Ausmed Publications.

Karchmer, T. B., Giannetta, E. T., Muto, C. A., et al. (2000). A randomized crossover study of silver-coated urinary catheters in hospitalized patients. *Archives of Internal Medicine, 160,* 3294–3298.

McDonald, L. (2001). Florence Nightingale and the early origins of evidence-based nursing. *Evidence-Based Nursing, 4,* 68–69.

Muir-Gray, J. A. (1997). *Evidence-based health care: How to make health policy and management decisions.* New York: Churchill Livingstone.

Pravikoff, D. S., Tanner, A. B., & Pierce, S. T. (2005). Readiness of U.S. nurses for evidence-based practice. *American Journal of Nursing, 105*(9), 40–51.

Rycroft-Malone, J., Buchnall, T., & Melnyk, B. (2004). [Editorial.] *Worldviews on Evidence-Based Nursing, 1,* 1–2.

Rycroft-Malone, J., Seers, K., Titchen, A., et al. (2004). What counts as evidence in evidence-based practice? *Journal of Advanced Nursing, 47,* 81–90.

Sackett, D. L., Rosenberg, W. M. C., Muir Gray, J. A., et al. (1996). Evidence-based medicine: What it is and what it isn't. *British Medical Journal, 312,* 71–72.

Wennberg, J. E. (2002). Unwarranted variations in healthcare delivery: Implications for academic medical centres. *British Medical Journal, 32,* 961–964.

CHAPTER 2

Elements of Evidence-Based Practice

Leslie Rittenmeyer

- Deconstruct the definition of evidence-based practice down to its core elements.

- Discuss the influence of evidence-based practice toward achieving desired patient outcomes.

- Discuss the meaning of *best available research evidence.*

- Explain a pluralistic approach to sources of evidence.

- Describe how clinical expertise, patient preference, and available resources influence clinical decision making.

Available resources	Meta-analysis
Best available research evidence	Meta-synthesis
	Patient preference
Clinical expertise	Pluralistic approach
Effectiveness	Questions of appropriateness
Expert opinion	Questions of effectiveness
Local data	Questions of feasibility
Meta-aggregation	Questions of meaningfulness

Clinical Story

To fulfill the requirements of their capstone course, senior nursing students Jeni, Maggie, and Henrik have teamed up to do an evidence-based practice project. Even though they have been learning about evidence-based practice throughout their curriculum, they feel their knowledge is somewhat fragmented. Because their project is comprehensive, they realize that they need to bring all the different components of evidence-based practice into a cohesive whole that they understand and apply. They decide as a group to start by deconstructing the definition of *evidence-based practice* to better understand the core elements. As they identify desired outcomes for their project and base them on the best available research evidence, they also need to learn how to use a pluralistic approach when locating the best sources of evidence. As they proceed with their project, they also learn how clinical decision making is influenced by clinical expertise and the preferences and values of the patient within the context of available resources. The group is very excited about this project and realizes going through this process will prepare them to implement the core principles of evidence-based practice when they graduate in just a few short months. ■

Introduction

At first glance, the definition of evidence-based practice (discussed in Chapter 1) does not appear complicated. However, when all of the elements are separated and the words and meaning are pulled apart, one begins to see the complexity. Sometimes, to understand things in their entirety, you have to deconstruct the whole into smaller pieces and then put the pieces back together again, much like a jigsaw puzzle. In doing so, you develop a better understanding of the big picture. When you understand the big picture, it then becomes easier to apply that knowledge to a variety of situations

Components of Evidence-Based Practice

Recall the definition of evidence-based practice from Chapter 1: "the conscientious, explicit and judicious use of current best evidence in making decisions about the care of individualized patients. . . . It means integrating individual clinical expertise with the best available external clinical evidence from systematic research" (Sackett, Rosenberg, Muir-Gray, et al., 1966, p. 971). It is important to realize that the nursing discipline has adapted this definition to include the components of best available research evidence, clinical expertise, resources, and patient preferences (DiCenso, Cullum, and Ciliska, 1998; Muir-Gray, 1997).

Best available research evidence is a term that suggests clinicians use the best evidence available to them to make informed clinical decisions. This is, of course, opposed to making decisions that are *not* based on the best evidence. The complexity of the workplace seldom allows nurses time to search for the latest synthesized evidence, and even if they could, there is such a large amount of information that it would not be a realistic activity. As alluded to in Chapter 1, many clinicians tend to practice using outdated or incomplete knowledge. Things are often done because people have always done them that way. There may be a noticeable gap between evidence and practice. Information becomes outdated quickly, and evidence-based practice attempts to place updated and synthesized information in the clinician's hand. Therefore, the emphasis of evidence-based practice is to bring a synthesis of the external available research evidence to the busy clinician to improve clinical decision making, thereby improving patient outcomes. Without question, clinical expertise, patient preference, and available resources influence how the evidence is used to make clinical decisions. Haynes, Devereaux, and Guyatt (2002) suggest that vital to evidence-based clinical decision making is the individualization of care to the context of the patient's situation. These ideas are discussed in more depth later in this chapter.

What Is Best Available Research Evidence?

As novice practitioners, the students in the opening clinical story ask themselves: "What constitutes best available research evidence?" Data and information that come from many different sources can become the evidence used to influence clinical decision making.

Randomized Control Trials

The gold standard for evidence is randomized control trials (RCTs). RCTs, very simply put, are clinical trials that involve at least one test treatment and one control treatment. This type of trial is most often used to test effectiveness or safety. For example, an RCT can determine how effective a particular drug is in reducing a particular symptom without causing dangerous side effects.

RCTs are not without some constraints and are sometimes subject to bias and chance. In all of the quantitative methods, there is an emphasis on measurement and statistical analysis. If a rigorous research method is used to generate data, other quantitative methods like cohort studies and case control studies can also be considered good sources of evidence. Quantitative methods are not appropriate for answering all research questions. Pearson (1998) suggests that RCTs are good for cause and effect questions, but not for all questions that are of interest to clinicians. The criteria used to appraise the rigor and quality of these types of studies are discussed in later chapters of this book.

Pluralistic Approach: Quantitative Versus Qualitative Research

Ask yourself the following: What if you had a pressing clinical question and, after searching the research literature, you come to find that there is not any quantitative work, including RCTs, in your area of interest? As a clinician, do you just forget about it and say, "Oh well, there isn't any evidence so I guess I'll just wing it?" That is why, when considering the best available evidence, nurses need to take a **pluralistic approach.** *Pluralism* is a philosophical term that posits that there is more than one way to look at something. Pearson (1999; 2004) contends that professionals and consumers alike have broad evidence interests, and therefore there is a need to be able to systematically synthesize both quantitative and qualitative works. He argues that each is of equal importance in influencing clinical decision making.

In the clinical story, Maggie has already taken a job on an oncology unit, and she wonders what it might mean to a person to be told that he or she has a terminal illness. She has completed her research course and knows she can answer this question by searching the qualitative research. She does a review of the literature and is surprised to find that there are numerous qualitative research studies on this subject. Seeing these studies, she realizes the importance of accessible synthesized qualitative research as well as quantitative research. Nursing is a human science, which means a great deal of research is framed within qualitative methodologies, and it is necessary to have a vehicle to synthesize and disseminate this evidence. Others in the nursing profession agree with this. Monti and Tingen (1999) believe having multiple paradigms in nursing reflects a robust scientific community that encourages creativity and debate. Jensen and Allen (1996), Sandelowski and Barroso (2003), and Walsh and Downe (2005) all advocate for the need to move beyond just meta-analysis of quantitative research and embrace meta-aggregation of qualitative work. **Meta-analysis** is a statistical method that allows for the combination of the results of many studies to aggregate the conclusions into data that are stronger than are those of just one study. **Meta-aggregation** (sometimes referred to as **meta-synthesis)** combines the findings of qualitative research and synthesizes them to create major themes that accurately depict the meaning of a particular experience.

Expert Opinion

Another source of evidence is expert opinion. **Expert opinion** is evidence that draws on the expert knowledge of individuals or groups; it is not research-based evidence. Although some clinicians believe this type of evidence is not credible, most maintain it is valuable when there is little or no other evidence available or as a supplement to synthesized research. There are times when the best available evidence will come from expert opinion because there is no other rigorously generated research.

Pearson (2003) advocates for a process that systematically examines expert opinion in various types of documents. These documents include books, conference proceedings, reports, and consensus clinical guidelines. Although not completely mainstream, the systematic review of text and opinion is gaining momentum.

Local Data

Knowledge from **local data** is gaining recognition as a legitimate source of valuable evidence. These data can come from a variety of sources and may be useful in improving clinical or organization outcomes. Rycroft-Malone et al. (2004) identify the following sources for local data:

- Audit data
- Performance evaluations
- Feedback from a wide range of stakeholders
- Information from social and professional networks
- Knowledge about the culture of an organization
- Patient stories and narratives
- Local and national policy

Stetler (2003) labels this evidence as "internal evidence." She asserts that these data are obtained systematically from local sources and then framed in a way to make improvements in patient outcomes. Rycroft-Malone et al. (2004) believes that locally obtained data will play a future role in evidence-based practice but believes more understanding is needed about how this type of data is systematically collected and appraised, how it will be integrated with other types of evidence, and what role it will have in informing clinical decision making.

What Types of Questions Does the Best Available Evidence Answer?

Pearson, Wiechula, Court, et al. (2005) contend that health practitioners seek evidence to address a wide range of issues and thus the type(s) of evidence that a practitioner needs depends on the nature and purpose of the activity. They propose four types of questions that might be asked by health-care professionals that would require different types of evidence (Box 2■1).

Questions of feasibility ask for evidence that addresses to what extent a particular activity would be practical or practicable. A feasibility question asks whether an intervention or activity is physically, culturally, or financially feasible within a given context.

Questions of appropriateness ask for evidence that addresses how appropriate a given activity or intervention is related to the context in which the care is given. In other words, is the activity appropriate to the situation?

BOX 2■1   Interdisciplinary Rounds

Questions of feasibility, appropriateness, meaningfulness, and effectiveness often address clinical questions that are of interest to more than one discipline. The same evidence can be framed by different disciplines to make clinical decisions that are appropriate to that discipline.

Example

An interdisciplinary team consists of a nurse, social worker, psychiatrist, and case manager. Their job is to provide support services to persistently mentally ill patients who reside in independent apartments. All of them want to know the most effective interventions to help these clients take their medications effectively. The psychiatrist wants to know because it influences his clinical decision about what medications to order. The nurse wants to know because she is to provide patient education about medications and is responsible for intervening in drug-related problems. The social worker wants to know because she is designing a program for support services. The case manager wants to know because she is to provide the day-to-day support for activities of daily living. Each of these disciplines will benefit from the same evidence but for different reasons.

Questions of meaningfulness look for evidence that addresses how people experience a particular phenomenon. This evidence explores opinions, thoughts, feelings, beliefs, and subjective interpretations of events.

Questions of effectiveness seek evidence that addresses whether an intervention, when used appropriately, achieves the desired outcome.

An easy way to remember these questions is with the acronym FAME.

The Influence of Clinical Expertise, Patient Preference, and Available Resources

Jeni, Maggie, and Henrik can now articulate their understanding of what evidence-based practice is, what constitutes best available evidence, and what questions can be answered. However, they believe there is one piece of the picture they need to explore further. They remain curious about the role that clinical expertise, patient preference, and available resources play in clinical decision making.

Clinical Expertise

Professional nurses, like other health-care professionals, are assumed to bring a certain amount of theoretical and clinical knowledge to their practice. Professional knowledge is respected because nurses are considered to be credentialed experts. Titchen (2000) labels this as "professional craft knowledge." Rycroft-Malone et al. (2004) acknowledge the importance of this knowledge in clinical decision making but also argue that for clinical experience or tacit knowledge to be credible, it must be made explicit so that it can be disseminated, critiqued, and developed. In other words, for tacit knowledge to be a source of evidence, it needs to be subjected to rigorous analysis and critique.

Haynes et al. (2002) view **clinical expertise** as an overlay to all other components of evidence-based practice because it is expected that nurses will integrate tacit knowledge automatically when making clinical decisions. Nurses' knowledge and clinical skills help in (1) accurately assessing the needs of patients' families, groups, communities, and systems; (2) better understanding the context or the circumstance of a particular situation; (3) creating a climate in which patients' values and preferences are considered more important than those of the practitioners; and (4) discussing how available resources influence health-care delivery. Haynes et al. state this model is prescriptive rather than descriptive. That is, it is a guide for "thinking about how decisions are made rather than a schema for how they are made" (2002, p. 36). Figure 2■1 depicts these relationships.

Patient Preference

The term **patient preference** refers to how involved a patient is in the clinical decision-making process. Some patients have definitive views about their health-care

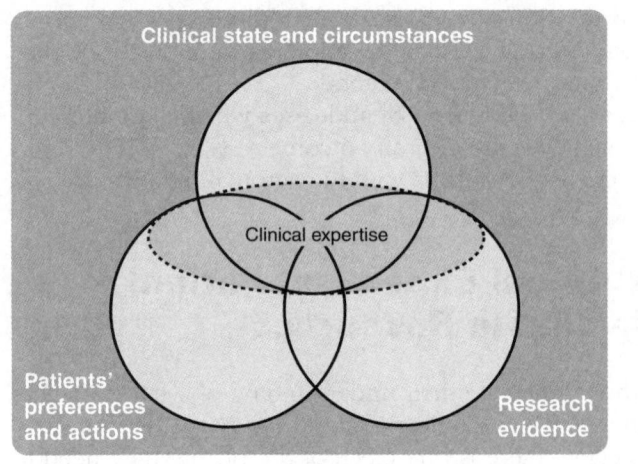

FIGURE 2■1 A model of evidence-based clinical decisions. (Reproduced with permission of the American College of Physicians, from Haynes, R. B., Devereaux, P. J., and Guyatt, G. H. (2002). Clinical expertise in the era of evidence-based medicine and patient choice. *ACP Journal Club, 136,* A11–A14.)

decisions, and others have less stringent views. Some want to receive a full disclosure of risk versus benefits, and others trust the clinicians to assess the risk of a given treatment. Haynes et al. (2002) suggest these choices are influenced by personal values, patient condition, available resources, aversion to risk, and amount of accurate or inaccurate information at hand.

Empowering patients to have a choice in their treatment sounds like an easy enough goal but the ways in which clinicians honor individual beliefs, values, past experiences, and knowledge and meld those into the other elements of evidence-based practice are less clear. There are times when patients make a decision that is contrary to the belief of the health-care provider. Some examples include a patient who decides to keep smoking after a heart attack, a patient who refuses lifesaving chemotherapy, or a patient who chooses to treat a condition with alternative methods. There is much to learn about what patient preference really means. More specific information about patient preference is addressed in later chapters.

Available Resources

There are clearly times and circumstances when the best available evidence points us in a direction that, when considering the circumstances, is not feasible or practical. For example, there might be evidence that recommends an intervention or activity that is very appropriate and feasible in one context, but because of a lack of **available resources** would not be appropriate in another. One of the goals of the evidence-based practice movement is to improve global health, and it is important to remember there are many health-care disparities caused by a scarcity of resources throughout the world. Residents of industrialized countries may not be familiar with the daily constraints faced by residents of less developed countries. What is important is that all informed health health-care decisions be made within the context of available resources (Box 2■2).

BOX 2■2 **Tools for Learning and Practice**

■ Go to Google Scholar (http://www.scholar.google.com) and search for the following article: Pearson, A., Wiechula, R., Lockwood, C., and Court, A. (2005). The JBI model of evidence-based health care. *The International Journal of Evidence Based Health Care, 3,* 207–215.

■ After reading the above article, look in the References list for this chapter and choose one other article that interests you.

■ Share what you have learned with a classmate.

■ Summary

Jeni, Maggie, and Henrik meet to review what they have learned through their exploration of the elemental components of evidence-based practice. They have come to appreciate that evidence-based practice provides a framework for clinical decision making and that better clinical decisions lead to better patient outcomes. The type of evidence needed to inform a clinical problem is driven by the type of questions asked. The types of questions we usually ask are questions of effectiveness, meaningfulness, appropriateness, and feasibility. The group now feels comfortable discussing how research evidence, clinical expertise, and patient values and preferences along with available resources provide the framework for evidence-based practice. They have learned that best available evidence can be gathered from different sources, such as synthesized qualitative evidence, quantitative research evidence, local data, and expert opinion. They also feel they can discuss how patient preference and available resources influence clinical decision making. Now that they have put all of the pieces of the puzzle together, Jeni, Maggie, and Henrik are ready to move on and start applying what they have learned toward the design of their project.

CHAPTER QUESTIONS

1. Discuss the relationship between evidence-based practice and clinical decision making.

2. Explain the meaning of *best available evidence.*

3. What type of evidence would a nurse look for in questions of feasibility, appropriateness, meaningfulness, and effectiveness?

4. Define *meta-analysis* and *meta-synthesis.*

5. Explain why the concept of clinical expertise overlays the clinical decision making model.

6. Discuss how patient values and preferences and available resources influence clinical decision making.

References

Dicenso, A., Cullum, N., & Ciliska, D. (1998). Implementing evidence-based nursing: Some misperceptions. *Evidence-Based Nursing, 1,* 38–39.

Haynes, R. B., Devereaux, P. J., & Guyatt, G. H. (2002). Clinical expertise in the era of evidence-based medicine and patient choice. *ACP Journal Club, 136,* A11–A14.

Jensen, L., & Allen, M. (1996). Metasynthesis of qualitative findings. *Qualitative Health Research. 6*(4), 553–560.

Muir-Gray, J. A. (1997). *Evidence-based health care: How to make health policy and management decisions.* New York: Churchill Livingston.

Monti, E.,& Tingen, M. (1999). Multiple paradigms of nursing science. *Advances in Nursing Science. 21*(4). 64-80.

Pearson, A. (1998). Excellence in care: Future dimensions in effective nursing. *Nursing Times, 3,* 25–27.

Pearson, A. (1999). Evidence based nursing: Quality through research. In R. Nay and S. Garnett (Eds.), *Nursing older people: Issues and innovations* (pp. 338–352). Sydney, Australia:

Pearson, A. (2003). Liberating our conceptualization of "evidence." *Journal of Advanced Nursing, 44,* 441–442.

Pearson, A. (2004). Balancing the evidence: Incorporating the synthesis of qualitative data into systematic reviews. *JBI Reports, 2,* 45–64.

Pearson, A., Wiechula, R., Lockwood, C., et al. (2005). The JBI model of evidence-based health care. *The International Journal of Evidence Based Health Care, 3,* 207–215.

Rycroft-Malone, J., Seers, K., Titchen, A., et al. (2004). What counts as evidence in evidence-based practice? *Journal of Advanced Nursing, 47,* 81–90.

Sackett, D. L., Rosenberg, W. M. C., Muir-Gray, J. A., et al. (1966). Evidence-based medicine: What it is and what it isn't. *British Medical Journal, 32,* 961–964.

Sandelowski, M., & Barroso, J. (2003). Creating meta-summaries of qualitative findings. *Nursing Research, 52*(4), 226–233.

Stetler, C. (2003). The role of the organization in translating research into evidence-based practice. *Outcomes Management for Nursing Practice, 7*(3), 97–103.

Titchen, A. (2000). *Professional craft knowledge in patient-centered nursing and the facilitation of its development* (Doctoral dissertation, University of Oxford, 2000). Kidlington, United Kingdom: Ashdale Press.

Walsh, D., & Downe, S. (2005). Meta-synthesis method for qualitative research: A literature review. *Journal of Advanced Nursing, 50*(2), 204–211.

CHAPTER 3

Global Perspectives and Borderless Knowledge

Alan Pearson

- Differentiate between local, national, and international sources of evidence for nursing.

- Describe and debate the role of international evidence in local clinical decision making.

- Develop a clinical question and source international evidence that addresses the question.

"Borderless" evidence/knowledge
Experience
Expertise

External evidence
Local evidence
Tacit knowledge
Tradition

Clinical Story

Mapani has been the head nurse on the cancer ward in the teaching hospital of a large government hospital in sub-Saharan Africa for 11 years. She is becoming increasingly worried about the number of patients with very sore and ulcerated mouths while receiving chemotherapy and radiotherapy. She knows that this has always been a problem, but as she begins her shift by looking through the care plans, she sees that of the 36 patients in the ward, 31 have moderate to severe mucositis. She knows the staff nurses and nurses' aides are meticulous in trying to ensure that every patient has a regular oral care with chlorhexidine, but the hospital budget is very small, and the staff is able to do this only once a day. This cannot, however, be the reason for this increase in sore mouths—Mapani and the ward nurses are practicing according to how things have always been done in hospital procedure—so she decides to press on with her work and hope for the best.

At the same time Mapani has these thoughts, Michael, the clinical nurse specialist (CNS) for the head and neck oncology unit in a prestigious academic health science center in the United States, is doing rounds at his hospital with the staff nurses on night duty. It is 2 a.m., and the unit is relatively quiet, so he and the two staff nurses sit at the nurse's station to review patients in the unit. They also notice the prevalence of mucositis in the current patient population and wonder about the change they have recently made from using chlorhexidine to using sunflower oil in their oral hygiene protocol. The change has increased the costs to the unit but occurred because the benchmarking exercise the hospital is involved in showed that the prevalence of mucositis in another, similar hospital in the same city runs at 5% less than their hospital. The only difference between the care delivered was found to be the substance used to clean the mouth.

For both of these nurses—living far apart from each other in very different cultures and systems—it is clear that their concerns and experiences are far more alike than they are different. What is also striking is their reliance on local evidence and their apparent indifference to the external, global evidence. In Mapani's case, her source of evidence is her own peers and the practices they have engaged in for years. Michael and his team compare their performance against that of another local team, without any thought that the hospitals they benchmark against may have much poorer outcomes than units across the rest of the world. Were both to explore the best available global evidence, they would find that evidence varies in strength and nine different treatments showed some effect. However, some were weak, and no single treatment is clearly supportable; frequent, gentle oral care with potable (drinkable) water and crushed ice may be as effective as any other intervention to prevent mucositis in patients undergoing radio- or chemotherapy (Worthington, Clarkson, Bryan, et al., 2010). ■

Introduction

Chapters 1 and 2 indicated that evidence-based nursing occurs when nurses make clinical decisions (with patients and the health-care team), taking into account the patient's values and preferences, the social and cultural context, their own judgment, and the best available global evidence.

The evidence-based practice movement had its genesis in the United Kingdom, Europe, Canada, and Australia—all countries that are closely aligned and where evidence sharing has been well established for centuries (Donaldson, 2007; Normand and Vaughan, 1993). Nurses in these countries are aware of international developments and either read journals from outside their country or search for information through PubMed (a database in the United States). This, to a large extent, explains why the concept of searching for and evaluating international literature and then developing appropriate local applications is now well understood in these countries.

The United States has an enormous population. U.S. health professionals publish frequently in a large number of U.S.-based journals, and the process of using local activity data from across the United States to establish benchmarks is more dominant in some regions of the United States than is the evidence-based approach. However, the escalating cost of health care is one of the greatest challenges in the United States. In 2008, $2.38 trillion was spent on health care in the United States, but 45.7 million citizens remained uninsured. The U.S. Census Bureau (2011) projects that the total health expenditure will climb to $3.225 trillion by 2014. Rapidly increasing cost of health-care delivery, critical staff shortages, and patient demand for more and better services all contribute to an increasing sense of urgency to improve access to quality care while reducing costs. Given these challenges, nurses and other health-care professionals are beginning to recognize the need to learn from the experiences and research of others, both in the United States and around the globe (Kuehn, 2010).

Whereas all nations focus on local problems and local solutions, the broader concerns of assessing health needs, surveillance, evidence-based decision making, and the social dimensions of health are truly global. The widespread movement of people and diseases across boundaries and the universal influence of the Internet serve only to emphasize how small the world really is. As society becomes knowledge-based, evidence is generated at ever-faster rates and exchanged in ever-larger networks. Evidence-based nursing is fundamentally embedded in these global developments. The process focuses on clinical decisions that are informed by the best available global evidence and is critically dependent on nurses' ability to access valid and reliable borderless evidence and apply it to the local context (Box 3■1).

What Is "Borderless Evidence"?

The concept of evidence is often misunderstood. A broad dictionary definition of the term *evidence* is: "the available facts, circumstances etc. supporting or otherwise

BOX 3■1   **Significance of Global, Borderless Evidence**

- Rapidly escalating costs of health care and calls for better, safer patient outcomes mean that the best evidence should inform clinical decisions.
- Research and evidence generation tend to coalesce in highly industrialized nations but scientific principles guide research in all countries that produce knowledge.
- Clinical problems are remarkably similar across the world; some solutions are setting independent, whereas others are context dependent.
- Internet availability and e-publication of evidence have created unprecedented access to international evidence.
- Best available evidence knows no national boundaries; to live up to the definition of evidence-based practice, clinicians must consider the international evidence.

a belief, proposition etc. or indicating whether a thing is true or valid" (Pearsall and Trumble, 1995, p. 487). Whenever nurses make clinical decisions with and for their patients, using local evidence is important. However, it is equally important to consider the external, global evidence that crosses borders of nations and disciplines. This is considered "**borderless" evidence** (or **knowledge**).

Local Evidence

Local evidence refers to the everyday knowledge nurses use within the local health system; this includes both **tacit knowledge** (implicit, unspoken) and more formally generated knowledge derived from local research studies. Tacit knowledge in nursing is largely associated with expertise, experience, and tradition. It represents the ideas, concepts, and understandings that are part of a knowledge-to-action continuum. This type of knowledge can be associated with the simple, everyday aspects of life such as eating and drinking; sleeping; mobilizing; and the experience of pain, suffering, recovery, and hope (Pearson, 2002; Pearson, Wiechula, Court, et al., 2005; Pearson, Wiechula, Court, et al., 2007). However, what appears simple on the surface actually hides the complexity and sophistication of expert nursing practice; it is hard to capture, evaluate, and report on in the formal research sense.

Local research is a more formal approach to evidence generation that involves the use of explicit methods of gathering and analyzing data. Increasingly, bedside nurses are engaging in local research efforts. These small-scale, locally generated studies play an important role in evidence-based nursing. However, if nurses base their practice solely on the findings of local research without accessing the global evidence, their practice will not reflect the intent of evidence-based health care and its interest in borderless knowledge.

Expertise

Expertise is highly regarded in nursing and is linked to the ability of a nurse to have relevant information in a given area of practice. Expertise is difficult to quantify and even more difficult to rank in terms of its reliability. Despite these difficulties, a large proportion of nursing practice relies on expertise. Furthermore, the opinions of experts often represent the best available evidence in areas in which research is limited or research on a specific question is difficult to conduct (Pearson et al., 2007).

Experience

Experience is knowledge and skill acquired through being involved in or exposed to practice over time. It is largely know-how, or procedural knowledge, rather than propositional knowledge, but it plays a major role in nursing practice. When nurses make clinical decisions, they often weigh external evidence with their own experience. Thus, experience in itself is a source of evidence in health-care practice (Pearson et al., 2007).

Tradition

Tradition plays a major role in nursing, largely because nurses are required to participate in an extended period of education and training to become familiar with the traditions of their profession and of the particular school they attended. **Tradition** is an inherited pattern of thought or action that leads to a specific, long-standing practice. Tradition may stem from logic and evidence from trial and error, but this is often not the case (Pearson et al., 2007).

In this chapter's clinical story, Mapani relies on the traditions of the unit. They have even been formalized into the plans of care. She begins to wonder if the methods they are using are correct, but she has stopped short of pursuing the question further because severely limited resources complicate her situation. Michael, however, has relied on local benchmarking to inform practice. Despite being in different hemispheres, both need to find better evidence to inform their practices.

External Evidence

Expertise and experience can be legitimate, internal sources of evidence for practice, and tradition can be seen as being not so legitimate. However, when the results of rigorous research are available, it is appropriate to weigh the results of external research against those internal sources of expertise, experience, and tradition. To date, much of the focus of evidence-based practice has been on determining the best available **external evidence** from research, almost to the exclusion of any other source of evidence. This is because evidence from rigorous research (external evidence) is least prone to bias.

Globalization and "Borderless" Knowledge

The desire to deliver the best possible care is a central concern of nurses across the globe, and an increased interest in improving health care is now universal. In diverse urban, suburban, rural, and remote communities across the world, there is a growing desire for a knowledge-based health-care system that is focussed on the individual and accessible to all.

Within nursing circles, Sigma Theta Tau International and the International Council of Nursing have developed mechanisms to support a global approach to evidence-based nursing practice. These include providing education, training, and resources to expand nursing's capacity for evidence-based practice in both developed and developing nations.

How can you, as a busy and time-poor nurse, ensure the knowledge you access and apply in local situations is the best available internationally and not limited to your state or your country—that it is, in effect, "borderless"? Fortunately, the evidence-based health-care movement has spawned accessible sources of information generated through global collaboration. The most notable collections are the Cochrane Library and the JBI Library and its evidence system, JBICOnNECT+. These sources draw together all of the world's best available knowledge/evidence to answer a specific clinical question and summarize it in a format that will inform nurses whenever they make a clinical decision.

Searching for the Global Evidence

The assumption of evidence-based nursing is that there is information nurses need to know in order to conduct practice professionally. There are, however, substantial gaps in available knowledge. Sackett, Rosenberg, Gray, et al. (1996) argue that almost every time a practitioner encounters a patient, new information is required about some aspect of the diagnosis, prognosis, or management. They note that there will be times when the question will be self-evident or the information will be readily accessible. This is increasingly the case as sophisticated information technology moves closer to the bedside.

Even so, there will be many occasions when neither condition prevails and there will be a need to ask an answerable question that will require the best available external evidence. This requires considerably more time and effort than most health professionals have at their disposal, and the result is that most information needs go unmet.

Asking Answerable Questions

The first step is to pose a question that is answerable. Asking answerable questions is a skill that can be learned. Sackett et al. (1996) offer useful advice in the context of evidence-based medicine and the effectiveness of interventions. These sources can be extended beyond questions of effectiveness to consider the appropriateness and feasibility of practices. The sources of a clinical question are the following:

- *Assessment*—how to properly gather and interpret findings from the history and physical examination and care
- *Etiology*—how to identify causes for problems
- *Differential diagnosis*—when considering the possible causes of a patient's clinical problems, how to rank them by likelihood, seriousness, and treatability
- *Diagnostic tests*—how to select and interpret diagnostic tests to confirm or exclude a diagnosis, based on considering, for example, their precision, accuracy, acceptability, expense, and safety
- *Prognosis*—how to gauge the patient's likely clinical course and anticipate likely problems associated with the particular disease and social context of the person
- *Therapy*—how to select therapies to offer patients that do more good than harm and that are worth the efforts and cost of using them
- *Prevention*—how to reduce the chance of ill health by identifying and modifying risk factors, and how to detect early problems by screening and patient education
- *Meaningfulness*—how to understand the experience of patients and the social context within which practice takes place
- *Feasibility*—how practical it is to implement a practice within a given clinical setting, culture, or country
- *Self-improvement*—how to keep your knowledge up to date, improve your clinical skills, and run a better, more efficient clinical service (adapted from Sackett et al., 1996)

Drawing on these factors, a clear, well-formulated question is developed to give focus to the search (see Chapter 8 for more detail on questioning). A clearly defined question should include specific details on the following:

- *The participants.* Participants should be clearly defined, including condition(s) (e.g., people with a confirmed diagnosis of emphysema), the population charac-teristics (e.g., females between 15 and 20 years), and the setting (e.g., in hospital medical wards).
- *The activities or interventions.* The question should specify the intervention or activity of interest (e.g., chest percussion or the administration of oxygen via a facemask).
- *The outcomes that are of interest.* The question should include the outcomes of interest to the review. The patient's satisfaction with care, peak flow, and oxygen saturation levels are examples of outcomes one might include in a review of interventions aimed at improving outcomes in people with emphysema.
- *The types of studies relevant to answering the question.* The question itself indi-cates the study designs that are most appropriate. When the question focuses on experiences of people or communities, interpretive studies are usually indi-cated, whereas questions of feasibility may warrant economic evaluations and/or critical designs or evaluative designs. When the focus is on the effectiveness of a

treatment, randomized controlled trials are considered to be the most appropriate, and questions relating to etiology or risk factors may be best addressed by case-control and cohort studies (see Chapter 11 for full explanations of these types of studies).

Generally speaking, although nurses often want to answer very broad questions, the narrower a question is, the easier it is to conduct the search. For example, if one is interested in determining the most effective, appropriate, and feasible way of improving the quality of life for people with emphysema, it is desirable to conduct a series of searches based on specific, focused questions. A well-formulated question will give direction to the search strategy.

Finding the Evidence: Global Evidence Sources

After you have identified the question, issue, or problem, the next step is to find the evidence. To do this requires knowledge about the techniques used to unearth the evidence and make it available. Systematic reviews and evidence-based practice guidelines are designed to save practitioners time by presenting condensed information, so they may be your the first preference in a search. Just as research—published or unpublished—varies in quality, so can a systematic review or guideline. Practitioners who want to base their practice on the best available knowledge need to learn new skills to access the resources available (Westbrook, Coiera, and Gosling, 2005).

Be open to the idea that evidence is generated throughout the world. Therefore, approach to evidence must not be limited to one country. Language may pose a barrier to finding (or using) evidence that is published only in a non–English-language journal. Increasingly, organizations are trying to use international collaborations and multilingual translations to break down language barriers and make evidence available to more clinicians.

In subsequent chapters, you will learn more details about searching. Here, it is important to focus on how to capture the international evidence in your effort to find the best available evidence.

- *What databases/resources do you have available in your setting?* Not all databases are accessible to clinicians, and databases may or may not search across languages and nations. Some resources are simpler to search and easily available in the clinical setting, whereas others are more complex and housed away from the point of care.
- *Who will do the search?* You may need to consult an expert to help find answers across a broad spectrum of international sources. That expert may be a librarian in your facility or an advanced practice nurse. See Box 3■2 for recommendations.
- *How can you seek help will from your librarian?* Although librarians may not be well versed in the substantive area of the clinical question, they are highly skilled in electronic searching and in the retrieval of papers. Be sure to communicate clearly what your question is and that you are interested in the global evidence.

BOX 3■2 **Interdisciplinary rounds**

■ Borderless evidence means gathering evidence from any nation and any discipline that produces high-quality, relevant knowledge for nursing practice.

■ Librarians can help find the international evidence and modify searches to accommodate different spellings and words for key terms of the search.

■ World health organizations that promote access to international evidence have come from many disciplines.

■ When you are considering treatments, traditions vary across nations as to whose role particular treatments belong; therefore, do not limit searches to a specific discipline when exploring the international literature.

Certain databases are large and most likely to yield international evidence. However, it may be difficult to find full descriptions of the national origins of the journals included in the index. These databases include (Box 3■3):

■ *CINAHL.* The Cumulative Index to Nursing and Allied Health (CINAHL) database provides authoritative coverage of the literature related to nursing and allied health. In total, more than 2,900 journals are regularly indexed.

■ *Medline.* Medline is widely recognized as the best source for bibliographic and abstract coverage of biomedical literature. It contains more than 9.5 million records from more than 3900 journals.

■ *The Cochrane Library.* The Cochrane Library is a collection of databases provided by the international Cochrane Collaboration (with over 20,000 contributors across the globe) and other organizations. At its core is the database of *Cochrane Reviews,* a database of systematic reviews and meta-analyses that summarize and interpret the results of research. The Cochrane Library aims to make the results of well-conducted controlled trials readily available and is a key resource in evidence-based health care. There are a number of Cochrane entities, including the Cochrane Nursing Care Field and the Cochrane Library of Systematic Reviews, both of which can be searched to find nursing-care relevant reviews. Because of the Cochrane approach, reviews are more likely to include global evidence in the library.

■ *The JBI Library/JBICOnNECT+.* The JBI Library of Systematic Reviews is a fully refereed library that publishes systematic reviews provided by the Joanna Briggs Institute, with an emphasis on nursing, the allied health professions, and medicine. JBICOnNECT+ (Clinical Online Network of Evidence for Care and Therapeutics) is an online, point-of-care evidence source that enables health-care practitioners to search for, critically appraise, summarize, embed, use, and evaluate evidence-based information. It is a service of the international Joanna Briggs Institute (with almost 70 collaborating centers around the globe), whose mission is to facilitate evidence-based health-care practice globally. Because of the underpinning international collaboration, these sources are likely to include international, multilingual evidence.

BOX 3■3   **Tools for Learning and Practice**

Evidence-Based Practice Organizations with an International Focus:

- **Joanna Briggs Collaboration (http://www.joannabriggs.edu.au):** An international collaboration of health-care providers representing 32 nations
- **Cochrane Nursing Care Field (http://cncf.cochrane.org):** An international group of nurses volunteering to support increased awareness and use of the Cochrane Library of international systematic reviews and other evidence sources
- **Contact, Help, Advice and Information Network (CHAIN) (http://chain.ulcc.ac.uk/chain/index.html):** An international community of people working in health care and social care
- **Guidelines International (http://www.g-i-n.net):** International members from 46 countries with a mission to lead; strengthen; and support collaboration and work within the guideline development, adaptation, and implementation community
- **Sigma Theta Tau, International (STTI) (http://www.nursingsociety.org):** An invitation-only international membership. STTI publishes *Worldviews on Evidence-Based Nursing* and sponsors books and meetings relevant to evidence based nursing
- **World Health Organization (http://www.who.int/en/):** Coordinating authority for health within the United Nations system. It provides leadership on global health matters, shapes the health research agenda, sets norms and standards, articulates evidence-based policy options, provides technical support to countries and monitors and assesses health trends.
- **Virtual Health Library (http://regional.bvsalud.org/php/index.php?lang=en):** An open network of literature databases and other resources. It includes a collection of multiple non-English-language databases.

- *Embase.* Excerpta Medica Database (Embase) is a biomedical and pharmacological database that contains over 23 million records from 1947 to the present. Embase covers over 7000 biomedical journals from 70 countries and is more likely to index European journals than other indexes.
- *Virtual Health Library.* The Latin America and Caribbean Center for Health Sciences Information developed this open network of literature databases and other resources. It includes a collection of multiple non-English databases that can be searched using English words. The search will return the original language abstract as well as a translated abstract. Databases include LILACS (Latin America and Caribbean Literature on Health Sciences) and international agencies such as the Pan American Health Organization (Virtual Health Network, n.d.).

Conducting the Search: Implications for International Sources of Evidence

In later chapters, you will learn more about conducting careful searches of electronic databases and other sources. If you work with skilled librarians, they can help you obtain international evidence if you emphasize that you would like to find all sources of evidence. For example, differences in spelling conventions such as "randomised" versus "randomized" and "paediatric" versus "pediatric" require expertise in searching. Similarly, different countries use different terms for the same condition (e.g., "mucositis" and "stomatitis'").

■ Summary

It is remarkable how practitioners, as global citizens, are concerned with many of the same health problems. Thus, practitioners share a similar desire to have the right information for the right people at the right time. For example, a simple search on CINAHL for "pressure ulcer" filtered to Middle East journals nets articles such as "Measuring the Quality of Pressure-Sore Prevention Cushions Through the Use of a Pressure Mapping System," published in the *Journal of the Israeli Physical Therapy Society*. Using the same search term but limiting the journal set to Australia yields a similarly focused article in the *Australian Journal of Wound Practice & Research*.

Of course, some health problems are unique or more pronounced in certain regions of the world because of environment, sociopolitical conditions, or other factors that contribute to unique risks. For example, searching "malaria" in the African subset of journals results in 46 hits for the period of 1986 to 2010, whereas the same search generates only 15 hits for the Mexico–South American subset. Certainly you need to determine if you can apply the results from any study in a local context, regardless of whether it was conducted in your own country or another. Remain open to all sources of evidence to determine the best available.

In this chapter's clinical story, the international evidence applied to both fully industrialized nations as well as less wealthy nations. The available resources influenced the questions and the balance of the costs and benefits of the solution, but the evidence was applicable to both.

CHAPTER QUESTIONS

1. What is meant by *evidence for nursing?*

2. What are the differences between local and global evidence?

3. In what situation would the use of local evidence be more desirable than external evidence?

4. What databases/electronic sources of information enable you to access international evidence?

5. Develop a clinical question and search a database first by limiting the search to just a few country journal subsets. Repeat the experiment but broaden your search to include all subsets of journals. How did your results compare? Do you think that it is important to include the international journals and databases in your search? Why or why not?

6. Think about a current issue or problem in your setting. Your search yields a systematic review that includes studies from India, Africa, the United Kingdom, and the United States. What will you consider to determine if these results have relevance to your local setting?

7. Consider this statement: "Health is global." How does this statement relate to your way of thinking or does it have any relevance to you?

References

Donaldson, L. (2007). *Health is global: Proposals for a UK Government-wide strategy.* London: Department of Health.

Kuehn, B. M. (2010). How the UK uses data on comparative effectiveness. *Journal of the American Medical Association, 304,* 1058–1059. doi:10.1001/jama.2010.1289

Normand, C. E. M., & Vaughan, J. P. (Eds.). (1993). *Europe without frontiers: The implications for health.* Chichester, United Kingdom: John Wiley.

Pearsall, J., & Trumble, B. (Eds.). (1995). *Oxford English reference dictionary.* Oxford: Oxford University Press.

Pearson A. (2002). Nursing takes the lead: Redefining what counts as evidence in Australian health care. *Reflections on Nursing Leadership, 28*(4), 18–21, 37.

Pearson, A. P., Wiechula, R., Court, A., et al. (2005). The JBI model of evidence-based healthcare. *International Journal of Evidence-Based Healthcare, 3,* 207–215.

Pearson, A. P., Wiechula, R., Court, A., et al. (2007). A re-consideration of what constitutes "evidence" in the healthcare professions. *Nursing Science Quarterly, 20,* 85–88.

Pearson, A., Field, J., & Jordan, Z. (2007). *Evidence-based clinical practice in nursing and health care: Assimilating research, experience and expertise.* Oxford: Blackwell.

Sackett, D. L., Rosenberg, W. M .C., Gray, J .A. M., et al. (1996). Evidence-based medicine: What it is and what it is not. *British Medical Journal, 312,* 71–72.

U.S. Census Bureau. (2011). Health & nutrition: Expenditures (Report No. 130). Retrieved from http://www.census.gov/compendia/statab/cats/health_nutrition/health_expenditures.html

Virtual Health Library. (n.d). Information sources. Retrieved from http://regional.bvsalud.org/php/index.php?lang=en

Westbrook, J. I., Coiera, E. W., & Gosling, A. S. (2005). Do online information retrieval systems help experienced clinicians answer clinical questions? *Journal of the American Medical Informatics Association, 12,* 315–321.

Worthington, H. V., Clarkson, J. E., Bryan, G., Furness, S., Glenny, A. M., Littlewood, A., et al. (2010). Interventions for preventing oral mucositis for patients with cancer receiving treatment. *Cochrane Database of Systematic Reviews, 12,* Art. No.: CD000978. doi:10.1002/14651858.CD000978.pub4

Models for Evidence-Based Practice

In this unit you will learn the different models of evidence-based practice that help structure the process of putting evidence into action. Some models are appropriate for individual nurses whereas others help groups or organizations transfer evidence into everyday practice. In Chapter 4 you will discover some of the controversies that surround evidence-based practice. Some nurse theorists have criticized the evidence-based practice movement, claiming it ignores nursing theory and regresses the profession toward an era of thoughtless, antitheoretical practice. You will find divergent points of view and then examine different conceptual models and frameworks and how they can increase the efficiency of integrating evidence into practice. You will connect the frontline nurses' critical role in moving evidence into

(continues on page 34)

practice and the emerging concept of "knowledge translation." In Chapter 5 you will explore a sampler of the many models of evidence-based practice and see how the models can be used in the clinical story. You will find tools to help you compare each to help you choose which model fits a particular clinical situation. In Chapter 6 you learn about the common principles among the models and find the key issues that emerge from the models.

Why Bother With Theory?

Leslie Rittenmeyer

- Explain the divergent points of view surrounding evidence-based practice.
- Describe the characteristics of a comprehensive model of evidence-based practice.
- Discuss how comprehensive models of evidence-based practice are congruent with the broader theoretical constructs important to nursing.
- Discuss the challenges and barriers that frontline nurses confront in moving evidence into practice.

Epistemology
Evidence-based practice movement
Evidence generation
Evidence/knowledge transfer

Evidence synthesis
Evidence utilization
Nursing theory
Systematic reviews
Theory-guided practice

Clinical Story

Arshay, Golda, Kyle, and Ruby are taking an introductory research course and are developing a presentation about certain aspects of evidence-based practice. In their presentation, they must address the divergent points of view and controversies surrounding the evidence-based practice movement. They also need to discuss the characteristics of comprehensive models of evidence-based practice and address whether those models are congruent with the broader theoretical constructs important to nursing. Finally, they must provide a broad overview of the challenges and barriers frontline nurses face when moving from best evidence to bedside practice. Even though the students have been learning about evidence-based practice since the beginning of their curriculum, they realize they need more depth to their knowledge to do this assignment. Their first step is to search the literature and start reading. ■

Introduction

As you have read in the previous chapters, evidence-based practice has been around many years and is far from a new notion. As far back as 1992, the Evidence-Based Medicine Working Group advocated for an approach to clinical decision making in medicine that used research evidence instead of pathophysiological rationales, intuition, previous clinical experience, and expert opinion to determine appropriate interventions for patient care. Early emphasis on randomized controlled trials (RCTs) as the gold standard of evidence set the tone for the initial **evidence-based practice movement.** Further, assigning a descending order of credibility to other forms of evidence spurred debate over what constitutes acceptable evidence.

Although some in nursing embraced the evidence-based practice movement early on, others feared it was atheoretical and was causing the profession to regress to an era of mindless, process-driven practice. The more narrow definitions of *evidence-based practice* continued to fuel the debate that continues today. However, expanded definitions of evidence-based practice and a wider understanding of what constitutes evidence in nursing have eased some of the discomfort with the evidence-based practice movement and has allowed for healthy academic debate. There is now a greater understanding of how the models of evidence-based practice are congruent with the broader theoretical constructs that are important to nursing.

Evidence-Based Practice: Historical Perspectives

Definitions

While beginning research for their presentation, Arshay, Golda, Ruby, and Kyle find that some of the earliest debates about the evidence-based practice movement in nursing began more than a decade ago. The team discovers that many of the concerns expressed about the evidence-based practice movement in nursing stemmed from the influences exerted by evidence-based medicine on evidence-based practice in general. One of the sources of conflict in the early debate was the presence of differing definitions of evidence-based practice in the literature. The definition proposed by the Evidence-Based Medicine Working Group (1992, p. 2420) stated that "evidence-based medicine de-emphasizes intuition, unsystematic clinical experience, and pathophysiologic rationale as grounds for clinical decision making and stresses the examination of evidence from clinical research." A later definition proposed by Sackett, Rosenberg, Gray, et al. (1996) did not restrict evidence to RCTs, which allowed for clinical expertise also to be used as evidence. This was an important departure in the evidence-based medicine movement, and it continues to be influential today.

Stelter, Brunell, Guiuliano, et al. (1998, pp. 48–49) proposed the following definition: "Evidence-based nursing de-emphasizes isolated, and unsystematic clinical experiences, ungrounded opinions, and tradition as a basis for nursing practices, and stresses instead, the use of research findings and, as appropriate, quality improvement data, other operational and evaluation data, the consensus of recognized experts and affirmed experience to substantiate practice." Gerrish and Clayton (1998, p. 58) stated that evidence-based practice "uses research findings derived from randomized controlled clinical trials or other experimental designs to evaluate specific interventions." Ingersoll (2000, p. 152) expanded Sackett's (1996) definition to the following: "Evidence-based nursing practice is the conscientious, explicit and judicious use of theory-derived research-based information in making decisions about care delivery to individuals or groups of patients and in consideration of individuals' needs and preference." Ingersoll conceptualized evidence to include information from theory and research and, more important, a consideration of patient preferences; you can see that Ingersoll's definition moved us a little closer to where we are today. In a similar way, DiCenso, Guyatt, and Ciliska (2005, p. 4) defined evidence-based practice as "the integration of best research evidence with clinical expertise and patient values to facilitate clinical decision making."

A comprehensive definition of evidence-based practice and its relationship to nursing is provided by the Joanna Briggs Institute, an interdisciplinary not-for-profit international research and development agency: "Simply defined, evidence-based practice is the melding of individual clinical judgment and expertise with the best available external evidence to generate the kind of practice that is most likely to lead to a positive outcome for a client or patient. Evidence-based nursing is nursing practice that is characterized by these attributes. Evidence-based clinical practice takes into account the context in which care takes place; the preference of the client; the clinical judgment of the health professional, as well as the best available evidence." (Joanna Briggs Institute, n.d.)

Controversies

The variability in the definitions of evidence-based practice, particularly early on, led to some criticism of the evidence-based movement by nursing theorists and scholars. With the emphasis on RCTs and a narrow definition of what constitutes evidence, some professionals failed to see how the evidence-based practice paradigm would benefit nursing. Some even argued that there was not enough empirical nursing research to embrace the model.

Some scholars questioned how well a fit the evidence-based medical model was for nursing's **epistemology** (foundations of knowledge). Carper (1978), in her classic article, and White (1995), in her expansion of Carper's work, provide an important framework for identifying the different forms of knowledge that reflect the ethos, or worldview, of nursing. They labeled these empirical, personal, ethical, aesthetic, and sociopolitical. In the earlier days of the evidence-based medicine movement, even though there was some room for clinical expertise to play a role in clinical decision making, emphasis was placed predominantly on the empirical way of knowing (e.g., RCTs). It was not that nurses devalued empirical knowledge but pointed to the value of other research paradigms to inform clinical decision making. Walker and Redmond (1999) suggest that medically dominated models, which value only empirical forms of evidence, present a threat to nursing's perspective of theory-guided practice. Mitchell (1999) recognizes the relevance of RCTs for providing directions for procedures, techniques, and protocols while also providing additional resources for clients and nurses about the latest developments in diagnosis and treatment, but she expresses several concerns about the evidence-based practice movement. She suggests that evidence-based practice constrains nurses from defining their own values to guide the nurse-person process and takes away from the humanness of that process. This creates a scenario that allows nurses to relinquish professional responsibility to patients and devalues nursing as a human science. She states strongly that nurses must choose a path that ensures a value-specific, theory-guided knowledge base, in which the client is considered the expert about his or her health and change. Her thoughts in 1999 provoked thoughtful reflection, and continue to do so today.

Fawcett, Watson, Neuman, et al. (2001), although not opposed to evidence-based practice, expressed concern that the art of nursing might be subjugated to an emphasis on the science of nursing, threatening nursing's holistic roots. They clearly acknowledge the connections among theory, research, and practice; in fact, they believe that theories provide a lens through which critique and interpretation of various types of evidence may be viewed, which is essential for theory-guided, evidence-based holistic practice.

Upton (1999) suggests that, despite the honorable goals of evidence-based practice, the concept has exacerbated an already existing theory-practice gap because there are fundamental differences in contexts and beliefs among what she calls the four pillars of nursing: management, practice, research, and education. She states that "the present principles of evidence-based practice threaten to continue to exacerbate the theory-practice gap by the recognition that some of the principle beliefs underpinning the concept are in direct contrast to contemporary nursing's opinion and subsequently limit practitioner's creativity and autonomy" (p. 554). She believes these inconsistencies need to be resolved before the concept of evidence-based practice can be successfully implemented.

Ingersoll (2000) contends that ethical issues are raised if reimbursement in health care is connected solely to documented sources of evidence. Nolan and Bradley (2008) express skepticism about the evidence-based practice movement as well, concluding that although evidence-based practice can play a role in improving the treatment provided to patients, nurses should be aware of other kinds of evidence and appreciate that any single approach to determining care, no matter how popular, is likely to lead to a service that does not truly meet the complex individual needs of the patient.

Although the evolution of the evidence-based practice movement has been a little rocky and messy at times, the clinical story students preparing their presentation are fascinated by the progress that evidence-based practice has made in just one short decade. In following the historical progression of the movement, they are able to see how much of the debate and criticisms came about, and how some of the criticisms have been addressed. The expanded definition that includes patient preferences, insight and clinical expertise, the consideration of context, the consideration of local data, and acceptance of a pluralistic approach about what constitutes evidence has made it possible to have rigorous academic dialogue. This is good both for health care and the discipline of nursing.

As the students prepare the next part of their presentation, they reflect on the key points they have just learned:

- It is in the interest of nursing as a discipline that practice be grounded in theory; some professionals in nursing fear that evidence-based practice is atheoretical and forces a "cookbook" approach to care that might cause nursing to lose its value of holism.
- The current definitions of evidence-based practice have expanded over the past decade to include patient preferences, context of care, and clinical expertise.
- There is an expanded conceptualization of what constitutes evidence, moving beyond randomized clinical trials to a more pluralistic approach.

The students now feel they understand the issues, and they are ready to tackle the last part of their presentation. This means looking broadly at what constitutes a comprehensive model of evidence-based practice and addressing whether it is congruent with the broader theoretical constructs of the discipline.

Comprehensive Models of Evidence-Based Practice

There are several models of evidence-based practice, which are discussed in Chapter 5. In general, any comprehensive model views evidence-based practice as aprocess, with the goal of informing clinical decision making to improve global health. For instance, the JBI Model of Evidence-Based Health Care (Pearson, Wiechula, Lockwood, et al., 2005) is organized to address evidence generation, evidence synthesis, evidence/knowledge transfer, and evidence utilization.

Evidence generation points to the best available evidence and indicates where there is a lack of primary evidence. It helps us to see where there are holes in the body of available research. **Evidence synthesis** is a pooling of available research findings through the process of systematic review. **Systematic reviews** include systematically searching international databases to identify and summarize the best evidence surrounding a clinical question. Because the JBI model is a pluralistic model, systematic reviews can focus on evidence from quantitative research, qualitative research, economic analysis, expert opinion, and text. **Evidence/knowledge transfer** is the part of the process that moves the evidence to where it needs to go. This may be accomplished through journals, clinical guidelines, electronic media, educational programs, other publications, and professional conferences. Knowledge transfer is also about targeting specific groups that should receive the information and packaging so it aids utilization and clinical decision making. The last part of the process, **evidence utilization,** is the use of evidence to bring about practice or system change. Evidence utilization is influenced by many outside factors such as the institutional culture, power structures, and available resources.

In summary, evidence-based health care is a process that begins with clinical questions and concerns or interests of clinicians, patients, or consumers. The process attempts to answer these questions by generating knowledge and evidence through the process of systematic review. The knowledge/evidence is then transferred to target groups of professionals who utilize and evaluate its impact on health outcomes, health systems, and professional practice (Pearson, Field, and Jordan, 2007).

Congruency of Evidence-Based Practice With Theoretical Constructs of Nursing

In an attempt to answer the question of how current comprehensive models of evidence-based practice are congruent with the theoretical constructs important to nursing, the students decide to start out by examining the word *theory*. The word *theory* stems from the Greek word *theoreo,* which means to "look at, to observe, to contemplate."

Theories are sets of interrelated concepts with propositional statements that describe or link those concepts (Fawcett, 1999). Chinn and Kramer (2004) state that theories are a creative and rigorous structuring of ideas that project a systematic view of phenomena. **Nursing theory** aims to describe, predict, and explain the phenomena important to nursing. Theories help organize knowledge. Theories also guide the research process and the development of research questions that are pertinent to nursing. Most important, theories are meant to improve practice, not by dictating specific actions but by providing an overreaching guide for action. This is accomplished through the relationship between theory and research.

As long as one adheres to the broader definitions of evidence-based practice, it is hard to see the conflict between the aims and structures of **theory-guided practice** and evidence-based practice. Theory-guided practice is based on the assumption that practitioners can describe, explain, or predict why they do things. Evidence-based practice is a set of tools, procedures, and resources used to find the most current, best available evidence from research or other sources (if research is not available). It also involves applying that evidence to clinical decision making, taking into account the situation, culture, resources, and common sense. The overarching aim is to improve global health.

Challenges of Evidence-Based Practice

Arshay, Golda, Kyle, and Ruby now believe they have a good understanding of the controversies and critiques surrounding evidence-based practice. Although they believe evidence-based practice will help them provide better care, the students want to understand some of the challenges and barriers they will confront when attempting to implement it.

As they finish preparing this last part of their presentation, the students realize that implementation of a comprehensive model of evidence-based practice is sometimes messy and almost always complicated. They begin to realize it might be difficult for frontline nurses to implement an evidence-based practice on their own.

Hannes, Vandermissen, DeBlaeser, et al. (2007) conducted a study of 53 Flemish nurses that attempted to identify the barriers to evidence-based nursing (Box 4■1). Melnyk and Fineout-Overholt (2005) also identified barriers to the implementation of evidence-based nursing practice (Box 4■2).

BOX 4■1   Research Finding on Barriers to Evidence-Based Nursing

- Known existing barriers to the use of evidence-based nursing include a lack of time, resources, evidence authority, and support.
- Known internal barriers include a lack of motivation and resistance to change.
- Nurses acknowledge a lack of responsibility in the uptake of evidence-based nursing.
- Elements of power are visible in nurses' relationships with physicians, managers, and patients, the latter being more outspoken with nurses providing home-based care who consider themselves "guests" in the patient's environment.
- Different education levels might lead to two-tier nursing practice.

BOX 4■2   Barriers to Evidence-Based Practice in Nursing

- Lack of knowledge in relation to evidence-based practice strategies
- Negative views and misperceptions about research and evidence-based practice
- Failure to believe that evidence-based practice will result in more positive outcomes than will traditional care
- Voluminous amounts of information in professional journals
- Lack of time to search for and appraise evidence
- Large patient loads
- Lack of administrative support
- Demands by patients for certain types of care
- Peer pressure to follow established conventions
- Inadequate content and skills regarding evidence-based practice in educational settings

As you can see, the evidence-based practice movement has come a long way in the last past decade. Many of the controversies are being addressed and resolved through a process of scholarly discourse. Obviously challenges and barriers still exist, but there is an increasing body of knowledge on how to address them.

■ Summary

As they prepare the final version of their presentation, this chapter's clinical story students have learned that the road to implementing evidence-based practice might be challenging. Despite that, they now have some insight on how to approach the process, and they are confident in their abilities to discuss the criticisms of the evidence-based practice movement (Box 4■3 and Box 4■4). They also embrace the concept of both theory-guided practice and evidence-based practice and see nothing inconsistent between the goals of both systems. They understand there are barriers and challenges to the implementation of evidence-based practice but feel they are prepared to face them now that they know what to expect.

BOX 4■3 **Interdisciplinary Rounds**

As stated in the work of Hannes et al. (2007), one of the barriers to implementing evidence-based practice is the power inequalities in the health-care system between physicians and frontline nurses.

Example

Nurses are often in a dependant position and contradicting doctors' opinions is hard for many of them. Some nurses reported that sometimes doctors would even do the opposite to reaffirm the dominant position. Many nurses feel that doctors will take advice from other professionals before they will do so from nurses. Some nurses in this study admitted that sometimes because they don't take initiative they automatically defer to physicians. How would you begin to address this in your practice?

BOX 4■4 **Tools for Learning and Practice**

■ Search the Joanna Briggs Institute Web site (http://www.joannabriggs. edu/au) and print out the Joanna Briggs Comprehensive Model of Evidence-Based Health Care.

■ Search Google Scholar (http://scholar.google.com) for the phrase "controversies in evidence-based nursing." Print out one article and read it in its entirety.

■ Reflect on the definition of the word *theory* and give some examples of the way in which nursing theory can provide an overreaching guide for action.

■ Explore the nursing theory Web site http://healthsci.clayton.edu/ eichelberger/**nursing**.htm

---

CHAPTER QUESTIONS

1. Discuss the belief by some that evidence-based practice is atheoretical

2. Compare and contrast earlier definitions of *evidence-based practice* with a more current definition.

3. Answer the argument that the evidence-based practice movement is incongruent with the epistemologies of nursing.

4. Compare and contrast the aims of theory-guided practice with the aims of evidence-based practice.

5. Explain ways in which evidence-based practice is congruent with the theoretical constructs of nursing.

6. Explain the process of knowledge transfer and how it is connected to knowledge utilization.

7. Explain how the barriers of lack of administrative support and unequal power structures might hinder a frontline nurse from implementing an evidence-based practice.

References

Carper, B. (1978). Fundamental patterns of knowing in nursing. *Advance in Nursing Science, 1*(1), 13–23.

Chinn, P., & Kramer,M., (2004). *Integrated knowledge development in nursing,* 6th ed. St. Louis, MO: Mosby.

DiCenso, A., Guyatt, A., & Ciliska, D. (2005). *Evidence-based nursing: A guide to clinical practice.* St. Louis, MO: Mosby.

Evidence-Based Medicine Working Group. (1992). Evidence-based approach to teaching the practice of medicine. *Journal of the American Medical Association, 268*(17), 2420–2425.

Fawcett, J. (1999). *The relationship of theory and research* (3rd ed.). Philadelphia: F. A. Davis.

Fawcett, J., Watson, J., Neuman, B., et al. (2001). On nursing theories and evidence. *Journal of Nursing Scholarship, 33*(2), 115–119.

Gerrish, K., & Clayton, J. (1998). Improving clinical effectiveness through an evidence-based approach: Meeting the challenge for nursing in the United Kingdom. *Nursing Administration Quarterly, 22*(4), 55–65.

Hannes, K., Vandermissen, J., DeBlaeser, L., et al. (2007). Barriers to evidence-based nursing: A focus group study. *Journal of Advanced Nursing, 60*(2), 162–171.

Ingersoll, G. L. (2000). Evidence-based nursing. What it is and what it isn't [Op-ed]. *Nursing Outlook, 48*(4), 151–152.

Joanna Briggs Institute. (n.d.). Definition of evidence-based practice and nursing. Retrieved September 24, 2008, from http://www.joannabriggs.edu.au/

Melnyk, B. M., & Fineout-Overholt, E. (2005). Making the case for evidence-based practice. In B. M. Melnyk & E. Fineout-Overholt,(Eds.), *Evidence-based practice in nursing & healthcare: A guide to best practice* (pp. 3–24). Philadelphia: Lippincott Williams & Wilkins.

Mitchell, G. J. (1999). Evidence-based practice: Critique and alternative view. *Nursing Science Quarterly, 12,* 30–35.

Nolan, P., & Bradley, E. (2008). Evidence-based practice implications and concerns. *Journal of Nursing Management, 16,* 388–393.

Pearson, A., Field, J., & Jordan, Z. (2007). *Evidence-based clinical practice in nursing and health care: Assimilating research, experience and expertise.* Oxford: Blackwell Publishing.

Pearson, A., Wiechula, R., Lockwood, C., et al. (2005). The JBI model of evidence-based health care. *International Journal of Evidence-Based Health Care, 3,* 207–215.

Sackett, D. L., Rosenberg, W. M. C., Gray, J. A. M., et al. (1996). Evidence-based medicine: What it is and what it isn't. *British Medical Journal, 312*(7023), 71–72.

Stelter, C., Brunell, M., Giuliano, K. K., et al. (1998). Evidence-based practice and the role of nursing leadership. *Journal of Nursing Administration, 28*(7–8), 45–53.

Upton, D. J. (1999). How can we achieve evidence-based practice if we have a theory-practice gap in nursing today? *Journal of Advanced Nursing, 29*(3), 549–555.

Walker, P. H., & Redmond, R. (1999). Theory-guided, evidence-based reflective practice. *Nursing Science Quarterly, 12,* 298–303.

White, J. (1995). Patterns of knowing: Review, critique, and update. *Advances of Nursing Science, 17*(4), 73–86.

CHAPTER 5

A Sampler of Conceptual Frameworks and Models

Lisa Hopp

- Differentiate evidence-based practice conceptual frameworks and models based on their focus, purpose, origins, and practical tools that help make the model operational.

- Given a clinical situation, apply a specific model to a patient problem using the model's way of relating concepts.

- Debate the practical usefulness of conceptual models to guide evidence-based nursing practice.

Conceptual framework	Model
Context	Ottawa Model of Research Use (OMRU)
Descriptive framework or model	PARIHS framework
Explanatory framework or model	Potential adopters
Facilitation	Practice environment
Heuristic	Predictive framework or model
Innovation	Worldview
Iowa model	
Joanna Briggs Institute (JBI) model	

Clinical Story

Jaspar, Mina, Alfredo, and Grace often work the night shift together in a medical intensive care unit, and they have become good friends. They often tease one another about how they represent the "United Nations of Nursing." Jaspar was raised in a small town in southern England, moving to the city to attend school; Mina emigrated from Morocco when she was a teen; Alfredo started his career in Italy and moved to the United States when he married; and Grace is a native of this U.S. city, having recently graduated from a nearby school of nursing. They care for one to three patients each night, depending on the patients' acuity, yet they often talk with one another about the correct approach to patient care.

Tonight the unit is at full capacity with 14 critically ill patients. Some of these patients are quite unstable, and others are physiologically stable but still require close nursing vigilance. The group members know that they cannot stop for a break, yet they consult with one another when they are unsure about the best way to assess or intervene with their patients and their families.

Jaspar's patient had a heart attack about 12 hours before he started caring for her. The patient, Mrs. B., is a 55-year-old woman whose husband and two grown children have not left the hospital since she was admitted. Jaspar is caring only for Mrs. B. because she has been very unstable, is on a ventilator, has several invasive catheters, and is on multiple intravenous medications. Her daughters and husband are at Mrs. B.'s bedside when her heart rhythm suddenly deteriorates to ventricular tachycardia. Jaspar and his colleagues begin resuscitation.

While the others continue to defibrillate and resuscitate Mrs. B., Mina attends to the family members. Mina gently draws them to the side, calmly tells them what they are seeing, and asks them if they want to stay by Mrs. B.'s side or if they wish to go to the waiting room. They decide that, for now, they want to stay. Mina stays by their side, explaining what they are seeing and how Mrs. B. is responding to the resuscitation efforts. Although the family members are clearly distressed that Mrs. B is so critically ill, they ask Mina questions and tell her that they are glad they are able to stay in the room. Mrs. B. improves and becomes more stable. Mina stays with the family until Jaspar is once again able to bring them closer to the bedside.

When the four nurses are finished with their shift, they have breakfast together and talk about their night. They realize the ways they were raised in households with different cultural backgrounds influence how they think about families being present during resuscitation. They also have their own clinical strengths and preferences concerning the manner in which they make decisions about their nursing care. Nonetheless, even though they have unique approaches to the how of nursing, they share a common what—the evidence base of their decisions. If they use a framework, they can integrate their unique worldviews, hows, and common whats to develop a shared roadmap for using evidence to help them make decisions about supporting families during the resuscitation of a loved one. ◼

Introduction

Sometimes students and clinicians find theory too abstract and impractical to help them in everyday nursing practice. Others claim that theory can stifle creativity and innovation when designing research about how to implement evidence into practice (Rycroft-Malone, 2007). Still others argue that if theory is neglected in the efforts to implement evidence, the theory-practice gap will expand and limit ingenuity (Upton, 1999). As you can see, these are nearly opposite opinions. As you read in the previous chapter, there is no need to approach evidence-based practice atheoretically. In fact, many would counter that theory is essential to advancing the evidence-based practice movement.

If you are new to using frameworks, theory, and models to shape how you use evidence in your practice, you need a good reason to pursue the challenge. In addition, you should remain open to different types before you select an approach. In fact, some models may be more applicable than others in different contexts and for different goals. We are not able to review all of the possible conceptual approaches to evidence-based practice in this chapter. Instead, we will offer you samples that we think are robust and practical. That means they should work in a variety of situations and guide you in sensible and functional ways.

Like the group of nurses in the clinical story, how one approaches nursing care and how one thinks about nursing is influenced by one's **worldview.** In other words, how you nurse is influenced by your frame of reference and how you fit your experiences into your representation of the world. We use a system of symbols that "allows us to integrate everything we know about the world and ourselves into a global picture, one the illuminates reality as it is presented to us within a certain culture" (Aerts, Apostel, De Moor, et al., 2007).

Why Bother Thinking Conceptually?

Before you read further, you may be asking, Why bother? Theory, conceptual frameworks, and models may simply seem like an academic exercise or an activity for people with extra time on their hands instead of a tool for busy clinicians. Consider the following analogy before you decide to stop reading: If you need to go somewhere but you do not know how to get there, you look at a map. Depending on the purpose of your journey, you use a certain type and scale of map. You can also use a map to generate what-ifs. That is, if you go in a specific direction, you can find certain points of interest, hazards, or other places of note. Using theories, frameworks, and models is like using various types of maps to help you understand where you are going, how the places along the way relate to one another, and to help you to generate hypotheses. They help you avoid getting lost in the process of moving evidence into practice (see Box 5■1).

In this chapter's clinical story, the four nurses come from very different cultural and family backgrounds and began their nursing careers in different contexts. These experiences shaped how they think about family members being present during

> BOX 5■1 **Significance of Frameworks, Theories, and Models**
>
> ■ Trying to use evidence in practice without a conceptual approach is like driving in a new area without a map or directions.
> ■ Frameworks, theories, and models provide practical and creative guidance for implementing evidence in your practice.
> ■ Using a conceptual approach can improve efficiency and speed the uptake of evidence.
> ■ Frameworks, theories, and models provide research questions to advance nursing practice and health-care agendas.

resuscitation and how they view the evidence related to the practice. Nonetheless, they all participated in helping Mrs. B.'s family through this very difficult experience.

Frameworks, Theories, and Models

Translating knowledge gained from evidence into action is complex. This complexity exists in the even more intricate context of nursing practice and the worldviews of those who do nursing. A variety of frameworks, theories, and models exist to help you navigate this complexity. They vary in their purpose, origin, how far along they are in their development, intended users, and scope. This chapter provides only a sample of frameworks and models that will be useful as you try to make evidence actionable. You may want to explore others that are beyond the scope of this book.

Definitions

Words and language are the building blocks of frameworks, theories, and models. Before exploring them, we need to be clear about the meanings of *conceptual framework, theory,* and *model* and how they relate to one another. Some people use these three words interchangeably, whereas others are very careful to differentiate each, even though they all represent some kind of "mental device" (Kitson, Rycroft-Malone, Harvey, et al., 2008).

Conceptual frameworks identify "a set of variables and relationships that should be examined in order to explain phenomena. They need not specify the direction of relationships or identify critical hypotheses. In contrast, a theory provides a denser and logically coherent set of relationships. Theories can offer views on the causal relationships and seek to explain the phenomena" (Kitson et al., 2008, p. 5). Several theories can be consistent with a single conceptual framework (Kitson et al., 2008).

Models are generally less ambitious than either theories or conceptual frameworks. They are still representations of a real phenomenon, but they are narrower, usually represent a specific situation, and are made of more precise assumptions (Rycroft-Malone and Bucknall, 2010b). Several models may fit a single theory.

Figure 5■1 may help you understand the relationship among conceptual frameworks, theories, and models and how worldview and context shape how they are used. Some people think of the relationship among conceptual frameworks, theories, and models in layers of specificity and scope.

In this chapter's clinical story, nurses in the critical care unit used a particular framework to guide how they approached developing their unit-specific policies as well as how individual nurses used evidence to make clinical decisions. Their unit practice council chose a conceptual framework because it was practical and clear and helped them structure the process of evidence utilization. It helped them choose appropriate tools to implement and evaluate evidence uptake.

Organizing Your Thinking About Frameworks, Theories, and Models

When you explore different conceptual frameworks and models, use a systematic approach to sort them. Much like organizing a closet, you will be able to select the right conceptual "clothes" for a particular situation if you understand their purpose, what situation they best fit into, what concepts they address, and how best to use them.

Rycroft-Malone and Bucknall (2010b) reviewed literature about theory use and developed a series of criteria to help organize your thinking and evaluate frameworks and models (see Table 5■1).

- Begin by determining the scope of the framework or model. Does it address a very broad, large range of abstract concepts, or is it more narrow and precise and perhaps more concrete in focus? Think about whether the framework or model aims to describe, explain, or predict.
- Consider how far along it is in its development by looking at how the authors designed the framework and model and if they provide evidence to support it. Have others tested the framework or model in a practice or a research setting?

FIGURE 5■1 Relationship of conceptual frameworks, theories, and models. A conceptual framework describes, explains, or predicts a set of variables and relationships to explain a phenomenon (shapes). Theories describe a denser, more logical, coherent set of relationships (set of ideas). Many theories may be consistent with a framework. Models are more narrowly focused but may be skeletal or precise; several models may fit one theory (schema sharing a theme such as triangles, arrows, or weather symbols).

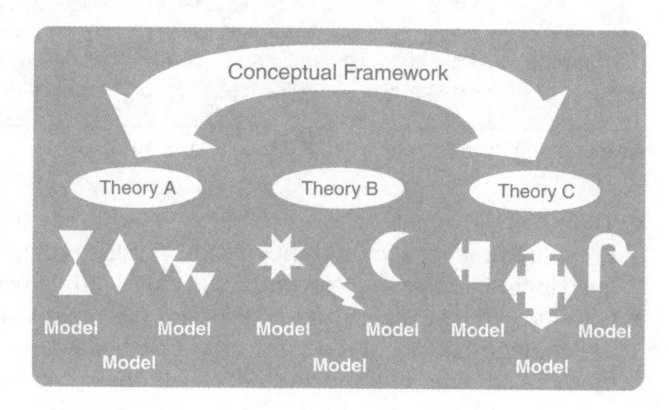

Table 5■1   **Criteria for Organizing Frameworks and Models**

Criterion	Comments
Structure	■ Frameworks vary in how extensive and abstract they are ■ Models tend to be more precise and prescriptive
Purpose	■ Descriptive—describes properties, characteristics, and qualities of a phenomenon ■ Explanatory—explains causal relationships and mechanisms of a phenomenon and relates it to other concepts ■ Predictive—predicts relationships through propositions or hypotheses
Development	■ Inductive approaches—generated from gathering information and building the model or framework ■ Deductive approaches—beginning with generalizations and gathering information to support the generalizations ■ Support sources—evidence from research, systematically derived consensus, or analyses to support or refute the framework or model
Theoretical basis	■ Theories provide a foundation for the framework or model. ■ One framework may borrow from several theories or be consistent with more than one theory. ■ May be implied or clearly identified.
Conceptual clarity	■ Definition of terms and how they relate to each other ■ Ability to identify differences and similarities among the theories that underpin the framework and model ■ Ability to promote new theoretical understanding
Users and context	■ Aimed at individuals, groups, or organizations ■ Intended for certain disciplines (nurses, medicine, or multiple disciplines) or groups of disciplines (all health-care providers or groups that create policy) ■ Real or simulated/hypothetical use
Functionality	■ Tools related to using the framework, such as assessment tools, implementation strategies, and evaluation methods ■ Ease of adoption or adaptation to clinical situations
Testability	■ Ability to generate and test hypotheses using a variety of research methods ■ Ability to use evidence to support or refute the framework or model

Adapted from Rycroft-Malone and Bucknall (2010a, 2010b).

■ Think about the intended users. How should they use the model or framework? For what functions should they use it? For example, is it intended to help a certain discipline assess, intervene, or evaluate implementation of evidence?
■ Consider if it is testable and how useful the model or framework is for you in the context that you intend to use it. In other words, think about the what, why, who, when, where, how, and how well of the framework or model.

Use these criteria to help you determine how well any particular model suits you, your setting, and need. We explore four models in more depth in this chapter and the next, but there are other models and frameworks that may interest you.

Specific Frameworks and Models for Evidence-Based Practice

Rycroft-Malone and Bucknall (2010a, 2010b) suggest the purposes of evidence implementation frameworks and models fall into one of three categories: descriptive, explanatory, or predictive. **Descriptive frameworks** or **models** describe the nature of the elements of a phenomenon or process without making claims about relationships. **Explanatory frameworks** or **models** specify cause-and-effect relationships and mechanisms. **Predictive frameworks** or **models** forecast how phenomena will behave and how they relate to one another, and tend to generate propositions and hypotheses (Rycroft-Malone and Bucknall, 2010a, 2010b). The purpose statement of the framework or model tells you what to expect of it and may help you make a decision about whether to use it.

Another way to sort frameworks, theories, and models is to analyze their intended use and users. For example, some are meant to guide individuals in making specific clinical decisions. Others are meant to guide groups or organizations in developing policy. Still others are aimed at enhancing the context to improve the chance that individuals and groups will use evidence in some way.

In the next section, you can review brief descriptions of frameworks or models that are best suited to help frontline nurses make decisions in clinical settings. Other excellent frameworks and models exist (e.g., the Stetler model, the Knowledge to Action model, and Dobbin's Dissemination model), but they are more complex and beyond the scope of this book. You can review more about them thorough descriptions in texts and journal articles related to these and other frameworks and models (e.g., Rycroft-Malone and Bucknall, 2010a). For each model discussed in this book, you will see how nurses can use each one to guide the policies related to family presence in the critical care unit, as illustrated in this chapter's clinical story.

Iowa Model

The **Iowa model** (Fig. 5■2) was developed at the University of Iowa hospital and was originally a guide to research utilization. The authors developed it further, based on feedback from staff nurses and nursing leaders. The model is popular in part because it is very practical and avoids abstract concepts. It is aimed at individuals or groups who collaborate within a system to change practice.

The purpose of the model is to guide practitioners through a series of decision points as they move through the evidence implementation process. The schema looks like an algorithm or flowchart of decision points that provides a linear process of putting evidence into action (Titler, 2010).

The process begins with a knowledge- or problem-focused trigger, something that motivates health-care providers to consider a change in practice. This might be

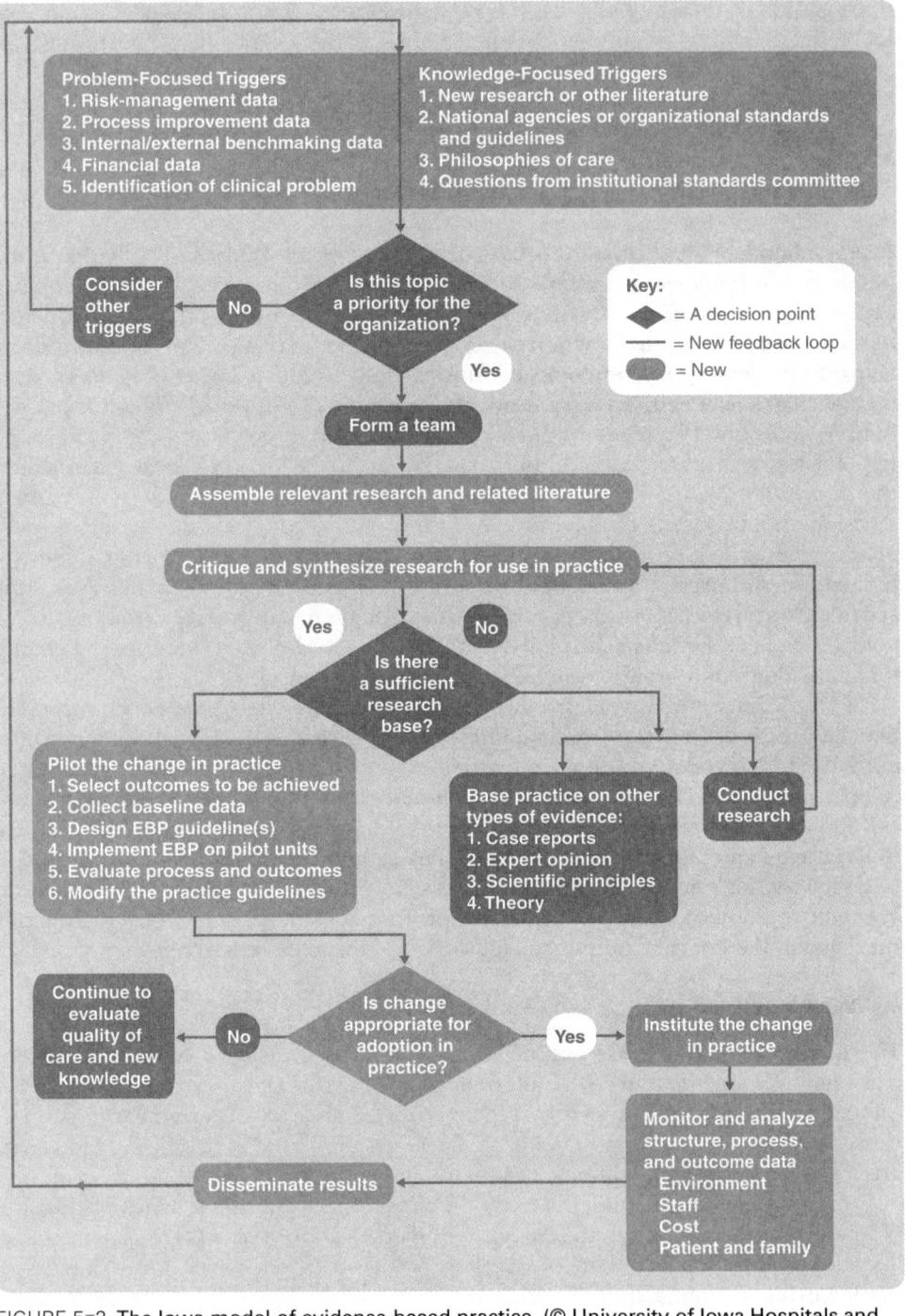

FIGURE 5■2 The Iowa model of evidence-based practice. (© University of Iowa Hospitals and Clinics, with permission.)

new research, a guideline, or change in philosophy of care, or providers may simply question current practice (knowledge-focused trigger). Alternatively, practitioners may recognize a problem based on internal data or an event. The first decision the practitioner or group must make is whether the issue is a priority for the organization. If it is not, then the model recommends that the practitioner refocus. If it is a priority, a team forms and its members search, appraise, and synthesize research and related literature. Next, the group decides if there is a sufficient research base to guide practice. If the group determines that there is not a sufficient research base, members can either rely on other types of evidence, such as case reports, expert opinion, scientific principles, or theory, or they can conduct further research. If they decide that the research base is adequate, they use a six-step process to create, pilot, and refine an evidence-based guideline. Based on the outcome of the design and pilot phase, the group decides whether the practice is appropriate for adoption or not. If it is not, the model returns to the beginning of the algorithm or continues to monitor the quality of care. If the change is appropriate, then the team takes the change to a broader implementation and monitors the outcomes and disseminates the results (Titler, 2010).

The model authors emphasize that the model indicates that evidence-based practice is a process that requires teamwork, multidisciplinary collaboration, and evaluation as keys to success (Titler, 2010).

In this chapter's clinical story, if the practice council used the Iowa model to develop a family presence initiative, Mina would begin with a knowledge trigger, such as reading a journal article about family presence. The article may have intrigued her because of her own view of the importance of supportive families in the critical care unit. In addition, close extended family relationships are at the center of her Moroccan heritage. She would then form a unit-based team if others validated that the initiative was aligned with the organization's goal of family-centered care. Once the unit leaders agreed that the initiative fit their strategic philosophy, Mina would seek the help of the unit practice council to search, appraise, and summarize the evidence. After Mina presented her findings, the council would decide if the evidence from research and other types of evidence was strong enough to proceed. Assuming it was, they may identify goals such as the following: (1) families express satisfaction, comfort, and support during witnessed resuscitation; (2) families experience no ill effects of witnessed resuscitation; and (3) health-care providers are able to complete resuscitation smoothly. Then they would adapt existing evidence by melding somewhat older Emergency Nurses Association guidelines with subsequent research findings to create their own unit policy, and conduct pilot tests to carefully evaluate the impact of the new policy on families and health-care workers by interviewing or surveying both groups. Finally, the team would analyze the findings from the evaluation to determine if they should make changes and institute the policy more widely and permanently. They may also present their findings to local groups or even more broadly at conferences and via publication.

The Ottawa Model of Research Use

Researchers from the Canadian province of Ontario developed the **Ottawa Model of Research Use (OMRU)** (Fig. 5■3) to help facilitators guide valid research

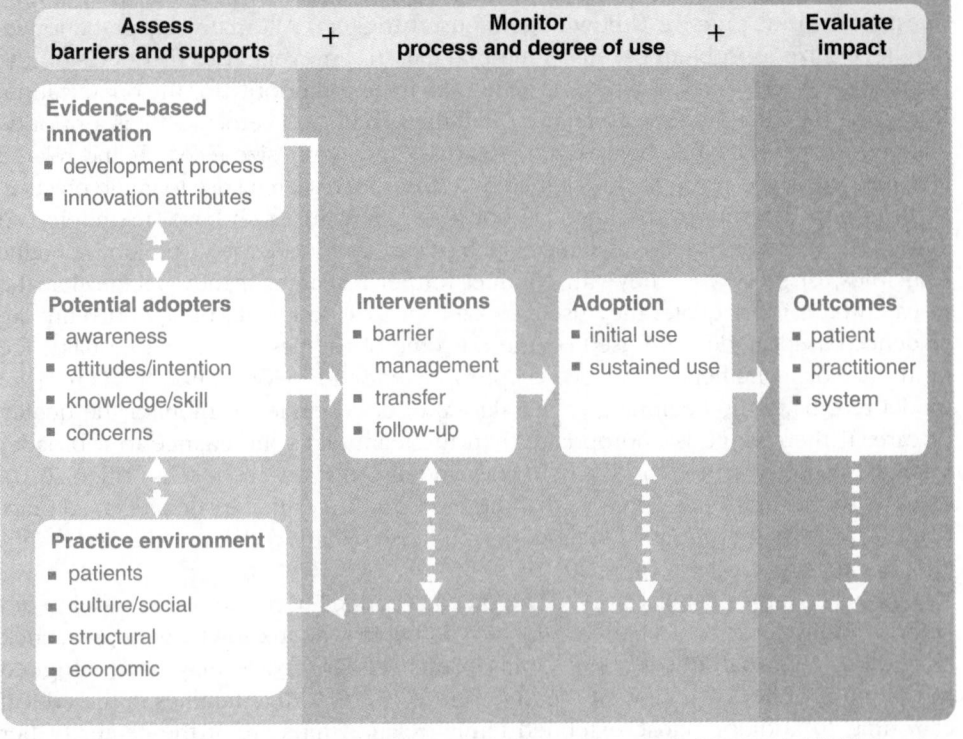

| Assess barriers and supports | + | Monitor process and degree of use | + | Evaluate impact |

Evidence-based innovation
- development process
- innovation attributes

Potential adopters
- awareness
- attitudes/intention
- knowledge/skill
- concerns

Interventions
- barrier management
- transfer
- follow-up

Adoption
- initial use
- sustained use

Outcomes
- patient
- practitioner
- system

Practice environment
- patients
- culture/social
- structural
- economic

FIGURE 5■3 The Ottawa Model of Research Use (OMRU). (Copyright © 2004 McGill University School of Nursing, with permission.)

implementation (Logan and Graham, 2010). It is descriptive and prescriptive as well as practical. The model reflects Roger's Diffusion of Innovation Theory because it focuses on six key elements:

- Research-informed innovation
- Potential adopters
- Practice environment
- Implementation strategies for transferring the evidence into practice
- Adoption of the innovation
- Health-related and other outcomes

Facilitators assess, monitor, and evaluate during a dynamic, interactive, multiple-feedback process (Logan and Graham, 2010).

During three prescriptive phases of the model, facilitators assess barriers and support, then monitor the process and degree of use during implementation, and finally evaluate the impact of the project. The assessment phase includes understanding the **innovation**—the new evidence-informed practice, policy, or change in practice—its quality (appraising the evidence supporting the innovation), and other attributes. Innovations that are based on strong evidence, simple, easily tried, user-friendly, compatible with current practice, and clear are more likely to be successful.

The assessment phase includes understanding the **potential adopters** of the innovation, such as practitioners, policy makers, patients, and other stakeholders. Adopters who are aware of the innovation have positive attitudes and intentions (perceiving fewer barriers and more facilitators), have the knowledge and skill necessary for the innovation, and are not concerned about the potential harm or work burden are more apt to adopt the innovation. Finally, the team or facilitator must assess the **practice environment,** the setting in which the change will occur. The practice environment includes parts of the implementation context such as the governing rules; cultural and social factors, such as local politics; power structures; resource availability; leadership approaches; peer groups; and other factors (Logan and Graham, 2010).

Based on a thorough assessment of the innovation, the adopters, and the environment, the facilitator and team can better target implementation interventions that maximize strengths and minimize barriers by using problem-solving and good management skills. However, Logan and Graham (2010) caution that the evidence about how to best target barriers and select effective implementation interventions remains in its infancy. Facilitators and teams should be flexible and experimental when they try implementation strategies, such as using prompts and clinical cues as reminders, opinion leaders (e.g., well-respected, expert nurses on a unit) to influence peers, or audit and feedback of clinical behaviors. Throughout the implementation process, the facilitators must monitor both the initial and long-term use of the innovation. Sometimes adopters will adopt a new practice but return to old patterns.

During the final stage of the model, the facilitator and team evaluate outcomes related to the patient, practitioners, and system once the new evidence-informed practice has been sustained. The schema for the model indicates that the stages are connected and bidirectional. This means that the stages are interactive, dynamic, and may not flow in a highly linear way (Logan and Graham, 2010).

If the Ottawa Model is used to implement the family presence in this chapter's clinical story, Mina, Jaspar, Alfredo, and Grace would all contribute to the implementation plan facilitated by their unit's clinical nurse specialist and a nurse researcher. The facilitators would appraise the evidence but invite the team to comment on what the evidence and innovation would mean to their work, how it relates to their values, worldviews, and prior experiences; what barriers they might anticipate; and concerns they may have for the families and their work. Jaspar and other staff may express certain fears about having family present during such a trying event: this may pose a risk to the family's psychological well-being, or it may disrupt the efficient flow of a resuscitative effort. The team may even fear litigation if the outcome had not been good. These are all very important indicators of potential barriers.

Conversely, the facilitators would also recognize that some of the staff, such as Mina, Alfredo, and Grace, are important role models and champions for change if they believe families can safely be present and gain a sense of intimacy with their loved one during a resuscitative effort. Jaspar may voice that he was not convinced that it is a good idea for families to witness resuscitation, even if the evidence seems to point in that direction. The facilitators may probe his resistance and use this information to plan for others with similar feelings. The team also needs to identify what support (e.g., clergy, grief counselors) could be available to families and health-care providers involved in the resuscitation so that both have a sense of safety. Finally, they would assess the structure of the intensive care environment for feasibility barriers (e.g., to see if there is enough room for the families near the bedside or chairs to sit in if someone became light-headed or could not stand).

During the preintervention phase, the team would likely engage many of the nurses and other professionals in education and discussion before starting a trial of the new policy; they may even use psychology professionals to role-play a simulated scenario to build the staff's confidence in supporting families. After trying to uncover all possible barriers and maximizing supports, they would decide on a clear start date for offering families the option of being present during resuscitation. The facilitators would be on hand to observe how the trial proceeded and to debrief the health-care team and family afterward to determine the intervention's degree of success or failure. Also, there may be additional changes, such as supplemental staff to support the family and those involved in resuscitation efforts. Facilitators would continue to monitor more episodes of family presence as they occur. To do this, they may conduct some guided telephone interviews with families of patients, survivors, and nonsurvivors, within a month or two of the event. These narrative stories could be analyzed to determine themes to help the team learn more about the experiences of families and health-care providers.

In this chapter's clinical story, the nurses adopted the practice, and the outcomes for the family, nurses, physicians, respiratory therapy, and clergy were positive. They modified the published guideline somewhat when they realized that there was not enough space at the bedside in all patient rooms during resuscitation. But they resolved to make sure the family could touch, see, and talk to their loved one as soon as possible, and stay in the room if there was a safe nook for them to stand or sit in. The nurses also made sure they stayed near the family members to monitor and support their coping in the period following the resuscitation in case intervention was necessary.

Promoting Action on Research Implementation in Health Services

In 1998, a group of nurse scientists from the United Kingdom involved in managing change and conducting research conceived the Promoting Action on Research Implementation in Health Services Framework, more commonly known as the **PARIHS framework,** to increase the uptake of evidence in various settings (Kitson, Harvey, and McCormack, 1998). Its purpose is to "serve as a practical and conceptual heuristic to guide and evaluate research implementation and practice improvement endeavors" (Rycroft-Malone, 2010, p. 110). **Heuristic** refers to a rule of thumb, or structure for problem solving. Unlike the Iowa and OMRU models, this framework does not describe the process, or how, of evidence implementation or practice improvement. Rather, the PARIHS framework deals with three key elements that contribute to the success of evidence implementation: evidence, context, and facilitation (Fig. 5■4). The authors characterized each element on a continuum from low to high or weak to strong. They expressed the framework simply as an equation: SI = f (E, C, F), where successful implementation (SI) is a function (f) of the level and type of evidence (E), the quality of the context (C), and the approach to facilitation (f) (Kitson

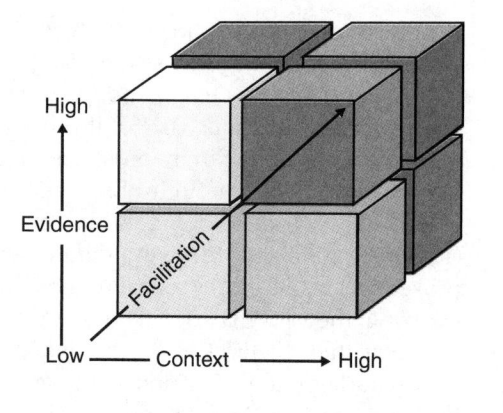

High

Evidence

Facilitation

Low ——— Context ———▶ High

FIGURE 5■4 Promoting Action on Research
Implementation in Health Services (PARIHS)
framework. (Rycroft-Malone, J., & Bucknall,
T. (Eds.), *Models and frameworks for implementing evidence-based practice: Linking
evidence to action.* Oxford: Wiley-Blackwell.)

et al., 2008). Successful implementation of evidence is more likely when the evidence
and context are strong and expertly facilitated.

Each key element of the framework is further defined by subelements and descriptions of each on a low-to-high continuum. Evidence includes knowledge from
research, clinical experience, patient preferences, and local data and information. An
example of high clinical experience is expertise that others have critiqued, is consistent and accepted among groups, and is relevant and appropriately weighted in the
decision-making process. At the other extreme, an example of weak clinical
experience is a single anecdote that lacks any critical reflection and cannot be
validated by others (Rycroft-Malone, 2010).

Context refers to the practice environment in which the change happens and
includes the subelements of organizational culture, leadership, and evaluation practices. A culture on the high end of the continuum is characterized as a learning environment with decentralized decision making, mutually respectful relationships
between the managers and staff, and facilitative leadership styles. Transformational
(rather than autocratic) leaders who make roles clear and promote effective teamwork
and structures are ranked on the high end of the leadership spectrum. The third
subelement refers to mechanisms and structures for evaluation. Strong evaluation is
characterized by many sources of information with straightforward feedback methods
for individuals, teams, and the organization. The framework predicts "that a conducive
context for evidence-based practice is where there is clarity of roles, decentralized
decision making, staff are valued, transformational leadership, and a reliance on multiple sources of information on performance" (Rycroft-Malone, 2010, p. 119).

The third element of the PARIHS framework is **facilitation,** or "the process of
enabling or making easier the implementation of evidence into practice" (Rycroft-
Malone, 2010, p. 119). The method of facilitation depends on the characteristics of
the evidence, the context, and the stakeholders. The mode of facilitation can vary
from technical, "doing for," task-driven support to a more holistic, enabling, coaching
approach. For example, "doing for" would be a facilitator who searches, appraises,
and develops a list of strategies for evidence implementation and hands this over to
a manager to enforce. An enabling facilitator would develop the skills in others,
coaching and engaging the ideas of all stakeholders rather than making all of the
decisions of implementation. Adept facilitators alter their approach based on their

expert assessment of those involved, the qualities of the context, and the stage of the implementation process (see Box 5■2 for interdisciplinary tips).

Jaspar, Alfredo, Grace, and Mina would work closely with a facilitator, such as a clinical nurse specialist (CNS), if the PARIHS framework was used to guide the implementation of the family presence initiative. The CNS would assess the qualities of the context, either through observations and insight or by using a tool that PARIHS researchers are developing to diagnose the strengths of the evidence and context (Kitson et al., 2008). Knowing that the evidence related to the effectiveness of family presence and its impact on families and health-care providers is positive yet still evolving, the CNS may decide to gather local data from interviews of staff and families to assess their feelings about the initiative.

In addition to the evidence, the facilitator would use any strengths he or she finds in the context, such as taking advantage of the decentralized decision making of the unit practice council and the staff's enthusiasm for learning from one another and the evidence. The CNS would enable the practice council by coaching them through the evidence selection and appraisal process if they need help. If the council is already skilled in appraisal and policy development, the CNS may focus more on supporting their teamwork rather than technical tasks such as searching for evidence, organizing, and summarizing the evidence. The CNS would adapt when staff need more technical support (e.g., determining how to delegate care during the resuscitation to ensure adequate staff and family support). During the evaluation process in a high context setting, the CNS would focus on helping staff reflect upon and refine their strategies.

Joanna Briggs Institute (JBI)

The last model examined in this chapter is the **Joanna Briggs Institute (JBI) model** (Fig. 5■5). In the last chapter, you were introduced to the key elements of the JBI model. You learned JBI is an international organization that has comprehensively addressed evidence-based practice since its inception in 1996. The model describes how the institute and its global collaborating groups work together to get evidence into practice to improve global health. This goal sets the JBI model apart from the other models and framework presented in this chapter because the other models aim only at the local level. Despite its very broad purpose, the JBI model

---

BOX 5■2 **Interdisciplinary Rounds**

- Multiple disciplines such as psychology and sociology as well as other health-care fields have contributed to the development of frameworks, theories, and models.
- Most frameworks, theories, and models related to evidence implementation can be used by many disciplines and promote collaboration among disciplines.
- Seek out the perspectives of other disciplines to understand how worldviews may be influenced by discipline.

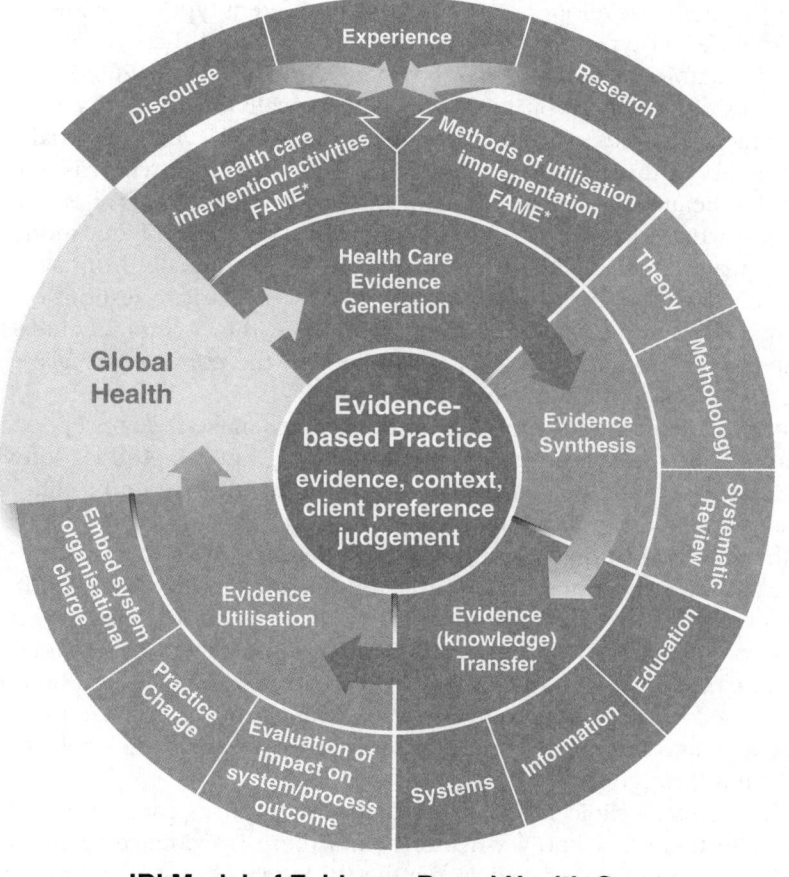

JBI Model of Evidence-Based Health Care

*FAME
Feasibility
Appropriateness
Meaningfulness
Effectiveness

FIGURE 5■5 Joanna Briggs Institute model. (From Pearson, A., Wiechula, R., Court, R., and Lockwood, C. [2005]. The JBI model of evidence-based healthcare. *International Journal of Evidence Based-Healthcare, 3*[8], 207–215.)

can be used to guide evidence implementation at a more local level as well by providing tools to that allow you to think globally and act locally (Pearson, Wiechula, Lockwood, et al., 2005).

To better understand the JBI model, picture it as a pie with five pieces, with evidence generation, synthesis, transfer, utilization, and enhanced global health in a circle clockwise (see Chapter 4 for definitions). JBI has developed methods and tools for each slice of the pie to enhance the chance that evidence will make its way into routine practice.

The JBI model developers emphasize that different types of evidence are used to inform different types of questions and the quality of the evidence varies in a way that is meaningful for the type of evidence (Pearson et al., 2005). For example, questions of effectiveness of interventions are ideally answered by systematic reviews or meta-analyses of well-conducted randomized, controlled trials (you will learn more about these types of evidence in later chapters), whereas questions related to the meaning of interventions or phenomena to patients should not be answered with experimental evidence. Rather, these kinds of questions are best answered from narrative data from qualitative studies, ideally from systematic reviews or meta-syntheses of these types of studies. Similarly, questions of feasibility (i.e., physically, culturally, or financially possible within a certain context) and appropriateness (if an intervention fits or relates to the context) are also questions that are important to making clinical decisions.

At each stage of the JBI model, methods exist to make the concept operational. For example, at the synthesis stage, JBI has developed methods, software, and training to support the production of systematic reviews and an online library to distribute them. During the transfer stage, knowledge is translated into accessible forms through education; training, and short, easy-to-use forms of predigested, ranked, and rated evidence. The transferred knowledge must be used if evidence is to be of any value. Utilization includes methods to embed evidence in practice manuals, to enhance use through process improvement methods of audit and feedback, and measurement of outcomes. To support both transfer and utilization, JBI has developed education, training, and tools, and over 60 affiliated groups work together to make the model practical and useful to meet the goal of improved global health through local efforts (Pearson, 2010).

In this chapter's clinical story, the group of staff nurses could use the JBI model tools to help them first know whether or not there is evidence to support family presence. Mina and Jaspar could search the JBI library of systematic reviews to find evidence about the experience of family presence from the perspective of both health-care providers and the families. Because of JBI's unique attention to questions of meaning, they could search for systematic reviews relevant to this question. The nurses would find a systematic review exists that would help them understand what both groups might experience if they implemented the program (evidence synthesis). The team could then summarize the systematic review into a shorter information sheet that includes a brief of the main methods and findings of the review so their fellow staff can more quickly and efficiently grasp the key aspects of the review (evidence transfer). Finally, they would need to embed the evidence through a process of assessing the readiness of the unit for the change, working with their leadership group to help identify potential barriers, and making baseline measurements of the way that families are cared for during resuscitation. They could use these baseline measurements and seek input from other staff and family members about what barriers exist to offer families the option to be present during resuscitation. In addition, Mina, Alfredo, Grace, and Jaspar each have a unique perspective about the initiative, which brings rich understanding to the potential ups and downs of the initiative. They would most likely develop multiple strategies such as speaking one-on-one with their fellow staff members, conducting role-playing educational sessions, and bringing an expert to the unit to discuss the best approaches to implementing the policy. Finally, after implementing the family presence initiative, the team would need to evaluate whether the barriers still exist, and should measure the impact of the project on families and staff (evidence utilization).

■ Summary

In this chapter, you were introduced to practical ways of using frameworks and models in everyday practice (Box 5■3). You learned about four quite different conceptual approaches to getting evidence into practice. The Iowa model focuses on step-by-step decision making when a problem or new knowledge triggers the beginning of a change process. Theories related to quality improvement could relate to this model. The OMRU is based on theories of planned action and diffusion of innovation. It directs facilitators to assess the qualities of the innovation, adopters, and practice environment before instituting the intervention; monitoring its use for adoption and sustainability; and finally evaluating the impact of the innovation on outcomes. The PARIHS framework diverges from these two models because it does not describe a process. Rather, it predicts successful implementation as a function of the quality and strength of the evidence, context, and facilitation. Finally, the JBI model describes the role of evidence generation, synthesis, transfer, and utilization in improving global health, with an emphasis on tools and strategies to make each phase operational for local providers. Finally, you learned that the nurses in the clinical story have unique worldviews based on their prior experiences, cultures, and family structures that shape their perspectives on nursing and patient care. These worldviews and the use of a particular model created distinct stories of implementing a family presence initiative.

BOX 5■3   Tools for Learning and Practice

- Select two frameworks or models and apply them to an evidence implementation project; compare the way the conceptual approach steered the process.
- Work with a practice council or other clinical group to select a model to guide evidence implementation.
- Use online resources to help you understand frameworks and models for evidence implementation:
  - http://www.parihs.org (presentations, tools, ongoing framework developments)
  - http://www.joannabriggs.edu.au/about/jbi_model.php (description, links to articles, tools, and ongoing development of the model)
  - http://www.kusp.ualberta.ca/knowledgeutilizationcolloquia.aspx
  - http://www.implementationscience.com (a free, full-text online journal publishing ongoing development of frameworks, theories, and models)

CHAPTER QUESTIONS

1. Compare and contrast a theory, conceptual framework, and model. How might these three ways of thinking abstractly fit together?

2. How is a road map like a framework or model?

3. You are having coffee with a fellow student or colleague who thinks that theory, frameworks, and models are a waste of time and have nothing to do with practical nursing care. How might you argue that they can help you in daily nursing practice?

4. What are the essential pieces of each of the four models/frameworks discussed in this chapter?

5. Which model or framework seems to fit your way of thinking best? Why?

6. In your opinion, what is the most important aspect of a framework or model?

7. Can you imagine different situations or contexts in which one model may fit better and another in which you might adapt another model? Explain.

8. Think about a recent practice change that occurred in your setting. Select one of the models or frameworks and apply it to what happened. Do you think that the implementation process may have gone differently if the model or framework would have been used to guide implementation?

References

Aerts, D., Apostel, L., De Moor, et al. (2007). *World views: From fragmentation to integration*. Originally published in 1994 by VUB Press: Brussels. Internet edition by Clement Vidal and Alexander Riegler. Retrieved from http://www.vub.ac.be/CLEA/pub/books/worldviews.pdf

Logan, J., & Graham, I. (2010). The Ottawa model of research use. In J. Rycroft-Malone & T. Bucknall (Eds.), *Models and frameworks for implementing evidence-based practice: Linking evidence to action* (pp. 83–108). Oxford: Wiley-Blackwell.

Kitson, A., & Brisby, M. (2008). Speeding the spread: Putting KT research into practice and developing an integrated KT collaborative research agenda. Alberta Heritage Foundation for Medical Research. Retrieved from http://www.ahfmr.ab.ca/download.php/fdb47de28f52562a0452b42534d33b39

Kitson, A., Harvey, G., & McCormack, B. (1998). Enabling the implementation of evidence-based practice: A conceptual framework. *Quality and Safety in Health Care, 7*, 149–158.

Kitson, A., Rycroft-Malone, J., Harvey, G., et al. (2008). Evaluating the successful implementation of evidence into practice using the PARiHS framework: Theoretical and practical challenges. *Implementation Science, 3*(1). doi:10.1186/1748-5908-3-1

Logan, J. & Graham, I. D. (2010). The Ottawa model of research use. In J. Rycroft-Malone & T. Bucknall (Eds.), *Models and frameworks for implementing evidence-based practice: Linking evidence to a ction* (pp. 84–108). Oxford: Wiley-Blackwell.

Pearson, A. (2010). The Joanna Briggs Institute model of evidence-based health care as a framework for implementing evidence. In J. Rycroft-Malone & T. Bucknall (Eds.), *Models and frameworks for implementing evidence-based practice: Linking evidence to action* (pp. 185–205). Oxford: Wiley-Blackwell.

Pearson, A., Wiechula, R., Lockwood, C., et al. (2005). The JBI model of evidence-based health care. *International Journal of Evidence-Based Health Care, 3*, 207–215.

Rycroft-Malone, J. (2007). Theory and knowledge translation. *Nursing Research, 56*(4S), S78–S85.

Rycroft-Malone, J. (2010). Promoting action on research implementation in health services (PARIHS). In J. Rycroft-Malone & T. Bucknall (Eds.), *Models and frameworks for implementing evidence-based practice: Linking evidence to action* (pp. 109–135). Oxford: Wiley-Blackwell.

Rycroft-Malone, J., & Bucknall, T. (2010a). Theory, frameworks, and models: Laying the groundwork. In J. Rycroft-Malone & T. Bucknall (Eds.), *Models and frameworks for implementing evidence-based practice: Linking evidence to action* (pp. 23–50). Oxford: Wiley-Blackwell.

Rycroft-Malone, J., & Bucknall, T. (2010b). Using theory and frameworks to facilitate the implementation of evidence into practice. *Worldviews on Evidence-Based Nursing, 7*. doi: 10.1111/j.1741-6787.2010.00194.x

Titler, M. (2010). Iowa model of evidence-based practice. In J. Rycroft-Malone & T. Bucknall (Eds.), *Models and frameworks for implementing evidence-based practice: Linking evidence to action* (pp. 137–146). Oxford: Wiley-Blackwell.

Upton, D. J. (1999). How can we achieve evidence-based practice if we have a theory-practice gap in nursing today? *Journal of Advanced Nursing, 29*, 549–555.

CHAPTER 6

Common Principles

Lisa Hopp

LEARNING OBJECTIVES

- Compare and contrast select models and frameworks for implementing evidence into practice.
- Using the principles common to select evidence implementation frameworks and models, construct a map to implement evidence in a particular context.

KEY TERMS

Complex problems
Complicated problems

Clinical Story

It is a quiet night in the intermediate care unit. Libbie, Alin, Enrique, and Lindsay have just received the handoff report from the evening shift and are organizing how they will care for the 28 fairly stable, monitored patients for the night. In this unit, nurses exchange the shift report in the nurses' station and structure the oral report around patient problems. Two and a half or three hours may pass before a nurse enters some of the patients' rooms. Nurses may not see patients because of the time required for nurses who are due to end their shift to finish their chart reviews and documentation; for the handoff itself; and for the oncoming nurses to prepare medications, find supplies, and otherwise plan for their shift.

The four RNs are crowded around the medication area, waiting their turn to dispense the medications they need for midnight doses when suddenly they hear a crash at the far end of the hall. They rush toward the noise, and they find Mrs. W., a frail elderly woman, on the floor by the door to the bathroom. Lindsay quickly assesses Mrs. W.'s neurological status and finds that her pupils are equal, round, and reactive to light, but she is not responding to their verbal commands. In the fall, her IV line was been pulled out, and the puncture site is bleeding slightly. Libbie also notices that Mrs. W. has been incontinent of urine, and the floor is slick. Enrique checks her vital signs. Mrs. W.'s blood pressure is elevated, but her heart rate is regular and only slightly elevated, and she is breathing normally. The nurses stabilize her spine and roll her onto a lift board; Mrs. W does not show any response during the movement. While two nurses stay with the patient, Lindsay calls the physician and the night nursing supervisor. Enrique makes a quick check of the other patients.

Mrs. W. suffers a broken hip and concussion from the fall. Eventually she recovers but her hospital stay is over 3 weeks longer, and she is transferred to an acute rehabilitation center to recover more fully before returning home. She can no longer live independently because of a decrease in her functional ability, so she lives with her daughter.

The incident prompts a full study of what happened and must be reported as a sentinel event to the Joint Commission (the accrediting agency for the hospital). Lindsay, Enrique, Alin, and Libbie are distressed by the incident. The investigation of the incident reveals the nurse reporting off to Alin had not indicated that this patient was at high risk for a fall. The team wants to take a look at the procedures during shift changes and determine how they can better recognize risk to prevent patient falls and injury.

Introduction

Conceptual models and frameworks are abstract representations of reality. They are useful because they can give us the big picture and guide our continued understanding of complex processes such as getting evidence into practice. In the previous two chapters, you learned about the debate between theorists and supporters of evidence-based practice, the value of theory, how to organize your thinking about models and frameworks, and some of the specifics of four models and frameworks of evidence implementation. These are the Iowa model, the Ottawa Model of Research Utilization (OMRU), the Promoting Action on Research Implementation in Health Services (PARIHS) framework, and the Joanna Briggs Institute (JBI) model (see Chapter 5 for descriptions and schema of each model). In this chapter, you will compare these four models/frameworks to better understand when to use a particular approach and examine their common principles to determine some universal features that are broadly applicable to your clinical practice (see Box 6■1).

In this chapter's clinical story, the four nurses face an all too common adverse event—a patient fall with injury. None of them was neglectful or uncaring, yet this patient fall may have been prevented. This is a real, concrete problem that can benefit from using a framework or model to uncover the best evidence and to put it into action.

On the surface, preventing falls in an acute care unit may not seem difficult. In fact, patients and their families fundamentally expect to be safe while in the hospital. But preventing falls is an example of a complex problem rather than a complicated problem, and there is a distinction. **Complicated problems** are usually made up of a series of simple problems. **Complex problems** tend to be unique, are associated with a great deal of uncertainty, and are less predictable. They cannot be solved with

---

BOX 6■1 **Significance Analyzing Evidence-Based Practice Models and Frameworks**

Before you buy a pair of shoes, you try them on for fit, style, comfort, and utility. Similarly, before you apply an evidence-based practice model or framework, you need to consider its fit and usefulness.
Consider the following factors:

- Who is intended to use it?
- What does the model or framework do?
- Where and at what level does the model or framework work best?
- What is its purpose?

When you have analyzed these factors, proceed to evaluate it based on the following criteria:

- Relevance
- Coherence
- Practicality
- Ability to structure messy or complex issues
- Fit with setting and user
- Effective visual representation
- Transferable to a variety of problems

rigid rules; the essence of the problem lies within the patterns and relationships (Lindberg, Nash, and Lindberg, 2008). Theories, frameworks, and models can help capture complexity yet provide some structure to problem solving.

In this chapter's clinical story, the four nurses are undoubtedly feeling responsible for the patient's fall. It is the unit's policy to "huddle" immediately after a fall to determine the details of what happened and to complete an incident report. Although these short debriefings help to capture the facts of the fall and may cause those involved to think about how to avoid the problem in the future, this method cannot address all of the multilevel issues related to preventing all falls. In fact, each fall presents unique issues and involves intersecting relationships, including the singular patient characteristics, the circumstances of the particular environment, the work load of the nurses, the processes of the unit (e.g., handoffs and placement of patients within the unit), the organizational supports and policy, and various other factors. Preventing all falls in all circumstances is a complex problem.

A Structure for Comparing Frameworks and Models

In the last chapter, you discovered you could compare models and frameworks using a simple journalist's approach. That is, you compare the who, what, where, when, why, and how well of each. There are certainly more sophisticated methods to analyze theoretical ways of thinking, but this approach is practical and easy to apply. It will allow you to determine your preference for a particular model and its fit to a particular situation, and to illustrate what is common and different among them. You may find one particular model or framework just makes sense to you so that you end up shaping your thinking to match that particular model. More likely, you will see that one framework or model will make more sense than another, depending on the nature of the problem, focus, setting, or other situational variable. Although each model is unique, there are some common principles that emerge with your analysis (see Table 6■1).

Who: Intended Users

Many frameworks and models are designed for multiple disciplines rather than for a single professional group. The four models discussed in Chapter 5 could be applied in any health profession. Despite this fact, some are more frequently used in nursing, whereas others are more commonly used in other disciplines. For example, the JBI model is appropriate for any group in healthcare and guides very diverse disciplines, including nursing, nurse midwifery, medicine, physiotherapy, radiological imaging, public health and occupational therapy (Pearson, Wiechula, Lockwood, et al., 2005). The Iowa model has been very popular for nurse-sensitive evidence-based practice and quality improvement programs and in nursing curricula. The OMRU model has been used across nursing, medicine, and allied health. The PARIHS model has been most popular amongst nurse-driven evidence-based practice and research applications, but it is intended to be applicable within and across many disciplines (see Box 6■2).

Table 6■1   **Comparison of Four Evidence-Based Practice Models/Frameworks**

	Iowa	Ottawa	PARIHS	JBI
Who: Intended Users	Interdisciplinary or single discipline teams at unit or agency level; the Ottawa model can be extended to networks and the JBI model to an international collaborative network			
What: Function	A decision-support schema with three major decision points: determining the priority of the problem or knowledge-focused trigger, readiness of the evidence, and outcomes of a pilot implementation to change practice	Three iterative phases: (1) assessment of barriers and supports of the innovation, adopters and practice environment; (2) monitor of the process and degree of use including barrier management; (3) evaluation of the impact on the patient, practitioner, and system	Successful implementation of evidence is a function of the strengths and weaknesses of the evidence, context, and facilitation. Skillful facilitators base their approach on the strengths and weaknesses of the evidence and context	Three phases beginning with synthesis of effect and meaning, moving to evidence transfer and utilization with tools for each phase; the goal is to improve global health through local implementation
Where: Settings	Units and systems	Individuals, units, systems, and networks	Units or groups of units	Units, systems, centers, global collaboration
Where: Level of Intended Users	Meso	Micro Meso Macro	Meso	Meso to macro
Why: Purpose	Descriptive and explanatory			Descriptive

What: Function of the Model or Framework

All four models under our consideration aim to enhance the implementation of evidence to improve patient outcomes. However, the functional aspects of each model are different. Each guides users to move evidence into practice in a different way. The Iowa model is a step-by-step decision aid with three key decision points: (1) whether the topic is a priority for the organization, (2) whether there is sufficient evidence to proceed, and (3) if change is warranted based on a pilot implementation. The model does not suggest ways of actually implementing the change. Rather one step of the pilot implementation is to "implement [evidence-based practice] on pilot units"

BOX 6■2   **Interdisciplinary Rounds**

- Negotiate using one of the models or frameworks to solve a complex clinical with a multidisciplinary team. Defend the team's choice to the chief operating officer of the institution (whose background is health-care administration).
- The quality assurance officer (who is not a nurse) does not believe that a model is necessary to address a clinical problem. Convince him.
- Ask someone from another discipline to tell you about a clinical problem and discuss how he or she would solve it. Explain how two of the models you studied would frame the problem. Negotiate a choice based on your shared evaluation of how well the model or framework would work to help you sort of the problem, the evidence, and its implementation.

(Titler, p. 138). The model does guide users through the common steps of the evidence-based practice process (identify the problem; assemble a team; review; critique and summarize literature; and develop, implement, and evaluate a plan). But it does not provide ideas about how to move the evidence-based innovation into practice.

In contrast, the OMRU is an iterative model that directs users to first assess barriers to and supporters of the innovation as well as characteristics of adopters and the practice environment to target change processes. For example, if one barrier is a lack of equipment for the evidence-based innovation, the change process would include acquiring the appropriate equipment. The second phase of the model is to monitor the process and degree of use by managing barriers, facilitating transfer, and doing the follow-up that leads to initial and sustained adoption. The third phase is evaluation of the innovation's impact on patients, practitioners, and the health-care system.

The PARIHS framework explains how to assess the key elements (evidence and context) to use facilitation skills, purposes, and roles to either offset weaknesses or reinforce strengths in the evidence or context.

The JBI model functions through the array of tools for evidence synthesis (software, training, and dissemination of systematic reviews), transfer (online evidence summaries for clinicians and consumers, training, and tools to embed) and utilization (software for evaluation).

Where: Levels and Settings

Generally, models are scoped for different levels of users such as the individual (micro), group or system (meso), or national/international level (macro). Some of the models and frameworks apply at all levels, whereas others are most suited for only one level. The Iowa model is best suited for teams working to influence clinical policy at the unit or within an agency (meso), rather than individuals using evidence to make nursing practice decisions (Titler, 2010). Individuals (micro), teams within a unit (meso), and even whole health systems or networks (macro) could use OMRU, because the potential adopters of the innovation include patients (if an individual practitioner uses the model), practitioners, and policy makers (if a team within a unit, system, or network of systems use the model) (Logan and Graham, 2010). It is best suited for teams who influence others to use evidence to impact patient, practitioner, and system outcomes.

The PARIHS framework best fits the meso level at the team, unit, and organization level. One domain in this model is context and the subelements leadership, organizational culture, and evaluation processes. The authors' definitions and tools were developed to measure context, and they seem to best fit the needs of meso-level intended users.

The JBI model is unique because its goal is to improve global health through international collaboration of all health-care disciplines. Even with the international focus, the intent is for implementation to occur at the local level and for it ultimately to impact global health (Pearson et al., 2005). The JBI and its collaborating centers use the model to frame the work at the macro level (international) and to guide the activities of the center. Because centers involve partner-clinical agencies, the model can apply at the unit level and at the health-care system level. Nonetheless, it is perhaps best known for its unique approach at the macro level.

Why: Purpose

All four of models discussed in this book are descriptive, and all but the JBI model are also explanatory. That is, they explain the relationships among the concepts or stages in the process (Rycroft-Malone and Bucknall, 2010). The Iowa model and OMRU describe a process. OMRU describes three phases of moving evidence into practice: (1) assessment of barriers and supports, (2) monitoring of the process, and (3) use of evidence and evaluation of the impact (Logan and Graham, 2010). The Iowa model describes a series of decisions in the process of moving from problem trigger to evidence assessment (Titler, 2010). Both of these models can be used to guide quality improvement.

The JBI model is unique because of its scope and because of how the model uses available tools to make the key phases (evidence synthesis, transfer, and utilization) operational. It has been used to structure collaborative work including the formation of academic and clinical partnerships around the elements of the model. Individuals can also use it to structure their thinking about the flow of knowledge, from generation to utilization.

How Well: Evaluating the Usefulness

If you are just beginning to use theories, frameworks, and models to better understand nursing practice, you will want straightforward criteria for evaluating them. Even as you become more experienced, you will return to these criteria because they address how sensible and practicable the framework or model is for you. These criteria include the following:

- Relevance
- Coherence
- Practicality

- Ability to structure messy or complex issues
- Fit with setting and/or user
- Effective visual representation
- Transferable to a variety of problems

As when you read the first few pages of a new book, you will probably look at a model or framework to see if it attracts you in some way. This means it needs to be relevant to your practice and to how you use information to inform decisions. The model or framework needs to make sense—it must be coherent. Even though conceptual frameworks and models are a bit abstract by nature, they still need to be understandable and logical.

For a framework or model to be usable, it needs to be practical at some level. That does not mean that you will necessarily understand all of the concepts and their relationships at first glance, but you should be able to generate ideas about how to apply the model or framework without too much strain.

Frameworks and models should help you sort and understand complex problems. If a framework or model only makes your understanding muddier, it is not helpful. Conversely, a model can bring clarity and insight. For example, in this chapter's clinical story, if the nurses are to implement evidence-based changes, they will need to understand the context, those involved in the change, and the dimensions of the change itself. They could use the OMRU model to help assess the barriers and promoters of the innovation, the adopters, and environment. Without this structure, they may not know how to begin the change process.

When you choose a model, it must fit the situation, the setting, the individual or team involved, and interpretation of both the problem and the model itself. This requires trying out a specific model or framework to determine if it fits your needs, just as you might try out a lens prescription to be certain it improves your vision. The one that fits correctly will help you visualize and decipher an approach to the problem.

Most models are depicted in a visual schema or picture to help users see how the concepts relate to one another. This serves as a map, and you can use the diagram just as you might chart a trip. However, that picture needs to make sense.

Finally, to be useful a model or framework needs to work for a variety of problems. It may fit best in one context, but it should also be widely applicable to a variety of problems. For example, a question might arise from something that happens in the clinical arena (e.g., an increase in the incidence of falls) or from reading about a new approach in the literature (e.g., a systematic review about hourly rounding's effect on fall rates). Looking at your four options, you can see that the Iowa model is transferable to many situations that can arise from either of these of triggers.

In this chapter's clinical story, the nurses work with a team that includes a clinical nurse specialist, quality improvement nurse, physiotherapist, frontline nurses from several units, risk manager, and gerontologist. The team initially is overwhelmed at the prospect of sifting through the assessment, intervention, and evaluation aspects of this very important problem. Then Alin remembers studying the PARIHS framework in his senior capstone course; he and his team implemented a small-scale evidence-based practice innovation. He shares this experience with the team. In addition, the quality improvement nurse has used the Iowa model, and the gerontologist is familiar with OMRU. The physiotherapist is aware of the JBI model and has used some of the resources from the physiotherapy node of JBI Connect+. As they begin unraveling the solutions to the problem, they realize that different aspects of each model and framework influence their decisions.

After they formulate questions related to fall assessment and prevention, they consult with their hospital's library scientist (see Chapter 8 for question development and Chapter 9 for searching). A review of the JBI model reminds them that synthesis of evidence of effect and meaningfulness is necessary to understand the full scope of the problem and its solutions. When they transfer the knowledge from synthesized sources, they need concise summaries if they expect their colleagues to have time to attend to the key aspects of the evidence.

Using the PARIHS conceptual framework, they next assess the sources and strength of the evidence. Then they use the context assessment index (CAI) to evaluate the strengths and weaknesses of the organizational culture, leadership characteristics, and evaluation practices (McCormack, McCarthy, Wright, et al., 2009). Based on these assessments, the team decides what type of facilitation (ranging from doing for to enabling others) is required for certain units. They select clinical nurse specialists from the pilot units to lead the facilitation efforts. Each unit has a unique subculture and leadership group, but they share the same evaluation processes.

Using the data from the CAI, the facilitators plan how to use facilitation tools and skills within and across the units to implement changes in risk assessment and fall prevention. One of the practice changes they plan to implement is bedside handoff. They realize this seemingly small shift in the location of the handoff report has reverberating consequences that will need skillful facilitation. They plan to use elements of the OMRU model to further assess the barriers and supports for changing practice in the affected units. In addition, they will employ audit and feedback to use (JBI) and monitor (OMRU) the key best practices defined by the evidence. The solutions will undoubtedly reflect both the best available evidence as well as the multidisciplinary team's varied expertise.

The patients' preferences will also inform the project in at least two stages. As they are developing a plan to implement the results of the evidence, the team grapples with how they can ensure that nurses, physicians, and physiotherapists consider individual patient preferences. Throughout the project planning, Enrique voices his lingering guilt that the fall had a profound effect on the patient's subsequent functional ability, and he and Lindsay pursue more information on the patient experience of a fall with injury. They work with the librarian to find qualitative evidence of patients' experiences with a fall, and they advocate for including what they learn from this evidence in the implementation plan.

This commonplace clinical story illustrates how a critical incident can uncover a complex problem. The framework/model "mash-up" application should help you understand how elements of each model can bring light to the problem. You can see how the different models can influence how you see and approach the situation. However, it is best to use just one model to frame a complex problem and its solutions to bring coherence and structure to the process (see Box 6■3).

BOX 6=3 **Tools for Learning and Practice**

- Explore the four models presented in Chapters 5 and 6 using the Reference lists.
- Search the bibliographic databases to find more models related to evidence and research utilization.
- Conduct a Google search to find Web sites dedicated to the following models and frameworks:
  - http://www.joannabriggs.edu.au
  - http://www.parihs.org/
  - http://www.ncddr.org/kt/products/ktintro/
  - http://www.uihealthcare.com/depts/nursing/rqom/evidencebased practice/iowamodel.html

Summary

In this chapter, you learned about the common and distinguishing principles of the four sample models and frameworks. Each model or framework brings a unique perspective to implementing evidence into practice. It is your job to decide which model or framework best fits your particular problem, setting, and team. The evaluation framework can help you determine which one will work best. This chapter's clinical story shows that models and frameworks can bring clarity to complex problems.

CHAPTER QUESTIONS

1. Have you ever used a model or framework in how you think about a problem in your clinical work? If you have, how did it affect how you framed the problem? If you have not, why not?

2. Describe a complicated problem from your clinical experience. Describe a complex problem in your clinical experience. What characteristics differentiated the complicated from the complex? What impact did the complicated and complex problems each have on how you, a team, or the organization approached the problem? Was the solution successful? Why or why not?

3. Describe the key aspects of each of the four frameworks and models (Iowa, OMRU, PARIHS, and JBI). What do they share in common? What is particularly unique about each model?

4. Describe a recent complex problem or issue that you have experienced in your clinical setting. Which of the frameworks or models do you think would fit best? Why?

5. Think about a situation that would potentially benefit from using a model or framework to guide the implementation of evidence. What would you want that model of framework to do for you to be useful?

6. Can you imagine using one of the four models or frameworks in your clinical practice? Using the evaluation criteria, justify your answer.

References

Lindberg, C., Nash, S., & Lindberg, C. (2008). *On the edge: Nursing in an age of complexity*. Bordentown, NJ: PexusPress.

Logan, J., & Graham, I. (2010). The Ottawa model of research use. In J. Rycroft-Malone & T. Bucknall (Eds.), *Models and frameworks for implementing evidence-based practice: Linking evidence to action* (pp. 83–108). Oxford: Wiley-Blackwell.

McCormack, B., McCarthy, G., Wright, J., et al. (2009). Developing and testing of the context of assessment index (CAI). *Worldviews on Evidence-Based Nursing, 6*, 27–35.

Pearson, A., Wiechula, R., Lockwood, C., et al. (2005). The JBI model of evidence-based health care. *International Journal of Evidence-Based Health Care, 3*, 207–215.

Rycroft-Malone, J., & Bucknall, T. (2010). Analysis and synthesis of models and frameworks (pp. 223–245). In J. Rycroft-Malone & T. Bucknall (Eds.), *Models and frameworks for implementing evidence-based practice: Linking evidence to action* (pp. 83–108). Oxford: Wiley-Blackwell.

Titler, M. (2010). Iowa model of evidence-based practice. In J. Rycroft-Malone & T. Bucknall (Eds.), *Models and frameworks for implementing evidence-based practice: Linking evidence to action* (pp. 83–108). Oxford: Wiley-Blackwell.

How to Do Evidence-Based Practice

In this unit, you will work through the evidence-based practice process step by step and relate it to the familiar nursing process. You begin with an overview of the process in Chapter 7 and then move to asking questions that lead to finding the best available evidence. You will be able to remember the process using a simple memory device of the "5 A's," meaning each step begins with an "A": Ask, Acquire, Appraise, Apply, and Assess.

Just like assessing patients is an orderly process of probing, the evidence-based practice process begins with asking questions using a systematic approach. The second step is to acquire evidence by searching bibliographic databases or other sources of evidence where the answers to your question will be if the evidence exists. This step relates to the diagnosis phase

(continues on page 76)

of the nursing process based on your assessment. After you establish a nursing diagnosis, you develop a plan by weighing your nursing care options and deciding what is important. This step in the nursing process relates to the important part of the process of appraising or weighing the quality of the evidence you find or using a system where someone else has appraised the quality of the evidence. Next you apply the evidence just like you implement your nursing care plan. There are three chapters related to applying evidence because it happens at multiple levels—by individual nurses, health systems, and national groups. Finally, just as you evaluate the impact of your nursing interventions, you must assess the impact of evidence implementation.

CHAPTER 7

Overview of the Evidence-Based Practice Process

Lisa Hopp

(continues on page 78)

PICo question	Research process
Preappraised evidence	Social contract
Problem solving	Strength

Clinical Story

Ali is student on a general surgical floor, and she has already received her assignment for the next day. She wants to be well prepared to provide care for a 70-year-old man who has had a bowel resection (removal and reconnection of part of the bowel). She will be caring for him on his first postoperative day. She anticipates he will experience postoperative pain. Although pain is just one issue that she will need to manage, she knows it will be one of her nursing care priorities. She thinks about how she will assess, diagnose, plan, implement, and evaluate her plan of care.

Because Ali wants to understand all aspects of caring for her patient's pain, she looks for a clinical practice guideline. She searches the Registered Nurses' Association of Ontario (RNAO) best practice guidelines first. She finds a comprehensive guideline on the assessment and management of pain that she can adapt for her patient's acute postoperative pain (RNAO, 2007). She plans to complete a comprehensive pain assessment when she first meets the patient and a standard quicker assessment to reassess his pain. Ali anticipates she will need to give the patient medication to relieve his pain, and she needs to be aware of possible adverse effects from the medication and how his other health problems may put him at higher risk for adverse reactions. Ali knows that she will need to make sure that the patient has adequate pain relief to be able to move and get out of bed to speed his recovery. She is aware that because her patient is older, he may react in a different manner than would a younger person to both the surgery and the analgesia. She reads the guideline to determine if she might offer other interventions in addition to medications, such as music and relaxation, to help reduce the patient's pain. Also, she must carefully evaluate and document the patient's response to her interventions. Ali is confident her plan is well supported with the best available evidence and she is ready to adjust it as she cares for her patient the next day. ■

Introduction

Some might claim that evidence-based nursing practice is nothing more than providing good care. In part, they are right. Evidence-based practice is about doing the right thing, for the right patient, from the right person, at the right time, and in the right way to achieve the right outcome at the right cost (Royal Colleges of Nursing, as cited in Livesley and Howarth, 2007). But how do you know the right way to assess, diagnose, plan, implement, and evaluate your care? Evidence-based nursing practice is not something that happens *in addition* to the nursing process. Rather, evidence should inform all aspects of nursing care (Fawcett and Garrity, 2009).

In this chapter, you will review the definition of *nursing* and reflect on what nursing means to you. You will compare three processes: the nursing, research, and evidence-based practice processes and relate them to basic problem solving. Each step of the evidence-based practice process will be defined to prepare you to learn more about each phase in subsequent chapters.

Essence of Nursing Practice

Busy clinicians juggle many competing demands while caring for a caseload of patients in a complex environment. In this chapter's clinical story, Ali anticipates many potential problems that her postoperative patient may have in addition to recognizing the importance of pain relief. She realizes that although her patient's comfort is a priority in and of itself, pain relief is linked to other aspects of the patient's experience in the first postoperative day, such as being able to move to avoid complications of immobility.

The clinical story captures the essential features of nursing. The goal of Ali's care is to help the patient regain health through a caring relationship in which she attends to a range of responses including pain, limited mobility, challenges to nutritional and fluid intake, elimination, and the social and emotional impact of surgery. She plans to gather data, such as the patient's report of pain, to integrate into the decisions she makes to intervene and alleviate the patient's discomfort and to promote mobility. She has the obligation to find and use the best information to care for the patient correctly —to provide the highest quality and safe care by using evidence to inform her decisions (American Nurses Association [ANA], 2010) (Box 7■1).

BOX 7■1 **Significance of Evidence-Based Practice**

- The American Nurses Association established the role of evidence-based practice in its 2010 Social Policy Statement; this policy statement ratifies using evidence to practice nursing as an expectation of every professional nurse in the United States.
- Registered nurses enter into a social contract with the public to use evidence to inform their nursing practice.
- Governing bodies in other countries such as the United Kingdom and Australia have explicitly committed nurses to using evidence in their practice.
- Evidence-based practice is integral to high-quality nursing practice; it is not an add-on or an academic exercise.
- Evidence informs each phase of the nursing process.

Like Ali, you make many decisions, often simultaneously and perhaps without being fully aware of how you make these decisions. Think about what sets your care apart from what others do for and with patients. Then think about how you "know" and compare that with how others define the essence of nursing practice.

Definition of Nursing

The American Nurses Association (2010) defines **nursing** for nurses who practice in the United States. The current definition evolved from the first Social Policy Statement written in 1980. The ANA states that "nursing is the protection, promotion, and optimization of health and abilities, prevention of illness and injury, alleviation of suffering through the diagnosis and treatment of human response, and advocacy in the care of individuals, families, communities and populations" (p. 3). When you become registered, you enter into a **social contract** with patients and families to uphold this definition of professional nursing. In the context of nursing, the code of ethics defines our social contract with the public, meaning the "profession's expression of the values, duties and commitments to the public" (p. 24). Through this social contract, society grants professional nurses the authority to practice.

Essential Features of Nursing

The ANA (2010) lists seven essential features of professional nursing. All of them relate to evidence-based nursing practice in some way if we heed the full definition of *evidence-based practice* (Table 7■1). For example, when nurses develop a caring relationship, they must embrace the patient's values and preferences and use effective interventions to facilitate health and healing. Similarly, when nurses influence public policy to promote social justice, they should advocate for decision makers to honor all patients' values and preferences and assure equal access to the treatments that work, regardless of the patients' ability to pay. If you think broadly and self-consciously, you will find a place for evidence in nearly every aspect of nursing.

Nursing Actions

When non-nurses discuss professional nursing, they generally talk about what nurses do. Nurses are known for **nursing actions.** Nursing actions are how nurses intervene to protect, promote, and optimize health and abilities. They act to prevent illness and injury; alleviate suffering; and advocate for individuals, families, communities, and populations to produce beneficial outcomes (ANA, 2010). These interventions are developed from knowledge gained from both theory and evidence (ANA, 2010).

The latest edition of the ANA's Social Policy Statement (2010) is the first time policy makers explicitly addressed the role of evidence-based practice in the definition of *nursing practice*. Previous editions in 1995 and 2003 did mention the role of research in informing nursing practice, but only the current edition features the role of evidence in all nursing actions (ANA, 2010). Now when nurses become registered, they enter into the social contract to use evidence to inform their actions.

Table 7■1   **Essential Features of Professional Nursing and Relationship to Evidence-Based Practice**

Essential Feature	Application to the Evidence-Based Practice Concept
Provision of a caring relationship that facilitates health and healing	Honoring patient preferences and values in shared decision making
Attention to the range of human experiences and responses to health and illness within the physical and social environments	Determining the applicability of evidence to an individual patient and his or her context
Integration of assessment data with knowledge gained from an appreciation of the patient or the group	Gathering individual or local data and situating them with evidence from the research of groups
Application of scientific knowledge to the processes of diagnosis and treatment through the use of judgment and critical thinking	Using clinical expertise and appraisal of the best available evidence of effectiveness to select the most appropriate nursing intervention
Advancement of professional nursing knowledge through scholarly inquiry	Using the evidence syntheses to identify gaps in knowledge and the need for further research
Influence on social and public policy to promote social justice	Advocating for policy that assures equal access to effective treatment and the incorporation of patient values and preferences in policy decisions
Assurance of safe, quality, and evidence-based practice	Questioning traditional practices and using the best available evidence to drive safe, high-quality care while discarding ineffective practices

From American Nurses Association. (2010). *Nursing's social policy statement: The essence of the profession*. Silver Spring, MD: Nursingbooks.org.

Problem-Solving Processes

In daily practice, nurses are continually preventing and solving problems related to both the patient's experience and nursing actions. For example, Ali anticipated the patient would experience surgical pain. Her plan of care includes her plan for managing this potential problem. She uses the nursing process as a way to avert or modify the problem of acute pain related to the patient's abdominal surgery, and she uses evidence to inform each step of the process.

Problem solving is a generic process that describes part of the thinking and doing of nursing practice. It is a step-by-step sequence of defining the problem, identifying the possible causes, generating possible solutions, selecting the best solution, implementing it, and evaluating the effect on the problem. Many disciplines use a problem-solving approach. In fact, people solve problems in their everyday life, but they do not pay close attention to how they approach problem solving.

In contrast, evidence-based nursing does require close attention to the decision-making process by first considering the problem and its potential etiology, or cause; generating questions that focus on the effectiveness, feasibility, or appropriateness of interventions; and understanding the meaning of the patient's experience. As part of the process, you will ultimately choose an intervention or use what you learn from evidence of meaningfulness to guide what and how you address the problem. Finally, you will evaluate the effectiveness of your interventions and how your patient experienced your intervention. As you can see, problem solving and evidence-based practice are closely connected (Fig. 7■1).

Nursing Process

Nursing's Social Policy Statement (ANA, 2010) defines the **nursing process** and links it with the definitions of *nursing* and *theoretical and evidence-based knowledge.* "Nurses use their theoretical and evidence-based knowledge of these human experiences and responses to collaborate with patients and others to assess, diagnose, plan, implement, evaluate care, and identify outcomes" (p. 14). This definition means that the nurse is obliged to use both theory and evidence to care for patients and to do the work of nursing. The nursing process employs critical thinking to assess, diagnose, identify outcomes, plan, implement, and evaluate. These actions may happen simultaneously or in a more sequential fashion (ANA, 2010).

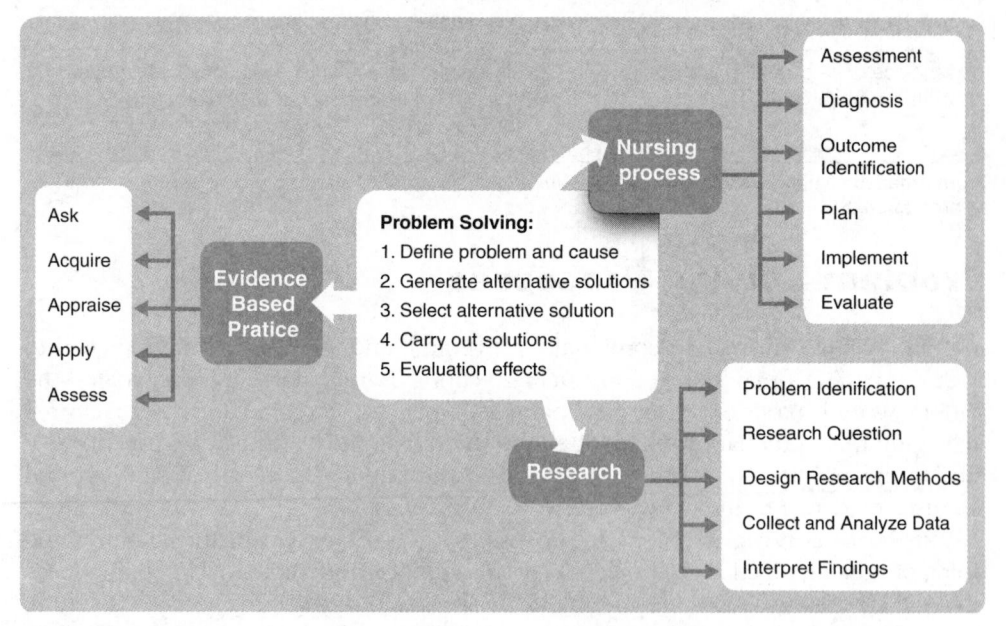

FIGURE 7■1 Concept map: Relating problem solving, nursing process, research and evidence-based practice.

The ANA has formed nursing standards for each phase of the nursing process. **Nursing standards** are an "authoritative statement by which the nursing profession describes the responsibilities for which its practitioners are accountable, the outcomes for which registered nurses are responsible, and by which the quality of practice, service, or education can be evaluated" (ANA, 2010, p. 42). In other words, a professional nurse has the responsibility to act competently in all six phases of the nursing process. In providing care, such as comfort measures to decrease pain, the nurse uses the best available evidence to inform how best to assess, intervene, and evaluate patient outcomes. You use evidence to understand how the patient experiences pain and discomfort.

Research Process

Ideally, research-based evidence will be available to answer the clinical question. Research-based evidence is stronger than other types of evidence because it is less susceptible to many types of bias, if the research is conducted in a rigorous way. If research is not available, the nurse will need to seek out other sources, such as expert consensus opinion. **Expert consensus opinion** occurs when experts in an area of science discuss and come to an agreement about the best approach to a problem. The best expert consensus opinion would involve a systematic and rigorous method to determine a conclusion that is then exposed to public opinion or external critique.

The **research process** follows the basic problem-solving methodology. Investigators begin by posing a specific question related to a problem. For example, Good, Albert, Anderson, et al. (2010) recognized that many people who have surgery have unresolved pain even though they receive IV medication through patient-controlled analgesia (patients trigger the IV dose on demand). They reviewed the literature to identify the unresolved issues related to successfully treating postoperative pain. They found questions remained about the effect on pain of combining relaxation and music during the immediate postoperative period. After narrowing their focus to this specific area, the authors designed a study to test hypotheses about the effect of patient teaching and relaxation plus music, both as single interventions and combined, on patients' pain ratings. They based these hypotheses on the underlying mechanisms of how music and relaxation might work to decrease pain. They planned the methods of study so that they could detect differences among the treatments. Then they implemented the study with four groups of patients; an experimental condition was randomly assigned to each group to receive one of the experimental conditions or standard pharmacological care. Throughout the study, they carefully measured the same outcomes in all subjects, analyzed the results, and came to the conclusion that that relaxation plus music therapy significantly decreased pain immediately after surgery, whereas patient teaching alone did not. Most single studies do not provide enough evidence to change practice, but you can see that the process of planning and conducting the research is systematic and logical.

The three processes—nursing process, problem solving, and the research process—share parallel phases. For example, in all three, the first step is uncovering and naming the problem. In problem solving, that is done by defining and stating the problem. In the nursing process, the problem is assessed and diagnosed. In the research process, the literature is reviewed, and the research question is stated (Table 7■2).

Evidence-Based Practice Process

The **evidence-based practice process** is problem solving that begins by identifying the problem, asking specific questions, acquiring evidence based on the specific question, appraising the evidence for its quality, applying the evidence, and assessing the outcomes of the intervention. A memory device is the five 5 *As*—Ask, Acquire, Appraise, Apply, Assess. This sounds very neat and straightforward. However, putting evidence into action may not happen quite so tidily. Nursing practice and patients' responses to health and illness are complex. However, if you take time to understand each step, you will begin to master the process despite the complexity of your work.

Ask

It may seem obvious that to find an answer, you need to ask the right question. Therefore, the first step of the evidence-based practice process is to **ask,** or pose a clear question that will lead to the right evidence for the problem. As in the research process, the question drives the rest of the evidence-based practice process. It forms the blueprint for the search for evidence by pointing to keywords and maintaining the focus on the key decision that needs to be made to solve the problem. Similarly, in the nursing process you first assess the patient to determine the problem.

Table 7■2   **Comparison of Processes**

Problem Solving	Nursing Process (ANA)	Research Process (Polit & Beck, 2008)	Evidence-Based Practice Process
Define problem and cause	Assessment	Problem identification and research question	Ask
Generate alternative solutions Select alternative	Diagnosis Outcome Identification Plan	Design research methods	Acquire Appraise
Carry out solution	Implement	Collect and analyze data	Apply
Evaluate effects	Evaluate	Interpret findings	Assess

From American Nurses Association. (2010). *Nursing's social policy statement: The essence of the profession.* Silver Spring, MD: Nursingbooks.org.

In the evidence-based practice process, the way you state the question depends on the purpose of your query. In future chapters, you will learn more about how to shape a general problem into either a **PICO** question (if you ask about the effectiveness of interventions) or a **PICo** question (if you want to understand the meaning of a patient's experience). This template approach ensures that you remember the important elements for specific, well-formed questions; each letter represents one part of the question. For questions of effectiveness (PICO), *P* represents *p*opulation; *I* equals *i*ntervention; *C* stands for *c*omparison intervention; and *O* is *o*utcome. For questions of meaning (PICo), *P* still represents *p*opulation; *I* refers to the phenomenon of *i*nterest; and *Co* means *co*ntext. When you use this simple memory device, you are more likely to develop solid, searchable questions.

The size of the problem will also influence how you ask the question. In the next chapter, you will learn more about scope and scale, two ways of thinking about the size of the question. For example, Ali may be interested in the best available evidence related to how patients experience acute, postoperative pain, and how to assess pain, intervene, and evaluate the effectiveness of her interventions. In this case, she would look for a very comprehensive source of evidence, such as a complete clinical practice guideline from the Registered Nurses' Association of Ontario or the American Pain Society. Alternatively, she may need information about only one very narrow part of her care, such as whether relaxation and music are likely to help limit the intensity and duration of pain during the immediate postoperative period. In this case, she may use evidence from a systematic review of all research trials that tested the effectiveness of these interventions. The size of these two problems is quite different. The way that Ali would seek evidence and use the evidence to inform her clinical decisions depends on how she asks the question.

Acquire

The next step of the evidence-based practice process is using the question to determine how to search for the evidence. That is, one **acquires** the best information that links the diagnosis of the patient problem with potential solutions. One needs to know where to look, how to access the source, and how to find the best available evidence. These are not trivial issues. Many nurses in the United States have limited access to the Internet at point of care, and a significant portion feel they do not have the right skills to search databases (Pravikoff, Tanner, and Pierce, 2005). Later in this book, you will find out more about the best way to approach the search process and when to seek the help of experts so you can avoid these barriers in your own practice.

The complexity or ease of the search process depends on the source you explore. As a novice, it may be helpful to know the best bet resources: the places where it is easiest to find the best available evidence published in a thorough, yet efficient manner. In this chapter's clinical story, if Ali searches individual organizations for the practice guidelines, she can simply browse the sites for the pages that house the practice guidelines. She may only need to use a key phrase search such as "pain guideline" to find a short list of pages within the site. However, if she searched a larger database, such as the Agency for Healthcare Research and Quality National Guideline Clearinghouse, a simple search using "pain" as the keyword would net more than 1000 guidelines, far too many to sort them easily for relevance to her problem. She would need to use advance search tools or work with an expert, such as a librarian, to narrow the search. If she wanted to search for systematic reviews or individual research reports for information that was not adequately covered in the guideline, she would need to use bibliographic databases and a structured search using the appropriate keywords and linkages.

Many students and bedside nurses find using bibliographic databases to be a significant barrier to using evidence in their practice. Practice leads to more confidence and expertise, and you should not be satisfied with a quick Internet search once you understand the importance of uncovering the best evidence. In some situations, you will need the help of a librarian or other expert to find the best information. In fact, librarians are integral members of strong evidence-based practice teams.

Appraise

The next step of the evidence-based practice process is to **appraise** the evidence; that is, critically evaluate the evidence for its quality. It is unlikely that you will find only a single source when you search for the best way to answer your question. In fact, if you settle for the first piece of information you find, you cannot be assured that it is the best available. Instead, you have to judge the quality of a variety of sources to determine what is truly the best available. In other words, nurses who use evidence to inform each aspect of the nursing process must be skeptical.

In cases of the effectiveness of interventions, one needs to evaluate both the **strength** and the **magnitude** of the evidence in the source. The strength of the evidence relates to the quality or believability of the evidence, whereas the magnitude of the evidence refers to the "so-what" factor, or how big an effect the intervention makes on the outcome. Similarly, when one appraises evidence of meaning, feasibility, or applicability, one evaluates the credibility of the source.

It may be easier to understand how important appraisal is if you examine a simple case of buying your next car. When considering your purchase, you will have criteria that are important to you. These might include cost, durability, appearance, fuel economy, comfort, and safety. Using these criteria, you can rate the quality of each car you are considering to help you make your decision. The difference among your choices may be large or small. When you judge the strength of quality of the cars, you rate each against your criteria, and the magnitude of the differences among the cars will help you finalize your decision, particularly if one costs a great deal more than another. You ultimately want to pick the one that is the highest quality for the best price. Selecting nursing interventions based on the evidence is quite similar. That is, you use a set of criteria to judge the quality and significance of the effectiveness of an intervention.

Some sources of evidence are **preappraised**. If this is the case, the guideline developers, reviewers, or publishers have already completed the hard work of evaluating the strength and magnitude of the evidence. However, you still need to understand what appraisal process the authors used to rate the evidence and if it was rigorous. In addition, you need to understand what the ranking system means. For example, you might choose to rely on the publication of a credible group, such as *Consumer Reports*, to conduct a thorough evaluation of the cars you are considering rather than completing the ranking yourself. *Consumer Reports* uses experts and a highly standardized approach to testing and rating the products it reviews ("How We Test," 2010). Not only do you save time by trusting the evaluation, you also benefit from the expert knowledge that backs the reports. Conversely, if you ask a salesperson in the showroom for an evaluation of a car that you are interested in, you may not receive a rigorous, unbiased rating of the cars—particularly if you ask about a car from another carmaker.

As the example shows, some preappraised evidence will save you time and produce a more expert ranking, whereas other sources might be biased. Later chapters discuss preappraised evidence, the systems used to rank strength and magnitude, and how to judge and use appraisal systems.

Apply

No matter how strong or large the effect, evidence is useless until put into action. To **apply** the evidence is to make it actionable. The way that evidence is applied can range in scope from influencing individual clinicians' decisions to national (and even global) health policy. Some of the largest challenges in the evidence-based practice movement relate to changing behaviors and application of the evidence. Systems are emerging that will ease and speed the integration of evidence into the everyday practice of health-care providers around the globe.

As an individual nurse, your goal is to use evidence to inform decisions throughout the nursing process. Once you have appraised and chosen the evidence based on its strength and magnitude, you need to decide how to use it.

In this chapter's clinical story, Ali wants to use the practice guideline to plan how best to assess the patient's pain and determine the appropriate intervention that will reduce the patient's pain while limiting side effects. She applies the evidence when she reviews the patient's record and sees that preoperatively, a nurse completed a comprehensive assessment of the patient's prior experiences, beliefs, and understanding of what to expect of his surgery. Ali knows the guideline made specific recommendations about tools to complete both comprehensive and ongoing assessments of pain intensity during the postoperative period. The guideline reinforced her understanding that the patient's self-report of pain is the ideal way to assess but that it requires the patient to be able to communicate (RNAO, 2007). She decides to use the numeric rating scale (rating pain intensity on a scale of 1 to 10) to assess the intensity of pain because it is valid, easy to use, appropriate to use with her patient who could communicate, and commonly used in the facility. Also, based on the guideline, Ali anticipates the pharmacological treatment and plans to offer music and/or relaxation as an adjunct to the medication. Ali feels confident about putting the evidence into action, especially when she realizes that the guideline developers preappraised the evidence and gave each of these recommendations their highest quality ranking. Although she already planned to use the evidence to influence her own actions, she discovers the guideline also provides evidence and tools to help apply the evidence in nursing units, organizations, and even at the national level (RNAO, 2007).

Assess

As in the nursing, problem solving, and research processes, the last stage of the evidence-based practice process is to **assess,** or evaluate, the outcomes. The method of assessment must be supported by evidence. That is, the measurement must be valid and reliable.

Some of the same tools are used to diagnose a problem and to evaluate the effect of interventions on outcomes. For example, Ali can use the same technique to assess her patient's level of pain before and after her interventions. However, additional tools can be sued to assess whether the interventions worked or if the interventions actually took place. In other words, one assesses and documents both the process and outcome of applying the evidence.

Process evaluation happens through an audit of whether the evidence-based interventions occurred. You may be part of an audit effort, or the quality team may conduct data collection. If quality officers or other facility staff audit and provide feedback about how frequently nurses use the evidence when providing care, then nurses have the opportunity to improve their care (Box 7■2). Although evidence is not always strong or well developed, audit and feedback remain common methods to enhance the uptake of evidence in practice (Cheater, Baker, Reddish, et al, 2006; Jamtvedt, Young, Kristofferson, et al, 2006).

Ali uses the guideline to plan to reassess the patient's report of pain at the appropriate time after both the medication use (based on the predicted peak activity of the drug) and the introduction of music and relaxation, as well as when the patient changed his activity. She will document her assessments and evaluation in the record and advocate for other treatments if his pain is not adequately relieved (RNAO, 2007).

Changing Practice Is Challenging

When you are new to nursing or to evidence-based practice, it is useful to deconstruct the process into its component parts. However, you will find that putting evidence

---

BOX 7■2 **Interdisciplinary Rounds**

- Librarians are part of the evidence-based practice team. Introduce yourself to the hospital or university library and discuss how you might work together to find evidence.
- Take a leadership role to work with librarians to identify best-bet resources and consult with an information technologist to make these online resources easily available on computers at the point of care.
- Evidence from many disciplines can inform nursing practice. Adopt an open, curious attitude when looking for evidence.
- Welcome and talk with members of other disciplines about how they use evidence to inform their practices.

into action is a messy process and often complex. Even when the issue and interventions seem quite straight forward, changing practice is challenging. You will find that although the steps of problem solving, the nursing process, and evidence-based practice process seem linear and can be neatly sorted on paper, in reality, they happen in cycles or in an iterative manner. Sometimes it will seem as though you take two steps forward and one step backward. However, that is often the nature of how people create change—in small steps, slowly nudging the process along. Despite the increased use of evidence in current nursing practice, more research is needed to better understand how to put evidence into action more reliably and more quickly (Box 7■3).

■ Summary

When you become a registered nurse, you enter into a social contract with the public to use evidence to inform your practice. The ANA and governing groups in other countries have developed standards of practice that explicitly state the role of evidence in nursing care. In this chapter, you were shown how the nursing, research, and evidence-based practice processes were all variations of problem solving; they share parallel and common structures and functions. When deconstructed, the evidence-based practice process resembles the nursing process.

BOX 7■3 Tools for Learning and Practice

- Read the American Nurses Association's Social Policy Statement. Highlight statements relevant to evidence-based practice.
- Ask your colleagues if they are aware of explicit role for evidence in the statement.
- Next time you care for a patient, ask yourself how you know what assessment techniques to use or what interventions you should use. Think about whether you know what evidence supports how you approached the patient.
- Check your hospital's mission and goals to understand how the organization values evidence. Talk about the role of evidence-based practice with the formal and informal leaders in your unit and hospital.
- Look around the clinical environment for "evidence of the evidence" in your organization. For example, look for how evidence is made explicit in policies, or if there posters or other displays that transparently communicate the evidence and its quality.
- Visit the library and explore what database, journal, and evidence resource subscriptions the organization maintains.
- Think about a problem you recently had to deal with. Review the steps of the problem solving and analyze how you defined the problem and its cause, generated alternative solutions, and selected from your alternatives and how you carried out and evaluated your solution.

In future chapters you will read more about asking questions, acquiring and appraising the evidence that addresses the question, planning how to apply the evidence, and assessing the effect of putting the evidence into action.

CHAPTER QUESTIONS

1. What are the key words in the ANA's definition of *nursing*? How does this definition reflect what you do in your nursing practice?

2. What nursing standards require you to understand evidence-based practice?

3. Using the following hypothetical situation, think as an adult child. Generate a list of problems and their cause. Generate alternative solutions and discuss your thinking about selecting a solution and how you would evaluate the effectiveness of your solution:

   Your elderly parents have generally been healthy in the past and have lived independently in their own home. Your father has had a stroke and is unable to walk or complete the usual activities of daily living and has difficulty speaking. He needs ongoing intensive rehabilitation to recover more function. His insurance will not pay for inpatient rehabilitation. Your mother, though highly functional, cannot drive a car.

4. Using the same scenario, think as a nurse. Generate a list of nursing care problems and apply the nursing process to generate at least one diagnosis and a plan to intervene and evaluate the effect of your interventions.

5. Now think about what you know and don't know about intervening. How might the evidence-based practice process help you be more confident in your assessments or interventions? Make sure you can name each step of the evidence-based practice method.

6. Finally, how might you use the research process to fill in the gaps that you might not know how to handle?

7. How did your problem solving, nursing process, evidence-based practice, and research steps relate to each other? How does thinking as an adult child versus thinking as a professional nurse compare?

8. What do you want to learn next about using evidence to inform your nursing actions?

References

American Nurses Association. (2010). *Nursing's social policy statement: The essence of the profession.* Silver Spring, MD: Nursingbooks.org.

Cheater, F. M, Baker, R., Reddish, S., et al. (2006). Cluster randomized controlled trial of the effectiveness of audit and feedback and educational outreach on improving nursing practice and patient outcomes. *Medical Care, 44,* 542–551.

Fawcett, J., & Garrity, J. (2009). *Evaluating research for evidence-based nursing practice.* Philadelphia: F. A. Davis.

Good, M., Albert, J. M., Anderson, G. C., et al. (2010). Supplementing relaxation and music for pain after surgery. *Nursing Research, 59,* 259–269.

How we test. (2010). ConsumerReports.org. Retrieved from http://www.consumerreports.org/cro/how-we-test/index.htm

Jamtvedt, G., Young, J. M., Kristofferson, D. T., et al. (2006). Audit and feedback: Effects on professional practice and health care outcomes. *Cochrane Database of Systematic Reviews, 2,* Art. No.: CD000259. doi:10.1002/14651858.CD000259.pub2

Livesley, J., & Howarth, M. (2007). Integrating research evidence into clinical decisions. In J. V. Craig & R. L. Smyth (Eds.), *The evidence-based practice manual for nurses* (pp. 209–233). Edinburgh: Churchill Livingston.

Polit, D. F., & Beck, C. T. (2008). *Nursing research: Generating and assessing evidence for nursing practice* (8th ed.). Philadelphia: Lippincott.

Pravikoff, D. S., Tanner, A. B., & Pierce, S. T. (2005). Readiness of U.S. nurses for evidence-based practice. *American Journal of Nursing, 105*(9), 40–51.

Registered Nurses' Association of Ontario. (2007). Assessment and management of pain: Supplement. [Nursing best practice guideline]. Retrieved from http://www.rnao.org/Page.asp?PageID=924&ContentID=720

Ask and Assess: Questioning

Lisa Hopp

- List and define the elements of questions that address issues that are relevant to evidence-based nursing practice.

- Using a clinical scenario, craft a PICO question about the effectiveness of a nursing intervention that includes all the elements of the properly framed question.

- Using a clinical scenario, craft a PICo question about the meaningfulness of a patient-centered phenomenon that includes all the elements of a properly framed question.

- Explain the usefulness of a PICO or PICo format to construct a question that leads to a successful search of the best available evidence.

- Debate the role of questioning and curiosity in everyday nursing practice.

Attitude of inquiry	Iterative
Comparison	Meaningfulness
Context	Meta-paradigm
Environment	Narrative data
Health	Nursing
Intervention	Outcome

Person   **Population**
Phenomenon of interest   **Qualitative research**
PICo   **Scale**
PICO   **Scope**

Clinical Story

Amanda has had a busy day in a long-term acute care unit caring for five patients with a variety of medical problems, including heart failure, chronic obstructive pulmonary disease (COPD), and stroke. All of her patients are older than 70 years of age, have limited mobility, and have a decreased ability to care for themselves. Each patient had at least one IV infusion, and four required an IV medication. Despite the increased difficulty, Amanda administered 30 doses of medication safely and on time.

Completely exhausted at the end of her shift, Amanda still has many questions about her approach and the decisions she made during the day. She wonders if some of the IV drugs should have been pushed the way she did it. She thinks some of her patients could have been more mobile if she had the right equipment to help them. She wonders if the patient who was going to have heart surgery should have been bathed in a different way from what is normally done. These are just some of the questions that run through her mind as she drives home. ■

Introduction

To find an answer, you must first ask a question. That seems self-evident. The evidence-based practice process welcomes and embraces a self-conscious curiosity about the daily decisions made by nurses. At its core, evidence-based practice requires an **attitude of inquiry.** As a practicing nurse, you should regard your practice with curiosity and a certain amount of skepticism. Conversely, you will become immobilized by indecision if you spend all day questioning every decision. In evidence-based practice, the process is similar to following a treasure map; you must ask questions in a specific way to arrive at the necessary answers. In this chapter you will learn how to develop different types of questions that point to evidence to inform your clinical practice.

What Is the Relationship Between Assessment and Questioning?

Before you can ask a question, you take stock of a situation. You may even do this instinctively. For example, by asking a teacher a question, you realized that there was a gap in your understanding. In nursing practice, this taking stock is known as "making an assessment." When nurses assess patients they gather and organize information to identify a state of health or illness. In the evidence-based practice process, you will assess a situation to formulate a question.

Questions relevant to nursing practice arise from the concerns of the nursing **meta-paradigm:** person, health, environment, and nursing (Fawcett & Garrity, 2009, p. 5). The meta-paradigm is used to define nursing practice and provides a foundation on which to build a conceptual understanding of nursing concerns. Although the elements of the meta-paradigm and their use can be debated, think about them in broad terms to help organize the types of questions that are relevant to nursing practice.

Within the meta-paradigm, **person** refers broadly to the individual as well as families, groups, and communities. It also includes the integrated aspects of the biophysical, psychological, sociological, and spiritual person/family/community (Thorne, Canam, Dahinten, et al., 1998). **Health** can exist on a continuum as a person subjectively experiences and defines their own sense of wellness and illness along a spectrum (Thorne et al., 1998). **Environment** includes the immediate surroundings of the individual but can be expanded to incorporate sociopolitical and economical context of person (Thorne et al., 1998). **Nursing** is the "protection, promotion, and optimization of health and abilities, prevention of illness and injury, alleviation of suffering through the diagnosis and treatment of human response, and advocacy in the care of individuals, families, communities, and populations" (American Nurses Association, 2003, p. 6). To apply elements of the meta-paradigm to the clinical scenario, consider this: Amanda may have questioned how she could have helped (nursing) her elderly patients (person) become more mobile (health) in the busy long-term acute care facility (environment).

Elements of the meta-paradigm provide a structure to organize your thinking about clinical questions in broad terms. However, to develop more specific questions that align with appropriate types of evidence, you will use a particular format that incorporates elements of the meta-paradigm (Table 8■1).

Why Question?

When nurses reflect on their practice, they can discover better ways to care for patients. Reflection can lead nurses to consider alternative interventions, linking care with outcomes and increased understanding of how the patients and families experience health and illness within a specific community or situation. By questioning practices in a self-conscious manner, nurses give themselves a chance to learn. Without this attitude of inquiry, their practice will more likely stagnate.

Questions need to progress from casual wondering to a specific search for particular information so that knowledge will transform into nursing action. In evidence-based practice, questions provide the basis for searching for the best available evidence, for understanding the patient or family experience, and driving the specific implementation and evaluation of nursing practice. The question is the point at which the evidence-based practice process begins, and the question drives the rest of the process—through finding the evidence, appraising the evidence, making decisions to implement, and finally evaluating the use of the evidence.

Table 8■1 **Nursing Meta-Paradigm and PICO Questions**

Meta-Paradigm Element	Definition	Question Element	Example
Person	Individuals; families; communities; and the integrated aspects of the biophysical, psychological, sociologic, and spiritual person/family/community	Population	Elderly people unable to move in bed
Environment	Immediate surroundings or sociopolitical or economical context of the person	Population (further specified) or context	Hospitalized in an acute care hospital
Nursing	Protection, promotion, and optimization of health and abilities; prevention of illness and injury; alleviation of suffering through the diagnosis and treatment of human response; and advocacy in the care of individuals, families, communities, and populations	Intervention Comparison	Repositioning with a slip sheet Repositioning using a "lift and push" technique
Health	How a person experiences wellness and illness along a continuum	Outcome	Incidence of pressure or shearing ulcers

Scope and Scale of Questions for Evidence-Based Practice

In this chapter's clinical story, Amanda cared for patients with many different nursing care issues. Because of this variety, she might ask questions that vary in scope. **Scope** relates to the breadth of the question. It might also be defined in terms of setting, population, age group, or other category. **Scale** relates to the how *much* of the scope one wishes to address. Amanda could think about the scope of questions related to the nursing care of adult patients who have limitations in mobility. Within this very broad scope, she might scale the question to include interventions that could help patients improve their mobility. Alternatively, she may scale the question to relate to how often patients with limited mobility may need to be turned to prevent pressure ulcers. The scale of these two issues is much different. The first is very large within the scope. To answer the question properly, Amanda needs to gather information about all interventions related to patient mobility and determine which interventions will improve the patients' condition. She also needs to investigate many kinds of mobility aids, such as gait belts, walkers, and canes, as well as methods of advancing mobility from bedrest to walking, and techniques for turning and moving patients in bed. The second question is much smaller in scale, and Amanda needs to focus only on turning frequency.

Finding the right scope and scale of the question will help you find the right information for the right patients. As you develop an effective question that leads you to a certain type of evidence, you may frequently change its scope and scale to reframe the question again and again in an **iterative** fashion. You will work and rework the question until you are satisfied that it asks what you want to know.

Elements of Questions of Effectiveness and Meaningfulness

Most leaders in the field of evidence-based practice agree that a structured approach will help you develop a well-built question. A proper question helps ensure a successful search of the literature. You begin by assessing the patient or situation. You deconstruct the problem into its smaller parts, and then you reconstruct the individual elements into a coherent question. Depending on the type of issue you are faced with, you will craft the question somewhat differently.

The kinds of questions that health-care providers ask depend on what is important to their practice. These differences in perspective have led to some debate related to what counts as legitimate evidence. Different disciplines and individuals have different ideas about the nature of evidence. Chapter 5 discussed the Joanna Briggs Institute (JBI) model. The model's authors argued that health-care professionals engage in a variety of activities and decisions, and interact with people in different ways. Therefore, their knowledge needs are diverse and the way they seek knowledge varies. When the authors described the model, they identified four categories of evidence—feasibility, appropriateness, meaningfulness, and effectiveness—and related questions that are particularly well suited for nursing practice (Pearson, Wiechula, Court, et al., 2007). Feasibility questions are related to whether an intervention is "physically, culturally or financially possible within a given context" (Pearson et al., 2007, p. 86). Questions of appropriateness are similar but focus on how the intervention fits in the context. Finally, questions of meaningfulness and effectiveness are the types of questions that relate to how people experience an intervention or phenomenon and how well the intervention works to achieve an outcome (Pearson et al., 2007). Questions related to feasibility, appropriateness, and effectiveness can use a similar structure but you will need to adapt the format somewhat to form meaningfulness questions.

Effectiveness Questions: PICO

When you want to find the best available evidence about the effectiveness of a nursing intervention, you will use the PICO format. **PICO** is an acronym and is an easy way to remember the important parts of the question.

- *P* stands for *p*opulation (person and perhaps environment in the meta-paradigm).
- *I* stands for *i*ntervention (nursing in the meta-paradigm).
- *C* stands for *c*omparison treatment (also nursing in the meta-paradigm).
- *O* stands for *o*utcome (health in the meta-paradigm).

Amanda can generate many PICO questions related to her patients' care. Questions come from surprising or unexplained events, unwanted outcomes, or even routine nursing care. Recall that Amanda wondered whether her elderly, chronically ill patients could have increased mobility. She begins by thinking, "I wonder what I could do to help my older patients get out of bed to walk in the hallway?" This is a worthy question but it needs to be refined to help her create an efficient search for related evidence (Box 8■1).

Population

Amanda starts by focusing on the **population** ("person" and "environment" in the meta-paradigm). In PICO, *population* is defined as the group of people that are of concern in the question. This group may be related by a disease, a health condition, risk profile, the environment in which they exist, age group, or any combination of these factors. As you define the population by introducing more factors, you limit

---

BOX 8■1 Significance of Questioning

- Being curious about your practice leads to questioning and having an attitude of inquiry.
- Wondering about the "rightness" of your practice provides an opportunity to learn and to advance the practice of others.
- Questions should come from everyday nursing practice issues and therefore are real and meaningful to clinical work.
- Questions are of large and small scope and scale and therefore their answers can affect groups of people (patients, nurses, systems) or individuals.
- A pluralistic acceptance of different types of evidence requires adaption of the PICO (population, intervention, comparison, outcome) to the PICo (population, phenomenon of interest, context) format for asking questions .
- A guide to asking PICO and PICo questions help to focus the question.
- The PICO or PICo question drives the entire evidence-based practice process and keeps you focused on the problem.
- The elements of the question lead to generating keywords and synonyms to form a search strategy and/or to use to consult with a librarian.

the scope and scale of the question. To define the population for Amanda's question, she begins very broadly with "elderly people." But this definition would not specifically target elderly patients in the hospital with limited mobility who also have special needs. Amanda begins to narrow the population of the question to "elderly patients with limited mobility." However, although she is specifically interested in the environment of a long-term acute care setting, this may narrow the question too much and may eliminate helpful evidence. She may need to revisit the issue of environment after she begins to explore the literature. Once she finds some evidence, she can make a judgment about how well the evidence relates to the specific setting. You will find that as you develop your questions, you may need to revise and refine as you test the breadth of the evidence.

Intervention

After population, address the **intervention** ("nursing" in the meta-paradigm). Intervention is the nursing treatment or action that is the focus of the question. Amanda considers a variety of interventions such as gait belts to assist walking, walkers, lift devices, physiotherapy consultation, or even prompts that remind nurses to help patients increase movement. She settles with a fairly general intervention, such as a transfer aid, or a very specific intervention, such as a transfer sling that will help her assist patients transfer out of bed.

Comparison

If you are interested in comparing one intervention against another, you will include a **comparison** intervention in your question. The comparison may be to any other nursing intervention or it may be to taking no action at all. In her question, Amanda can compare using a transfer belt against a transfer sling, or she may be interested in comparing a slip-sheet to a lift device. However, comparisons are not essential to the evidence-based practice process. A comparison may not be necessary if you are interested in effectiveness regardless of the testing of any other intervention.

Outcome

Finally, you specify the **outcome**(s) ("health" in the meta-paradigm) that you want to know about. The outcome is the specific effect(s) of the intervention or what matters to the nurse and patient. It is what the nurse would use to evaluate whether the intervention had a beneficial or harmful effect on the patient, nurse, or organization. When developing her question about increased patient mobility, Amanda needs to address issues related to her patients' safety; how quickly patients mobilize; or complications of immobility, such as venous thromboembolism, pressure ulcers, fatigue, or discomfort. Like the other elements of the question, the degree of specificity or generality of the outcome will influence the scope and scale of the question and the breadth of your search.

Creating a PICO Question

After you determine the four important items, you glue the pieces together to form a complete PI(C)O question. Most questions of effectiveness can take the following form: What is the effectiveness of [insert intervention] versus [insert comparison, if there is one] in patients with [insert population/environment] on [health outcome]?

Table 8■2 **PICO Questions of Effectiveness**

General question: What is the best way to care for urinary catheters in patients with a stroke?
Narrower question: What is the best way to remove catheters in patients who have had a stroke and who have a urinary catheter?

	Element	Definition	Example
P	Population	Who in what circumstance is at the center of the issue?	Adult patients after stroke with an indwelling catheter
I	Intervention	What is the intervention of interest?	Clamping the catheter before removal
C	Comparison	What is the alternative intervention (if there is one)?	Gravity drain before removal
O	Outcome	What are the benefit(s) or harm(s)?	Time to first void Incidence of urinary tract infection

Final PICO: What is the effectiveness of clamping versus gravity drain prior to removal of an indwelling urinary catheter in patients after a stroke?

When thinking about patient mobility, Amanda can ask, "What is the effectiveness of a transfer sling (I) versus a transfer belt (C) in elderly patients in long-term acute care (LTAC) with impaired mobility (P) on patient comfort and incidence of nurse back injury (O)?" Another question Amanda might develop is "What is the effectiveness of using a turn schedule (I) versus an audible public address reminder (C) on the incidence of pressure ulcers (O) in elderly patients in LTAC who require turning (P)?" She could also generate many questions related to the effectiveness of various interventions for her elderly hospitalized patients with impaired mobility. Following the PICO model, Amanda starts with broad questions and develops more specific questions to focus her search. You can use these sample questions to help you formulate your own questions related to the effectiveness of interventions (Table 8■2).

Meaningfulness Questions: PICo

Nurses have broader concerns than merely the effectiveness of interventions. Leaders in evidence-based nursing practice have advocated for a pluralistic view of what counts as evidence (Pearson et al., 2007; Rycroft-Malone, Seers, Titchen, et al., 2004). Legitimate evidence arises from many sources including both quantitative and qualitative research. If we claim that as nurses, we are person centered, then we must care about how people experience their health. As a result, we are interested in **meaningfulness** of health-related phenomena. Pearson et al. (2007) define *meaningfulness* as "the extent to which an intervention or activity is positively [or negatively] experienced by the patient. Meaningfulness relates to the personal experience, opinions, values, thoughts, beliefs and interpretations of patients or clients" (pp. 86–87).

Evidence-based health care recognizes that patient preferences and values are important to decision making. Nurses and other health-care providers can use evidence of meaningfulness from **qualitative research** to help understand patient preferences and values. Qualitative research is a "systematic, subjective methodological approach used to describe life experience and situations and to give them meaning" (Burns & Grove, 2007, p. 151). Certainly it is inappropriate to seek meaningfulness knowledge from quantitative or experimental studies because meaning comes from the story, the **narrative data** gathered through qualitative research or discourse. According to Sandelowski (1994), a leading American qualitative research expert, "narratives are generally understood to be stories with a certain dynamic structure and shape directed toward achieving wholeness, or health" (p. 23).

To accommodate meaningfulness in the development of your question, you will adapt the PICO format to the **PICo** approach for questions related to meaning. That is, *P* still reflects the *p*opulation of interest but *I* refers to the phenomenon of *i*nterest and *Co* refers to the *co*ntext (Joanna Briggs Institute, 2008).

Phenomenon of Interest

Phenomenon of interest is the part of the patient's experience that you want to understand. Although they can vary in scope, the phenomena of interest tend to be broad. Like her curiosity about the effectiveness of the nursing interventions, Amanda has questions about many phenomena related to the meaning of the patients' experiences. She wonders about the meaning of impaired immobility, the experience of being dependent on someone else for mobility, or losing independence in general. If one of her patients has acquired a pressure ulcer, she will want to understand the meaning of having a pressure ulcer or being in pain.

When you consider the phenomenon of a patient's experience, the words associated with that experience must have meaning to the patient and be part of the patient's vocabulary. You would not ask the question about the patient's experience using a term that has meaning only to nursing or another health-care professional. For example, you would not ask the question "What is the meaning of the experience of continuous lateral rotation?" The term "continuous lateral rotation" has meaning for professionals. Instead of using unfamiliar terms, you need to find what the patient calls that experience. The patient may experience the treatment as helplessness (a more negative response) or comfort (a more positive response), but the experience is wholly of the patient, not the nurse. You may think that the treatment is effective and helpful but it may mean something entirely different to the patient.

Context

Context is important to how a phenomenon is experienced; it is the surroundings of the phenomenon or person. A patient experiences comfort while hospitalized in an intensive care unit differently from how he or she experiences comfort at home under usual circumstances. The context may be the environment, particular cultural factors, the community, the setting, or a health problem. In this chapter's clinical story, if Amanda wants to know about an elderly patient's experience of helplessness, she could use the general context of an acute care hospital unit. Alternatively, she can specify the context as the patient's experience within a particular health problem,

Table 8■3 **PICo Questions of Meaningfulness**

General question: What is it like to experience a stroke?
Narrower question: What does it mean to lose motor function after a stroke?

	Element	Definition	Example
P	Population	Who in what circumstance is at the center of the issue?	Patients with a stroke
I	Phenomenon of Interest	What is the patient-centered experience you want to understand?	Loss of control over movement
Co	Context	What is the environment, particular cultural factors, timing, community, setting, or health problem influencing the situation?	Early phase of hospital-based rehabilitation

Final PICo: How do people experience losing control of movement in the early phase of a stroke while they remain hospitalized for rehabilitation?

such as the recovery phase from a stroke that leaves residual paralysis. Finally, she may combine both contexts to determine the patient's experience during acute care hospitalization and the recovery phase from a stroke that leaves residual paralysis.

Creating a PICo Question

As with effectiveness questions, you may find it helpful to use a template approach for your meaningfulness questions. For example: How do patients [insert population] experience [insert phenomenon] in the context of [insert context]? You can imagine a variety of questions for Amanda's practice (Table 8■3).

Much like the research process, the question posed to the evidence-based practice process drives the rest of the course of action. The next section shows how Amanda prepares to take her questions to the next phase—searching.

Taking Questioning to Searching

The next step in the evidence-based practice process is to search for and find the best available evidence. This is the first job for your newly formed question. Regardless of whether you will consult a librarian or if you will construct your own evidence search, you need to deconstruct the question to identify keywords related to each element. Even if you are consulting with a librarian, you will need to know what synonyms are most likely associated with each element of your question. You will want to approach the librarian with a clear idea of what you want to know; it is best to go well prepared (Box 8■2).

Consider Amanda's next question: "What is the effectiveness of using a turn schedule versus an audible public address reminder on the incidence of pressure ulcers in elderly hospitalized patients who require turning?" To begin her search for

BOX 8-2 **Interdisciplinary Rounds**

- Questions provide a common ground for collaboration among disciplines.
- Multiple disciplines may have an interest in the same interventions and phenomena.
- Librarians are key to successful searches for the best available evidence.
- Take your PICO or PICo question to consult with your librarian and generate keywords and their synonyms.

Example:

A nurse on a long-term acute care unit takes the following PICO question to the library scientist: What is the effectiveness of a bladder-training program on incontinence in female patients recovering from a stroke?

The keywords and phrases include "bladder training," "urinary incontinence—control and prevention," "bladder retraining," "bladder program," "bladder management" "prompted voiding" "continence care" "incontinence," "continence." "urinary continence," "stroke," "cerebral vascular accident."

appropriate evidence, Amanda should begin by unpacking her PICO question again. Then she should determine synonyms for each of the *P, I, C, O* elements. For the population Amanda would use the keywords "aged," "elderly," "older adult," or other related term. For the intervention of "turn schedule," she would need to think about all words that could be used to describe a reminder system representing a schedule. These might be short phrases such as "turn clock" or "reminder clock." For her comparison, she could use terms such as "audible signal," "public address," or "audible reminder." Finally, for the outcome, she would use "pressure ulcer," "decubitus ulcer," "pressure sore," and other terms. Although developing a list of synonyms is time-consuming, the next step in the process is easier if you have synonyms for each element of the question. If you carefully use the most meaningful terms to represent what you want to know, your selection of key terms for the search will be easier and more effective (Box 8-3).

BOX 8-3 **Tools for Learning and Practice**

- Ask yourself what you need to know to provide the best possible nursing care to your patients. Think through a typical day and ask yourself, "Do I know what the best evidence is to...?" "How do I know if this is the right thing to do this?"
- Move from big questions to smaller questions (think of pouring all your questions through a funnel), particularly when you are a novice.

BOX 8■3   **Tools for Learning and Practice** (continued)

- Think about each element of a good question and identify what you want to know.
- Use a PICO approach for effectiveness questions or PICo for questions of meaning to help you build each part of the question.
- Glue the elements together to create a full question.
- Use this format to formulate effectiveness questions: What is the effectiveness of [insert intervention] versus [insert comparison, if there is one] in patients with [insert population/environment] on [health outcome]?
- Use this format to formulate meaningfulness questions: How do patients [insert population] experience [insert phenomenon] in the context of [insert context]?
- Tear the question apart again to identify keywords and their synonyms.
- Practice writing questions and ask someone else to make sure the questions contain all of the correct elements.
- Find out the names of your librarians, their contact information, and the process for working with them.
- Take your question, keywords, and synonyms with you when you meet with the librarian.

■ Summary

Finding the right answers requires the right questions. Questions relevant to nursing practice emerge from reflection on your daily work and relate to the meta-paradigm. The PICO and PICo formats will help you construct questions that will likely lead to effective searches and to the best available evidence of effectiveness of interventions and meaningfulness of patient experiences, respectively. If you adopt an attitude of curiosity and inquiry, you will find an abundance of questions as you think more self-consciously about your practice. With a little practice, you will be able to form questions that lead to effective searches and interpretation of the evidence.

CHAPTER QUESTIONS

1. What is meant by an "attitude of inquiry"?

2. Where do questions about nursing practice come from?

3. What is the purpose of asking questions in a particular format before proceeding with the evidence-based practice process?

4. Examine a typical day in your nursing practice. What types of questions can you ask about your day?

5. What do PICO and PICo represent?

6. Identify the *P, I, C* (if identified), and *O* in the following questions:
   a. What is the effectiveness of 2% chlorehexidine-impregnated wipes versus a traditional soap and water basin bath on the incidence of surgical site infections in adult patients who receive cardiothoracic surgery?
   b. What is the effect of using bar coding on medication errors in patients receiving oral medications in an acute care medical-surgical hospital?
   c. What is the effectiveness of using moisture-barrier products versus not using a moisture barrier on the rate of skin breakdown in incontinent, bed-ridden patients?

7. Develop a PICO or PICo question to fit the following issues:
   a. How well a smoking-cessation program works in adults with at least a 20-year pack-a-day history of smoking
   b. The impact of various dressings for IV catheters on phlebitis
   c. How a patient with end-stage heart failure experiences hopefulness

8. Identify what element is missing in the following questions and then improve them:
   a. What is the experience of family presence?
   b. What is the effect of open visiting hours?
   c. What is the optimal frequency of assessing risk for pressure ulcers?
   d. Do pressure-reducing mattresses work?

9. What are key terms that you would ask your librarian to use to search for evidence related to this question: What is the effect of suctioning a tracheostomy every 2 hours versus on an as-needed basis on secretion clearance in patients with a new tracheostomy?

References

American Nurses Association. (2003). *Nursing's social policy statement* (2nd ed.). Silver Springs, MD: Author.

Burns, N., & Grove, S. K. (2007). *Understanding nursing research: Building an evidence-based practice* (4th ed.). St. Louis, MO: Saunders-Elsevier.

Fawcett, J., & Garity, J. (2009). *Evaluating research for evidence-based nursing practice.* Philadelphia: F. A. Davis.

Joanna Briggs Institute. (2008). *Joanna Briggs Institute reviewer's manual: 2008 edition.* Adelaide, South Australia: Joanna Briggs Institute.

Pearson, A., Wiechula, R., Court, A., et al. (2007). A re-consideration of what constitutes "evidence" in the healthcare professions. *Nursing Science Quarterly, 20,* 85–88. doi:10.1177/0894318406296306

Rycroft-Malone, J., Seers, K., Titchen, A., et al. (2004). What counts as evidence in evidence-based practice? *Journal of Advanced Nursing, 47*(1), 81–90.

Sandelowski, M. (1994). We are the stories we tell: Narrative knowing in nursing. *Journal of Holistic Nursing, 12,* 22–33. doi:10.1177/089801019401200105

Thorne, S., Canam, C., Dahinten, S., et al. (1998). Nursing's metaparadigm concepts: Disimpacting the debates. *Journal of Advanced Nursing, 27,* 1257–1268.

CHAPTER 9

Acquire and Diagnose: Linking the Problem With Finding Best Sources of Evidence

Kim Whalen

- Distinguish among types of summarized sources of evidence.
- Generate key words for searching.
- Conduct a bibliographic database search using Boolean operators.
- Identify the best available resources for locating evidence.
- Describe how to communicate and partner with a librarian or information scientist.

KEY TERMS

Bibliographic databases
Boolean operators
Centre for Reviews and
    Dissemination (CRD)
Clinical practice guidelines
Cochrane Library
Critical appraisal
Cumulative Index to Nursing
    and Allied Health Literature
    (CINAHL)

Embase
Google Scholar
Hand searching
Joanna Briggs Institute (JBI)
    Library of Systematic
    Reviews
Keywords
Literature review
MEDLINE
MeSH subject headings

KEY TERMS (continued)

Peer-reviewed journals
Primary source
PubMed Central
PubMed Central's Clinical
    Queries

Secondary sources
Standardized subject headings
Systematic review
Truncation
Wildcards

*C*linical *Story*

Mark is in his final semester of his BSN program, and he is excited to participate in the capstone project that focuses on improving hand hygiene among nurses at the local community hospital. The team plans to conduct a literature review to locate the best available evidence, summarize their findings, and propose an educational intervention to the nursing leadership team at the hospital. To begin, Mark and his teammates read their project outline and start to divide up their tasks. One teammate suggests using Google, Bing, or another Internet search engine to gather all the information they need for their literature review. Because of the extensive research that he completed for his nursing theories course, Mark knows not to rely only on Internet sources, and he suggests they meet with their nursing librarian, Mrs. Daniels. She can provide advice on using journals and bibliographic databases available through their university library and help them identify the key words that can improve their search results from the databases and from the Internet. Mark quickly e-mails Mrs. Daniels to set up a time for them all to meet. ▪

Introduction

Seeking the best available evidence for clinical decisions is like a treasure hunt: you need a map to hunt for the most valuable prize. You use your question and the structured search strategy as your map to search for the best available evidence. Remember, the ideal evidence is the highest quality information that answers your question.

Whether you are preparing an academic paper or simply trying to find the answer to a clinical question in the middle of your clinical day, you need to develop some basic search skills and know when to seek help from a professional knowledge seeker: your librarian. Before beginning your search, you must be clear about what type of information you need. For example, if you have a very narrow question, you should start your search with clinical practice guidelines or a high-quality systematic review. If you are unable to find your answer in either option, you will need to search for articles and primary source documents. In this chapter, you will learn the differences between types of information; the basics of conducting a search of bibliographic databases; where to search for clinical practice guidelines, systematic reviews, and primary sources; and the importance of forming a partnership with professional librarians.

Sources of Evidence

With health-care information being published in books, journals, magazines, news-papers, bibliographic databases, and the Internet at such a rapid pace, staying on top of the latest findings can be difficult. When you are a busy clinician, making many decisions every day, the ideal source of evidence is one in which someone else has completed the difficult work of searching, appraising, and synthesizing the evidence. To be efficient in your search, you need to be able to distinguish among many types of evidence, know where to find the "best bet" sources of evidence, and how to get to those sources.

You may be familiar with the term **literature review.** It is often the first step in writing a paper or developing a research proposal. Its purpose is to summarize information from various authors and sources. As Timmons and McCabe (2005, p. 42) stated, "This information can be used for a variety of purposes, including uncovering gaps in research literature and identifying areas for further study." Literature reviews help you to understand background issues and determine the scope of an area of literature. However, because they lack the rigor of other types of reviews, you should not directly inform your clinical decisions with casual literature reviews. Authors of these kinds of informative articles usually do not explicitly communicate the methods they used to find their information, nor do they use a highly structured approach to the search strategy or explain how they selected the information included in the literature review.

Another type of review is a **systematic review.** This is a very different source of evidence from a casual literature review. Systematic reviews are a meta-synthesis or meta-analysis of evidence on a topic. They involve "the application of scientific strategies, in ways that limit bias, to the assembly, critical appraisal, and synthesis of all relevant studies that address a specific clinical question" (Cook, Mulrow, and Haynes, 1997, p. 376). Qualitative systematic reviews summarize study findings without using statistics; therefore, they are known as meta-synthesis. Meta-synthesis is the "process of combining the findings of individual qualitative studies (i.e., cases) to create summary statements that authentically describe the meaning of these themes (or cross-case generalisations)" (Pearson, Wiechula, Court, et al., 2005, p. 212). A meta-analysis, or quantitative systematic review, uses statistical methods to summarize study findings, and according to Pearson et al. (2005, p. 212), "key outcomes of the meta-analysis are the measure of effect, the confidence interval and the degree of heterogeneity of the studies synthesized." Although systematic reviews are "often a better place to start looking for answers to clinical questions than original studies" (McKibbon and Marks, 1998b, p. 105), systematic reviews have not been developed for every clinical question.

Clinical practice guidelines are another form of synthesized evidence designed to provide comprehensive recommendations about the diagnosis, management, or treatment of a particular condition or clinical question. Based on systematic reviews and adapted to local circumstances and values, (Cook et al., 1997), guidelines assist practitioners and patients with making decisions about care. High-quality clinical practice guidelines represent the synthesis of the best available evidence, clinical expertise, and consumer and stakeholder input. In addition, they contain practical tools to help you use the evidence. Many organizations, governments, and health-care specialty societies produce clinical practice guidelines.

During your time in school, or during your nursing practice, there will be occasions when you will conduct your own primary research. Literature reviews, systematic reviews, and clinical practice guidelines are different from primary research articles because they all offer analysis of already completed work, and they are not new research. Despite that, all reviews should be conducted with the same rigor that is applied to a primary research project (Evans, 2000). In this chapter you will learn how to develop an effective search strategy to identify relevant evidence for a literature review. You will also learn about the resources to use for efficiently locating evidence including clinical practice guidelines, systematic reviews, and primary research articles (Box 9■1).

Begin With a Good Question

With all the health-care information available, where do you begin? The previous chapter stressed, and Jones and Smyth (2004) agree, that the first step in locating the best available evidence is the development of a focused PICO or PICo question (Table 9■1). In this chapter's clinical story, Mark and his capstone project team begin by brainstorming their assignment and identifying their *p*opulation, *i*ntervention, *c*omparison, and *o*utcome. The team was charged with improving hand hygiene among nurses at the local community hospital. They were also charged with developing an educational program that would increase adherence to the hospital's hand

---

BOX 9■1   Significance of Acquiring the Best Sources of Evidence

- Use of incomplete or out-of-date information could affect patient safety.
- Gaining experience in identifying the best available information resources will make you a more effective and efficient researcher as well as nurse.
- A thorough search will provide the best available evidence for an informed clinical decision.
- Clinical practice guidelines, systematic reviews, and other synthesized evidence are important information tools.
- Individual articles and primary sources of information are also important but used independently do not always provide the best available evidence.
- Hospital and university librarians, also known as library scientists, are available to help you access the information you need—take advantage of their expertise and assistance.

Table 9■1   **Development of PICO Question**

General question: What is the best way to improve hand hygiene among nurses at the community hospital?
Narrower question: What is the best way to increase nurses' adherence to the community hospital's hand hygiene protocol?

	Element	Definition	Example
P	Population	Who in what circumstance is at the center of the issue?	Nurses in a community hospital
I	Intervention	What is the intervention of interest?	An educational program
C	Comparison	What is the alternative intervention (if there is one)?	A marketing campaign
O	Outcome	What are the benefit(s) or harm(s)?	Increase adherence to the current hand hygiene protocol

Final PICO: What is the effectiveness of offering a mandatory training session or posting written marketing materials throughout the hospital on improving adherence to the hospital's hand hygiene protocol among nurses on the ICU floor?

hygiene protocol among nurses. As a result of the assignment, the team initially asks, "What is the effectiveness of an educational program (I) or marketing campaign (C) on nurses in a community hospital (P) adherence to the hospital's hand hygiene protocol (O)?" After a bit of discussion, the team decides to further focus their question to ask, "What is the effectiveness of offering mandatory training sessions (I) or posting written marketing materials throughout the hospital (C) on improving adherence to the hospital's hand hygiene protocol (O) among nurses on the ICU floor (P)?"

While developing the PICO question, the team may find that they are interested in comparing a very specific type of educational program, a mandatory in-person session, or an online seminar, to a very specific type of marketing campaign, an email reminder system, or print posters displayed throughout the hospital. Rephrasing and refining their question will result in a more effective search.

Generating Keywords

While rephrasing their question, the team develops **keywords** and phrases to use to search the library's bibliographic databases and the Internet. Although it seems simple, selecting useful keywords is often the most time consuming and difficult part of an effective search (Timmins and McCabe, 2005). Mark's team begins by generating synonyms and related terms for each PICO element. For example, for the outcome of "adherence to the hand hygiene protocol," they think about all the other words and phrases used to describe a hand hygiene protocol. These include words such as "handwashing" or phrases such as "hand washing," "hand sanitation," "hand cleaning," and "hand hygiene." For the intervention of educational program, they list words and phrases such as "seminar," "workshop," "orientation session," "in-person workshop," and "online workshop." Armed with their PICO question and a set of synonyms, keywords, and phrases, the team is ready to move on.

Setting Limits

Before implementing their search, Mark and his team agree on the information resources they plan to use in their research. One of Mark's teammates thinks information found on the Internet would be sufficient. However, other teammates are aware of quality health-care information available in books, journals, magazines, trade publications, newspaper articles, dissertations, and library bibliographic databases. It is important for the team to agree on the types of information appropriate for their assignment. At the same time, the team must focus on accessing the best available evidence to answer their question.

Popular magazine articles, newspaper articles, and trade publications are valuable information resources but more practical in nature. They are typically not written by researchers or experts, nor do the articles go through a rigorous review process before publication. Useful for current awareness of health-care issues, procedures, equipment, and professional events, these types of publications are not sufficient resources for Mark's capstone assignment (Taylor, 2007). Although books and textbooks are also valuable sources of information, it is more appropriate for Mark and his team to search scholarly journals and other sources of evidence for their assignment. Scholarly, **peer-reviewed journals** publish results more quickly than books and textbooks. They report original research findings as well as synthesized analysis to professionals within the field. Before being published, most scholarly articles are approved through a peer-review process. This process involves multiple reviewers who hold advanced degrees within the discipline, teach within the field, are experts in the profession, and are very knowledgeable about the topic. Each reviewer evaluates the article, the research conducted, and the findings represented to determine whether the article warrants publication within that specific scholarly journal. Scholarly journals are often referred to as peer-reviewed, juried, refereed, or academic journals.

Scholarly, peer-reviewed journals publish primary sources of information as well as secondary sources of information. According to Stebbins (2006), a **primary source** is one created by the witness of the event. Taylor (2007) defines primary sources as those that have not been edited, interpreted, condensed, or evaluated, by someone else. She states, "Primary sources also present original thinking and observations, such as the original research used to write journal articles reporting on original scientific studies, experiments, or observations" (p. 38). An article written by a nursing student in a DNP program summarizing the results of her online survey of nurses about their preferred method of hand sanitation in their academic health center would be a useful primary source for Mark's assignment.

Secondary sources report on the work of others, not on the author's own original research findings. Although often easier to find, secondary sources need to be critically appraised to ensure that the information presented maintains the integrity of the original research findings and it has not been misinterpreted or altered (Taylor, 2007). Literature reviews and systematic reviews are considered secondary sources of information because they synthesize previously reported findings of others. A quantitative systematic review analyzing the research conducted on educational interventions found most influential in improving the rate of hand washing among hospital staff is an excellent secondary source for Mark's assignment (Box 9■2).

It is important that Mark and his teammates know the parameters of their assignment to discern if they can use both primary and secondary sources of information. If they are unable to use secondary sources, they can use the references cited or bibliography published within a literature review or systematic review to locate the primary sources identified by the review's author. **Hand searching,** the term used

---

BOX 9■2   **Interdisciplinary Rounds**

Reading multiple articles on a specific topic can seem overwhelming. Imagine being handed a stack of articles on a specific topic and having to take the time to appraise the studies conducted, analyze the reported findings, and compare the results. A goal of evidence-based practice is to synthesize the best available evidence so that students, clinicians, and patients can effectively access the information available and efficiently put the information to use.

Example:

A patient asks two different orthopedic nurses for information on the treatment of rotator cuff tears. Both nurses enjoy regularly reading nursing journals and both had read recent articles on the topic. One journal contained an article reporting that rotator cuff tears are best repaired through all-arthroscopic surgery. Another journal published an article reporting that cuff tears are best repaired with mini-open surgery. Yet another journal, not read by either of the two nurses, contained an article on the success of nonoperative treatments for rotator cuff tear repair. Which article or articles would be the best evidence to share with the patient?

Reading individual articles and independent primary sources of information can yield different reported results. Synthesized evidence, including systematic reviews, provides a summary of individual articles and primary sources of information related to a specific topic. Some systematic reviews use statistics to summarize findings and limit bias, whereas others create summary statements describing study findings. Systematic reviews appraise the studies conducted, the findings reported, and compare the results. Searching for a systematic review of the best treatments for rotator cuff tears would provide both the patient and the nurses with the best available evidence on the subject.

to describe looking through the references cited or a bibliography, is a very efficient way to locate relevant citations of usable primary sources of evidence. Mark and his team must also know if there is a time limit on the information they can use for their assignment. Some assignments require sources used to be published within the last 5 or 10 years; some assignments have no publication time limits. Keep in mind that limiting a search by time frame can help control the amount of information retrieved but it can also eliminate seminal pieces of information that were published outside of the time frame. Other limitations include limiting information published by language or by publication type. Limiting the search to only the information published in English or to only those studies conducted in the United States can help control the amount of information identified but can also eliminate key findings from the global health-care community. Limiting a search by publication type can focus findings only on scholarly, peer-reviewed journal articles and eliminate information published within magazines, trade publications, and other sources. After confirming the assignment, Mark and his team use their knowledge of the project and the required quality of information to determine which, if any, publication type limits they want to apply to their search.

Get Ready, Get Set . . .

Scholarly, peer-reviewed primary and secondary sources of information are most readily located within the **bibliographic databases** made available by academic and public libraries as well as from government and professional organizations on the Internet. Bibliographic databases contain abstracts, a synopsis of the article, and some contain the full text of articles including graphics, images, tables, and charts. Many databases are subscription-based so a fee must be paid to access. Bibliographic databases commonly used by nursing students include Medical Literature Online (MEDLINE), PubMed, Cumulative Index to Nursing and Allied Health Literature (CINAHL), the Cochrane Library, Embase, and the Joanna Briggs Institute (JBI) Library of Systematic Reviews.

Although bibliographic databases are offered by various providers, the user-friendly interfaces are designed in a similar way. Searches can be focused on a specific subject term or expanded through the use of keywords and phrases. Specific subject terms, otherwise known as **standardized subject headings,** were developed by the Library of Congress to organize large subjects logically into categories. Medical subject headings, known as **MeSH subject headings,** were designed as a controlled vocabulary for medicine by the United States National Library of Medicine. Arranged in an alphabetical and hierarchical structure, MeSH subject headings allow for more organized and accurate searching. According to the National Library of Medicine (2010), the MeSH heading of "handwashing" is defined as "the act of cleansing the hands with water or other liquid, with or without the inclusion of soap or other detergent, for the purpose of removing soil or microorganisms." Based on the definition, Mark and his team could choose to search using the MeSH subject heading for "handwashing" instead of the other phrases they had considered (see Box 9■3 for links to find subject headings).

The team could also choose to search the bibliographic databases or the Internet using keywords and phrases. Keywords and phrases can be combined using the

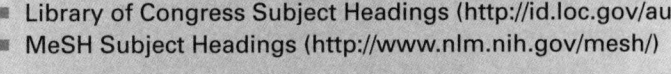

BOX 9■3   **Subject Heading Sources**

■ Library of Congress Subject Headings (http://id.loc.gov/authorities)
■ MeSH Subject Headings (http://www.nlm.nih.gov/mesh/)

Boolean operators AND, OR, and NOT to broaden or narrow a search. These operators can be used within most bibliographic databases as well as with most search engines. Mark and his team could choose to search using the search string handwashing OR "hand washing" OR "hand sanitation" OR "hand cleaning." This string will locate all the articles that contain at least one of these words or phrases (Fig. 9■1). Adding the Boolean operator AND will narrow the search. The team could search using the string (handwashing OR "hand washing" OR "hand sanitation" OR "hand cleaning" OR "hand hygiene") AND nurse. Placing quotation marks around a phrase ensures the results will include the entire phrase together and not each word separately. Like a mathematical equation, the parentheses enclosing a set of words and phrases allow the results within the parentheses to be combined with additional words and phrases outside the parentheses. The end result of the search string with the AND nurse would locate all the articles that contain at least one of the listed handwashing words or phrases as well as the word "nurse." Adding the NOT operator eliminates specific keywords or phrases from the search. Incorporating Boolean operators with subject headings, keywords, and phrases will shape the search strategy and result in the identification of more relevant information results.

Additional tools that can assist in shaping a search include **truncation** and **wildcards.** A truncation symbol, typically an asterisk (*) in bibliographic databases, can be applied to the end of a keyword to retrieve all the words beginning with that word. Nurs* would result in identifying articles that include the word "nurse," "nurses," "nursing," and so on. Wildcards, typically a question mark (?) in bibliographic databases, can be inserted within a word to retrieve all the words with alternate spellings. Randomi?ed would result in identifying articles that include the word spelled "randomized" or "randomised."

As previously discussed in this chapter, bibliographic databases are designed to enable a search to be limited by many elements including publication type, publication

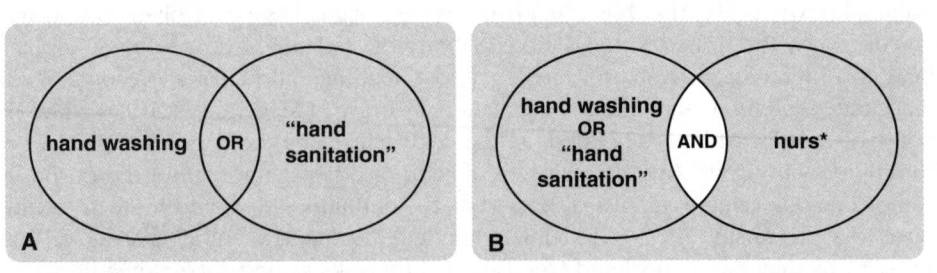

FIGURE 9■1 **(A)** Using the OR Boolean operator (results will include articles with both keywords or phrases). **(B)** Using the AND Boolean operator (results will include articles with both keywords and phrases).

date, and published language. Bird (2003) stated, "Databases are structured in a similar way so once you figure out the best search strategy it can easily be applied to numerous bibliographic databases and the Internet" (p. 57). In the meantime, do not give up—developing a useful search strategy can take some work.

Now Search

Clinical Practice Guidelines

Mark and his team start their search for information with a search of the synthesized evidence. If you are interested in knowing all aspects of care, often your first search is for a comprehensive clinical practice guideline. Quality clinical practice guidelines are often built off of systematic review findings. As with all sources of evidence, however, you need to be a good, critical consumer as clinical practice guidelines vary a great deal in their rigor.

It is difficult to know whether a clinical practice guideline might have the useful information embedded in it; therefore, always consider searching practice guideline sources first (Box 9■4). Mark's project covers a question in which evidence will not likely be available within a guideline. The team should focus their search more on systematic reviews and peer-reviewed journal articles.

Databases of Systematic Reviews
Systematic reviews, another form of synthesized evidence, might provide the ideal evidence needed for this assignment (Box 9■5).

The Cochrane Library
The **Cochrane Library** comprises the following six databases:

- The Cochrane Database of Systematic Reviews (CDSR)
- Cochrane Central Register of Controlled Trials (CENTRAL)
- Cochrane Methodology Register (CMR)
- Database of Abstracts of Reviews and Effects (DARE)

BOX 9■4   Clinical Practice Guideline Sources

- Agency for Healthcare Research and Quality-AHRQ (http://www.ahrq.gov/)
- Canadian Medical Association-CMA (http://www.cma.ca)
- Center for Disease Control and Prevention-CDC (http://www.cdc.gov/DiseasesConditions/)
- Guidelines International Network-GIN (http://www.g-i-n.net/)
- National Guideline Clearinghouse-NGC (http://www.guideline.gov/)
- National Institute for Health and Clinical Excellence-NICE (http://www.nice.org.uk/)
- Registered Nurses' Association of Ontario-RNAO (http://www.rnao.org/Page.asp?PageID=861&SiteNodeID=133)

BOX 9■5   **Systematic Review Subscription Databases and Internet Resources**

- Centre for Reviews and Dissemination-CRD (http://www.york.ac.uk/inst.crd)
- Essential Evidence PLUS—Daily POEMS (Patient-Oriented Evidence that Matters) (http://www.essentialevidenceplus.com/index.cfm)
- Cochrane Library (http://www.cochrane.org/cochrane-reviews)
- Joanna Briggs Institute-JBI (http://www.joannabriggs.edu.au/)
- PubMed Central's Clinical Queries (http://www.ncbi.nlm.nih.gov/corehtml/query/static/clinical.shtml)
- UpToDate (http://www.uptodate.com/home/index.html)

- Health Technology Assessment (HTA) Database
- NHS Economic Evaluation Database (EED)

The Cochrane Library is viewed as one of the most comprehensive collections of systematic reviews, controlled trials, and evidence-based health-care sources (Box 9■6). There is a cost to subscribe to the Cochrane Library, so Mark's team will need to check for availability at their library.

Joanna Briggs Institute

The Joanna Briggs Institute (JBI) is a global membership-based organization and members have access to a variety of evidence sources. One of the sources is the **JBI Library of Systematic Reviews**, which, as does the Cochrane Library, contains rigorous, peer-reviewed systematic reviews. In addition, members have access to a Database of Evidence-Based Care Bundles, a Database of Evidence Summaries, and over 10 full-text journals. Even if your hospital or university does not have a membership to JBI, you can freely access the full text of all the JBI systematic review protocols. Protocols, another term for systematic review proposals, can provide basic information about the systematic reviews that have already been published or are in process. In addition, nonmembers can find brief summaries of many systematic reviews combined with clinical recommendations in the form of the full-text JBI "Best Practice Information Sheets."

Additional Subscription Resources

Busy clinicians sometimes have access to additional synthesized resources not available within university libraries. Essential Evidence PLUS with its Daily POEMS (Patient-Oriented Evidence that Matters) database and Evidence Summaries database make synthesized information available to clinicians at the bedside via handheld mobile devices. UpToDate, another resource available to clinicians and patients online and on handheld mobile devices, synthesizes evidence to provide answers to clinical questions and treatment recommendations at the bedside. Check with your university or hospital librarian to find out what synthesized resources are available to you.

Additional Resources Containing Systematic Reviews, Literature Reviews, and Primary Source Articles

Systematic reviews might also have been published within journals accessible through other bibliographic databases, so the search for synthesized information is not over.

BOX 9▪6 **Search Tips for the Cochrane Library**

Tip 1—As Mark and his team have already identified the appropriate MeSH subject heading of "handwashing" they can use this to target their search. Selecting Cochrane's Advanced Search will enable the team to search using the MeSH search option. Limiting the search to only those pieces of information with the pre-determined MeSH "handwashing" subject heading will lead to very targeted results.

Tip 2—To make sure you've located the best available evidence, try another search with keywords and phrases. The Cochrane Library's Advanced Search option incorporates a useful Boolean operator structure to the interface. Limiting results to those with the keywords and phrases only in the abstract or only in the title, abstract, or keywords can also be useful. A targeted search, as in the example below, incorporates a combination of keywords, phrases, truncation symbols, and limiters.

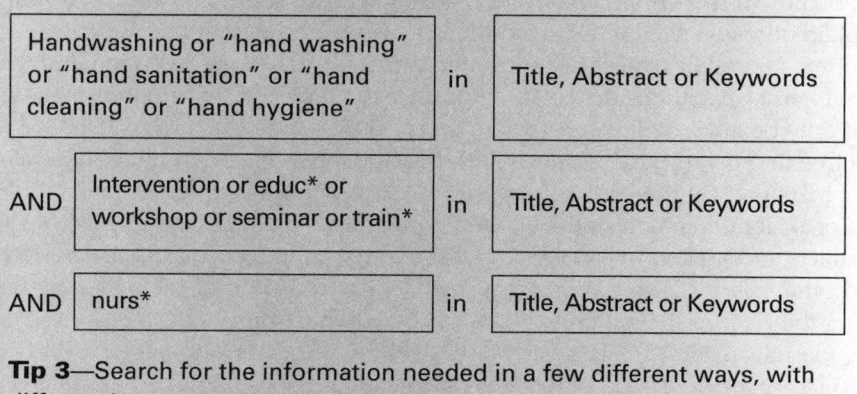

Handwashing or "hand washing" or "hand sanitation" or "hand cleaning" or "hand hygiene"	in	Title, Abstract or Keywords
AND Intervention or educ* or workshop or seminar or train*	in	Title, Abstract or Keywords
AND nurs*	in	Title, Abstract or Keywords

Tip 3—Search for the information needed in a few different ways, with different keywords, phrases, and limiters before moving on to another resource.

Mark and his team move on to search other bibliographic databases for systematic reviews, literature reviews, and primary source articles (Box 9▪7). Remember, many of the most commonly used bibliographic databases for evidence-based nursing practice require a subscription for access.

- **MEDLINE,** the National Library of Medicine's bibliographic database, is available by subscription through most nursing school libraries. It contains over 18 million abstracts and full-text journal articles from over 5,400 global journals published since 1947.
- **CINAHL,** the **Cumulative Index of Nursing and Allied Health Literature,** contains over 2 million abstracts from nearly 3,000 English-language journals and full-text English-language journal articles from over 600 journals published since 1981 (see Box 9▪8 for search tips).
- **Embase** contains over 20 million abstracts and full-text articles from over 7,000 peer-reviewed global journals published since 1974. Embase Classic

BOX 9■7 **Additional Sources Containing Systematic Reviews, Literature Reviews, and Primary Source Articles**

■ CINAHL (http://www.ebscohost.com/cinahl)
■ Embase (http://www.embase.com)
■ Google Scholar (http://scholar.google.com)
■ MEDLINE (http://www.nlm.nih.gov/databases/databases_medline.html)
■ PubMed Central (http://www.ncbi.nlm.nih.gov/pmc)

provides access from 1947–1973. Viewed as one of the most global sources of abstracts and full-text articles, Embase has limited availability in U.S. nursing school and hospital libraries.

Free Resources

In addition to subscription-based resources, there are some free Internet resources that contain peer-reviewed scholarly journal citations, abstracts, full-text articles, systematic reviews, and other quality health-care information. However, keep in mind that many free Internet resources do not provide access to the full text of articles. Rather, you will only be able to view or download abstracts or article citations. **PubMed Central** is a free Internet resource made available by the U.S. National Institutes of Health (NIH) and managed by the National Center for Biotechnology Information (NCBI) at the National Library of Medicine. PubMedCentral provides access to MEDLINE's 18 million abstracts and limited full-text articles from participating journals, publisher Web sites, and other Internet sites. You can supplement your search of bibliographic databases using the Internet search engine **Google Scholar.** Google Scholar search results only include information freely available from the Internet, so the results do not include abstracts or articles found only within subscription-based bibliographic databases. You must use caution and understand that results will not be comprehensive and often do not freely link to the full-text journal articles. Again, check with your university or hospital librarian to find out what Internet resources he or she recommends for your research.

Mark's team can also search for free, full-text systematic reviews via **PubMed Central's Clinical Queries** interface. In addition, internationally developed systematic reviews can be found at the highly respected **Centre for Reviews and Dissemination (CRD),** made available from the National Institute for Health Research (NIHR) and the University of York. Keep in mind that not every review is available in full text on the Internet, so work with your librarian to access the full text from another source.

Tracking Search Results

While Mark and his team search bibliographic databases and the Internet, they should also keep track of the search terms they used and the corresponding results. Keeping track of the most useful search string developed and the limits applied within each database will ensure that the same effective search can be reproduced in another

BOX 9▪8   Search Tips for CINAHL

Tip 1—As do the Cochrane Library, JBI, and other database interfaces, CINAHL's interface offers Basic Search and Advanced Search options. CINAHL's Advanced Search option incorporates a useful Boolean operator structure to the interface. Using the interface, searches can be limited to peer reviewed sources, nursing journals, practice guidelines, or systematic reviews, or searches can be conduction by publication date and many other useful elements.

Tip 2—CINAHL also offers the ability to search using MeSH and CINAHL subject headings. When using the EBSCOhost interface, place a checkmark in the "Suggest Search Terms" box and place the phrase "hand hygiene" in the search box. CINAHL will direct you to use the CINAHL term "hand-washing" instead. The search can be expanded to include results for the "handwashing" subject heading as well as its first layer of narrower terms. Narrowing to "Major Concept" will return only those results in which the "handwashing" subject heading is the major point. No matter which vendor provides your access to CINAHL, practice using MeSH and CINAHL subject headings to target your search.

Tip 3—Try using the Advanced Search option to combine MeSH or CINAHL subject headings with keywords and phrases. Also try limiting results to those with the keywords and phrases only in the abstract instead of throughout all text. A targeted search, such as the example below, incorporates a combination of subject headings, keywords, phrases, truncation symbols, and limiters.

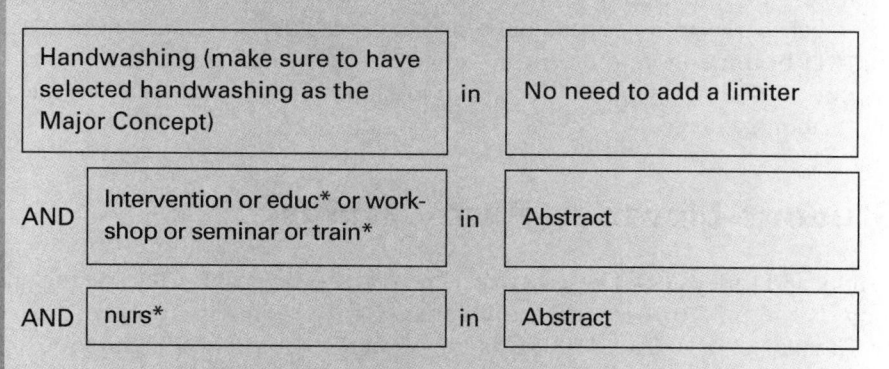

	Handwashing (make sure to have selected handwashing as the Major Concept)	in	No need to add a limiter
AND	Intervention or educ* or work-shop or seminar or train*	in	Abstract
AND	nurs*	in	Abstract

Tip 4—Do you notice how similar the search example above looks to the search example for the Cochrane Library? Once you figure out a search structure that returns relevant results, use that same structure to search other resources.

Tip 5—Search for the information needed in a few different ways, with different keywords, phrases, and limiters before moving on to another resource.

database. Tracking the number of relevant articles located from a specific database, an Internet source, or a specific journal will make it easier to revisit the most useful resources again, if needed.

Library Services

As Bird (2003) states, "Unfortunately, there is no single super discovery tool that will, by itself, search all the relevant literature for health care" (p. 58). A comprehensive search requires searching multiple sources of information to locate the best available evidence. If you find an abstract or citation mentioned on the Internet or within the references list or bibliography of a journal article, check to see if your library subscribes to the full-text journal within a bibliographic database or in print. Believe it or not, there are still some peer-reviewed nursing and health-care journals available only in print. If your library does not have the journal in electronic or print form, ask if a copy of the article is available through interlibrary loan or through a relationship with another library. Most university libraries will acquire full-text articles for students for free or a nominal fee. Hospital libraries vary in their ability to provide these types of services.

Diagnosing the Quality

Developing a successful search strategy and retrieving the full-text information is just part of the evidence-based practice process. The next step is the **critical appraisal** of the evidence once it's found. That means you need to judge if the information is relevant, and valid, and if the findings will help you answer your question. McKibbon and Marks (1998a) point out, "Despite the peer review process, not all research studies published in journals are methodologically sound, and some may be more sound than others" (p. 69). As you get more comfortable with keywords and practice searching, you will become more efficient in your knowledge-gathering skills. Nonetheless, as you will find in Chapter 11, it is your job to always be a critical consumer of the information gathered.

Student–Librarian Partnerships

Hendry and Farley (1998) suggest that after you have been able to define the question, "now is the time to befriend the librarians" (p. 3). This useful advice is echoed by Timmins and McCabe (2005), as they found that "establishing a good working relationship with librarians is an integral part of any successful literature search. They are an invaluable learning resource in getting to know the library and learning how to conduct a successful electronic search of the literature" (p. 44).

In this chapter's clinical story, Mark is wise to suggest a meeting with the school's nursing librarian. Librarians and information scientists are trained to assist with identifying relevant keywords, phrases, and subject headings. They are educated in the organizational structure of bibliographic databases and the Internet and are knowledgeable in using Boolean operators, truncation, and wildcards to locate relevant electronic information. They are also trained to identify relevant print and electronic resources and have the ability to acquire needed resources from others. Partnering with a librarian will result in a more effective search and more efficient information retrieval.

Visit your university or hospital library's Web site to find out the best way to contact your librarian. Many librarians prefer that students, especially a team of students like Mark's, make an appointment to meet. This ensures that the librarian and the group are available and prepared for the meeting. At the initial meeting with your librarian, be prepared to discuss your project and the types of evidence resources that you need to ideally address the problem. Bring your PICO or PICo question and an initial list of synonyms and keywords that you know might relate to the question's key components. In most cases, do not expect your librarian to do the searching for you; he or she will help fine-tune your search strategy and introduce you to the resources that will enable you to locate the best available evidence (Box 9■9).

■ Summary

The best available evidence can be found in many forms. There will be times when a synthesized form of information, including a systematic review, a clinical practice guideline, a Best Practice Information Sheet or a summary of the evidence, will be the best evidence. Other times, a handful of individual journal articles, or just one journal article, will be the best available evidence. Evidence can be found within bibliographic databases, Internet resources, journals, magazines, and books. Evidence can also be found

---

BOX 9■9 Tools for Learning and Practice

■ Locate your hospital or university library's list of available information resources. Look for sources of synthesized information as well as primary sources of information. Spend about 5 minutes in each resource becoming familiar with the interface and doing a quick search to see what kinds of information can be retrieved.

■ Use Google to search the Internet for "clinical practice guidelines" and "systematic reviews." Explore the sites. Pay particular attention to the original author and source of the information. Take note of the domain from which the information is available, for example, .edu, .gov, .com, .net.

■ Search the Internet for PubMed Central. Search the site for "clinical queries" and bookmark for later use.

■ Search the Internet for the U.S. National Library of Medicine (http://www.nlm.nih.gov/) for Medical Subject Headings (MeSH). Use the MeSH browser to search the controlled vocabulary for a term used to describe a topic of research interest. Bookmark the page for later use.

■ Find out the name of the hospital or university librarian who can work with you to locate information. Contact him or her to set up a time to talk or meet face to face.

by having conversations with experts within the field. Through practice you will learn how to wade through the wealth of information that exists, and ultimately identify and access the best available evidence for your question. In the meantime, contact your hospital or university librarian for help along the way.

CHAPTER QUESTIONS

1. Why is it important to be able to identify the best available evidence? Describe how you use evidence to make clinical decisions.

2. Name at least two types of synthesized evidence.

3. Define what a systematic review is. Explain the difference between a meta-synthesis and a meta-analysis.

4. Explain how a systematic review is different from a literature review.

5. What is a primary source of evidence?

6. Generate keywords, phrases, and MeSH subject headings to use for researching evidence for the following:
   a. The effect complementary medicines have on the treatment of chronic pain
   b. What diet and exercise interventions work best for adults with type 2 diabetes
   c. Effective treatments for pressure ulcer prevention in hospitalized older adults

7. What is the definition, also known as scope note, for the MeSH subject heading of "Health Literacy"?

8. What are the three common Boolean operators used to structure a search?

9. How would you use a truncation symbol, the asterisk, with the keyword "nurse" to ensure that the information in your search results would contain the keywords" nurse," "nurses," and "nursing"?

10. How would you use the question mark wildcard to find information containing the phrases "complimentary medicine" and "complementary medicine"?

11. List the bibliographic databases, Internet resources, and print resources available through your hospital or university library that contain the best available evidence for the questions listed in question 6.

12. Identify the names of the librarians and information scientists within your university or hospital library who can work with you to find the information you need. How do you think they can help you find the evidence needed to answer your question?

References

Bird, D. (2003). Discovering the literature of nursing: A guide for beginners. *Nurse Researcher, 11*(1), 56–70.

Cook, D. J., Mulrow, C. D., & Haynes, R. B. (1997). Systematic reviews: Synthesis of best evidence for clinical decisions. *Annals of Internal Medicine, 126,* 376–380.

Evans, D., & Kowanko, I. (2000). Literature reviews: Evolution of a research methodology. *Australian Journal of Advanced Nursing, 18,* 33–38.

Hendry, C., & Farley, A. (1998). Reviewing the literature: A guide for students. *Nursing Standard, 12*(44), 22–28.

Jones, L. V., & Smyth, R. L. (2004). How to perform a literature search. *Current Paediatrics, 14,* 482–488.

McKibbon, K. A., & Marks, S. (1998a). Searching for the best evidence. Part 1: Where to look. *Evidence-Based Nursing, 1,* 68–70.

McKibbon, K. A., & Marks, S. (1998b). Searching for the best evidence. Part 2: Searching CINAHL and MEDLINE. *Evidence-Based Nursing, 1,* 105–107.

Pearson, A., Wiechula, R., Court, A., et al. (2005). The JBI model of evidence-based healthcare. *International Journal of Evidence-Based Healthcare, 3,* 207–215.

Stebbins, L. F. (2006). *Student guide to research in the digital age: How to locate and evaluate information sources.* Westport, CT: Libraries Unlimited.

Taylor, T. (2007). *100% information literacy success.* Clifton Park, NY: Thomson Delmar Learning.

Timmins, F., & McCabe, C. (2005). How to conduct an effective literature search. *Nursing Standard, 20*(11), 41–47.

CHAPTER 10

Appraise and Plan I

All Evidence Is Not Created Equal

Leslie Rittenmeyer

LEARNING OBJECTIVES

- Explain the purpose of critical appraisal of evidence.
- Explain the skill sets needed to carry out critical appraisal activities.
- Discuss the critical appraisal of qualitative evidence.
- Discuss the critical appraisal of quantitative evidence.

KEY TERMS

Animal-assisted therapy (AAT)
Bias
Credibility
Critical appraisal
Crucial Appraisal Skills
   Program (CASP)
Dependability

Joanna Briggs Institute (JBI)
Public Health Resource Unit
   (PHRU)
RAPid
Rapid critical appraisal
Skill set
Transferability

Clinical Story

Kristin is in her last semester of a baccalaureate-nursing program. She is conducting a clinical preceptorship with Nicole, a team leader on the psychiatric unit of a community hospital. Nicole and Kristin have discussed their observation that many patients on the psychiatric unit seem to experience high levels of anxiety, regardless of their diagnoses. Kristin remembers reading about the use of **animal-assisted therapy (AAT)** to reduce anxiety in patients with Alzheimer's disease, and she wonders if this treatment might be as effective in the psychiatric setting. She shares her thoughts with Nicole, and after discussing it with their evidence-based practice mentor they decide to search for evidence on this subject. To focus their search, they write the following PICO question: "How effective is AAT as compared to other group therapies in reducing anxiety in patients with a psychiatric diagnosis who are hospitalized on a psychiatric unit?"

In conducting a search of the literature, they are disappointed that they do not find any synthesized sources of evidence, for instance, systematic reviews or meta-analysis of randomized clinical trials (RCTs). They know that systematic reviews and RCTs represent a higher level of evidence, but when none is accessible, you pick the best evidence that is available. After completion of their search they find only one **primary study** (research studies that collect original data) that directly addresses their PICO question. They also find a qualitative study that explores the meaning of the AAT experience for hospitalized psychiatric patients, and although their PICO question was framed as an effectiveness question, they decide to look at that research, too. They know the next step in the process, after question development and searching for evidence, is the critical appraisal process. They decide to critically appraise both the quantitative and qualitative study but feel they need to assess their skill set before starting. ∎

Introduction

In the evidence-based practice environment it is expected that clinicians possess rudimentary knowledge of research methods and the skills to critically appraise sources of evidence to determine their usefulness for practice. Knowledge of evidence-based practice is now considered a baccalaureate degree competency by the Commission on Collegiate Nursing Education (CCNE), and more schools are integrating these concepts and skills into their curricula. This speaks well for the future generation of nurses who will be well versed on the processes of evidence-based practice.

When you want to access information about a particular clinical problem, you would most likely start with a literature search, just as Kristin and Nicole did in this chapter's clinical story. Following that, you would probably identify reports that you believe would be helpful in answering your questions. However, once you have them, what do you do with them? Do you read them and just assume that the con-clusions are accurate or do you introduce some healthy skepticism into the process? A healthy skeptic would ask the following questions:

- How do I judge the quality of the research?
- How much confidence can I have that the evidence is of high enough quality to merit suggesting practice change?
- When should I be seeking further evidence?
- What criteria should I use to make these judgments?

These are all appropriate questions, and each can be answered by applying the step of **critical appraisal** to the evidence-based practice process. Critical appraisal is a process in which evidence is systematically evaluated to judge its quality and trustworthiness in informing practice change.

Whether you are a student or a practicing clinician, you need to develop critical appraisal skills. Studies are often subject to **bias.** Bias can come from distortions in the research process, for instance, how data are collected, number of subjects, or how data are analyzed. This is true in both quantitative work and qualitative work, and there is a danger of bias when the study is conducted in a way that might lead to a particular conclusion. Good researchers attempt to minimize bias by applying certain research methods. Unfortunately, some research work is conducted with more rigor than others, and you will have to decide whether the studies you are appraising are trustworthy and reliable enough to inform your practice.

The focus of this chapter is to help you become a skeptic by providing you the skills to make a competent critical appraisal. Be aware that there are many tools to guide critical appraisal. In a systematic review of critical appraisal tools conducted by Katrak, Bralocerkowski, Jassy-Westropp, et al. (2004), there were 121 published instruments to conduct reviews. For the purpose of illustration, the focus of this chapter is on two groups of tools: (1) RAPid by the Joanna Briggs Institute (JBI), which is just as the name implies, a tool to perform rapid appraisals; and (2) the Critical Appraisal Skills Program (CASP) from the Public Health Resource Unit (PHRU). Both groups of tools are explained in more depth later in the chapter. These two appraisal systems have been selected because of their reliability and validity, and they are user-friendly for students and clinicians alike.

How to Begin

There are some **skill sets** that you must develop to implement a systematic critical appraisal. A skill set is a set of basic techniques you need to carry out a task. In the case of critical appraisal, a basic understanding of research language, methodologies, and methods is needed. In addition, an understanding of basic statistics is helpful in the evaluation process. Different research paradigms call for different skill sets. For example, criteria for appraising research carried out in qualitative methodologies are different from the criteria for appraising research conducted in quantitative method-ologies. This is further complicated by the fact that there are differences in criteria for appraising research from different types of quantitative studies (e.g., RCTs), case control studies, cohort studies, diagnostic test studies, prognostic studies, and economic studies. There are also tools to appraise the quality of systematic reviews and clinical guidelines. An example of this type of appraisal can be found in Chapter 20. It is most important that the appraisal criteria in the tool match the research design.

For you to assess your own skill set for doing critical appraisal, Tables 10■1 and 10■2 provide a short description of the most common quantitative and qualitative study designs, and Box 10■1 provides a list of common statistical concepts that you should know. The content from your baccalaureate research course should be adequate to allow you to do a basic critical appraisal. It is very important that you maintain your basic research skills so that you can gather and appraise information

Table 10■1   **Selective Quantitative Study Designs**

Quantitative Study Designs	Description
Systematic reviews (meta-analysis)	The application of strategies that limit bias in the assembly, critical appraisal, and synthesis of all relevant studies on a particular topic
Meta-analysis (quantitative)	Use of statistical methods to pool the results of independent studies.
Meta-synthesis (qualitative)	Qualitative analysis of a group of individual studies in which the findings of the studies are pooled.
Randomized clinical trials	A true experimental design in which there is randomization, control, and manipulation.
Cohort study	A form of longitudinal study that is used to examine exposure disease associations; can be retrospective or prospective (observational study design)
Case control study	A study design that uses patients who already have the disease and looks back and analyzes if there are characteristics of these patients that differ from those who do not have the disease (observational studies)
Case series/case report	Case series (also known as a clinical series) is a research design that tracks patients with a known exposure given similar treatment or examines their medical records for exposure and outcome; can be retrospective or prospective (observational studies)
Cross-sectional studies	Cross-sectional studies involve data collected at a defined time, providing a snapshot of a disease in the population (observational studies)
Diagnostic studies	A study design that evaluates the accuracy of a diagnostic test
Prognostic study	A study that measures the possible outcomes of a disease and the frequency in which they occur

Table 10■2   **Selected Qualitative Study Designs**

Selected Qualitative Study Designs	Description
Phenomenology/hermeneutics	A study design that aims to describe the meaning of a phenomena for persons (either through participant voice or text)
Grounded theory	An inductive study design that uses systematic procedures to arrive at a theory (either through participant voice or text)
Participatory action research	A study design in which researchers and the study participants enter into an equal partnership to study a problem and then plan action based on the research findings, resulting in a difference in the lives of the participants
Ethnography	A research method whose major aim is to study persons in their cultural context
Focus groups	A research method that asks groups of persons about their opinions, attitudes, and beliefs about a particular topic

---

BOX 10■1 **Statistics to Review**

- Mean (X)
- Standard deviation (SD)
- Odds ratio (OR)
- Risk
- Relative risk (RR)
- Confidence interval (CI)
- Numbers needed to treat
- Mean difference
- Weighted mean difference
- Standardized differences in mean

---

that informs your clinical decisions. To inform your clinical decisions with the best available evidence, you need to be able to judge the quality of that evidence for application to your practice.

Critical Appraisal Tools

Feeling confident in their basic research and statistical knowledge base, Kristen and Nicole are ready to explore the tools they will use to conduct their critical appraisal.

With the help of their evidence-based practice mentor, the students are able to identify the skill set they need. As was stated earlier, it is important that you use an appraisal tool that asks the right questions for the particular research methodology. It is also important to keep in mind that no matter which tool is used, the purpose of critical appraisal is threefold:

1. To assess if the study is valid or of high enough quality to consider using to inform practice change
2. To determine if the results fit into a local context (your own)
3. To judge whether the results will help your patients

RAPid and CASP Critical Appraisal Tools

Melnyk and Fineout-Overholt (2005) discuss a method they refer to as **"rapid critical appraisal."** They contend that clinicians should be able to quickly appraise evidence to determine its validity and applicability to practice, and critical appraisal approaches should be user friendly so that busy clinicians can swiftly appraise a piece of research. The **Joanna Briggs Institute (JBI)** supports this stance and developed the critical appraisal system called **RAPid**. The JBI program, with its accompanying software, is intended to help students and clinicians develop skills in critical appraisal, allowing them to quickly exclude papers that are of inadequate quality to inform practice, enabling them to focus on the salient factors of high-quality research. The RAPid appraisal system has multiple tools that provide appraisal criteria for a variety of study designs. To access the software program, you or your institution must be a member of the Joanna Briggs Institute. This membership also allows access to a library database of completed RAPid summary reports. These reports are reviewed by a review board whose members are content experts. Even if you are not a member, you can readily access the RAPid critical appraisal criteria in the *RAPid Appraisal Users Manual,* which is easily downloaded in PDF format by going to JBI (http://www.joannabriggs.edu.au), clicking on "Evidence-Based Resources and Services," and choosing "RAPid" from the drop-down menu. Although providing an example of the complete array of RAPid appraisal criteria for all research designs is beyond the scope of the chapter, Box 10■2 lists the available tools from the Joanna Briggs Institute RAPid program. Later in the chapter, Kristin and Nicole will use the RAPid Tool for Intervention Studies to appraise one of their primary studies.

BOX 10■2 Joanna Briggs Institute RAPid Appraisal Tools

- Critical appraisal for a prognostic study
- Crucial appraisal for an intervention study
- Critical appraisal of risk study
- Critical appraisal for the cost study
- Critical appraisal for an experience study (qualitative)
- Critical appraisal for diagnosis two-level and multilevel studies
- Critical appraisal for systematic review of intervention

The **Crucial Appraisal Skills Program (CASP)** from the United Kingdom provides a set of tools appropriate for critical appraisal of both quantitative and qualitative methodologies. These tools come from the **Public Health Resource Unit (PHRU)** of the National Health Service (NHS). The aim of CASP is to enable both students and clinicians to develop the skills to find and make sense of research evidence, helping them to put knowledge into practice. The CASP tools can be easily downloaded from the PHRU Web site (http://www.phru.nhs.uk/pages/phd/resources.htm), and Box 10■3 lists the available CASP tools. A little later, Kristin and Nicole will use the CASP Tool to appraise their qualitative study.

Appraisal of Quantitative Research

When designing a study, researchers make well-thought-out decisions about what methods they will employ to decrease the possibility of bias. Box 10■4 reviews the key item a researcher may consider when designing a study. When the design of the study is well thought out there is less chance that the study will be flawed in some way, therefore making the results suspect.

The first step in the critical appraisal of quantitative studies is to identify what research design was used so you can choose the correct appraisal tool. (See Table 10■1 for a description of various research designs.) Once you have chosen the appropriate tool, you can then proceed to evaluate the study or systematic review. If you are working with another person, both of you should appraise the study independently.

BOX 10■3   Public Health Resource Center CASP Tools for Critical Appraisal

- Appraisal tool for systematic reviews
- Appraisal tools for randomized clinical trials
- Appraisal tool of qualitative studies
- Appraisal tool for cohort studies
- Appraisal tool for case control studies
- Appraisal tool for diagnostic studies

BOX 10■4   Planning a Good Research Study

- Possible threats to external and internal validity
- The sources of possible bias
- The best design to measure the research question
- The sampling strategy to be employed
- Possible legal/ethical concerns
- Appropriate data collection methods
- Methods needed to test reliability and validity of instruments
- Correct statistical methods for data analysis

This creates a system of checks and balances, making the process transparent and open. Kristin and Nicole are ready to appraise their study on the effects of **AAT** on anxiety ratings of hospitalized psychiatric patients. They have already labeled this study as an intervention study so they choose to use the RAPid tool for intervention studies. Remember that no matter what appraisal tool you use it must match the research design of the study. Table 10■3 demonstrates the appraisal criteria and how Kristen and Nicole apply the appraisal process to this particular study.

Appraisal of Qualitative Research

Qualitative evidence plays an important role in informing clinical decision making. It is also valuable in informing health services policy and planning. The data from qualitative work show how individuals and groups perceive health and health-related phenomena. Qualitative methodologies provide insights into topics that are difficult to measure quantitatively. Whereas quantitative paradigms attempt to control and predict, qualitative paradigms attempt to illuminate meaning and promote understanding.

Just as appraising quantitative evidence for quality, it is equally important to be able to judge the quality of qualitative evidence. Traditionally the concepts of reliability, internal validity, and external validity are used to judge the quality of quantitative evidence. Lincoln and Gruba (1985) suggest that the words *dependability, credibility,* and *transferability* are more suited to qualitative paradigms. Whereas the quantitative word *reliability* speaks to achieving the same results time and time again, in the qualitative world, **dependability** speaks to whether the results are logical, transparent, clearly documented, and consistent similarity in the quality of results is achieved.

Table 10■3 **A RAPid Critical Appraisal**

The patients were randomized to study groups	**Indicators:** the method of patient allocation is detailed sufficiently to demonstrate that it was without bias. Note that in some cases, full randomization might be either unfeasible or inappropriate for the intervention of interest.	Patients were not randomized in this study. The study was a pre- and post-treatment crossover design.
Allocation to treatment groups was concealed from the allocator	**Indicators:** in an attempt to eliminate selection bias, the person allocating each participant to treatment groups was unaware of which participant was allocated to which group.	All patients in this study received the same intervention. There were no control groups in this study.
Other than for the intervention/s of interest, participants were treated the same	**Indicators:** there were no additional treatments given to one group in comparison to another, apart from that treatment being tested.	All participants were treated the same.

(continues on page 132)

Table 10■3   **A RAPid Critical Appraisal** (continued)

The groups were comparable at entry	**Indicators:** there were no measurable differences in the characteristics of the different treatment groups. For example, in the examination of a new wound dressing, it is not appropriate to have a treatment group of young, healthy participants, and a control group of elderly participants with peripheral vascular disease.	All participants were hospitalized with a psychiatric diagnosis.
Those assessing outcomes were blinded to the treatment allocation	**Indicators:** those assessing participant outcomes were unaware of the treatment group that the participants were allocated to. Concealing allocation from the assessors further reduces the chances of bias. In certain situations it may be impossible to blind the assessor to the treatment allocation.	The assessors were not blinded to the treatment conditions but steps were taken to minimize bias by training the assessors in standard data collection procedures.
The outcomes were measured in a reliable manner	**Indicators:** a recognized, validated tool was used for measuring the outcomes. For example, when measuring a patient's level of consciousness, the Glasgow Coma Scale is a widely recognized tool.	The study utilized the state scale of the State-Trait Anxiety Inventory to measure patients' level of anxiety before and after AAT and recreational therapy. The internal consistency for the state scale of the State-Trait Anxiety Inventory is high: median alpha coefficient is 0.93. Construct validity is supported by studies showing that the state scale scores are higher under stressful conditions.
The statistical analysis used was appropriate for the data presented	**Indicators:** there are several statistical analyses available; the one(s) chosen were appropriate to the data being presented.	Instruments were scored twice for accuracy by one of the researchers using scoring keys for the State-Trait Anxiety Inventory. A mixed-models repeated measure was used to compare pre- and post-treatment differences in anxiety scores between and within the AAT condition and the therapeutic recreation condition by diagnostic category.

| The dropout rate was not significant | Indicators: generally a dropout rate of 15% or less is considered insignificant. A rate of 20% or greater is considered to significantly impact on the validity of the study. | Although the N for this study was 230, only 50 participants completed a pre and post-treatment measure for both types of sessions. Failure to complete all four measures was primarily due to time conflicts with medical treatments and patient discharges. A power analysis of the magnitude of differences between the change scores for AAT and therapeutic recreational therapy indicated that larger samples would be needed to achieve an 80% power level at an alpha of 0.05: of 300 patients with psychotic disorder, 125 patients with substance disorders, and 61 patients with other disorders. The fact that only 50 participants completed all four tools out of 230 is a major limitation of the study. Their findings are in line with this limitation, suggesting only promise for the intervention and the need for more research. |
| The rate of patient follow-up was adequate | Indicators: at least 80% of patients were followed up. | There was no statement that patients were followed up after completion of the study. |

From Barker, S., & Dawson, K. (1998). The effects of animal-assisted therapy on anxiety ratings of hospitalized psychiatric patients. *Psychiatric Services, 49*(6), 797–801.

Credibility refers to proof that the researcher made every effort to report an honest representation of the true voices of the participants. Finally, **transferability** refers to the degree to which the results of the study can be applied to other contexts or situations.

After updating their skill set to appraise qualitative research, Kristin and Nicole are ready to appraise their qualitative research article. They use the CASP criteria for qualitative research (Public Health Research Unit, 2006). Table 10■4 illustrates how Kristin and Nicole apply the CASP criteria to their qualitative study.

Table 10■4   **CASP Criteria**

Was there a clear statement of the aims of the research?	Consider: ■ The goal of the research ■ Why it is important ■ Its relevance	The goal of the research to explore the meaning of the experience of AAT was clearly stated. The topic is important because it provides insight into this experience. It is relevant to the research question.
Is the qualitative methodology appropriate?	Consider: If the research seeks to interpret or illuminate the actions and/or subjective experience of research participants	This was a phenomenological study and the methodology was appropriate to the research question.
Is it worth continuing?	Two over-reaching questions to decide if the research is worthy of appraisal	YES
Was the research design appropriate to address the aims of the research?	Consider: ■ If the researcher has justified the research design (e.g., have they discussed how they decided what methods to use?)	The research design was appropriate to address the aim of the study of exploring a lived experience. The researchers justified the research design and explained why they chose the design.
Was the recruitment strategy appropriate to the aims of the research?	Consider: ■ If the researcher has explained how the participants were selected ■ If they explained why the participants they selected were the most appropriate to provide access to the type of knowledge sought in the study ■ If there was discussion around recruitment (e.g., why some people choose not to take part)	The researcher used a purposive sample that is appropriate for this type of research. Participants were chosen because they had knowledge of the phenomena. They did not discuss why some participants chose not to participate.
Were the data collected in a way that addressed the research issues?	Consider: ■ If the setting for data collection was justified ■ If it is clear how data were collected (e.g., focus group, semistructured interview) ■ If the researcher has justified the methods chosen ■ If the researcher has made the methods explicit ■ If the methods were changed during the study how so and did the researcher explain why and how ■ If the form of data is clear (e.g., recordings, video, notes) ■ If the researcher discussed saturation	The setting for data collection was explained in detail. Open-ended interviews were employed to gather rich narrative data. Data collection methods were described explicitly. There was no evidence that any of the methods were changed during the course of the study. Interviews were taped and transcribed verbatim. Saturation was not discussed.

Has the relationship between researcher and participants been adequately considered?	Consider whether clear:
	
	■ If researchers critically examined their own role, potential bias, and influence during:
	  ■ formulation of research questions
	  ■ data collection, including sample, recruitment, choice of location
	■ How the researchers responded to events during the study and whether they considered the implications of any changes in the research design
		There was a short statement locating the researchers culturally. They provided a sound rationale for bracketing their presuppositions They spoke to the phenomenological technique of phenomenological reduction. There did not appear to be any unusual events the occurred during the course of the study.

Have ethical issues been taken into consideration	Consider: ■ If there are sufficient details of how the research was explained to participants for the reader to access whether ethical standards were maintained ■ If the researcher has discussed issues raised by the study (e.g., issues around informed consent or confidentiality or how they have handled the effects of the study on the participants during and after the study) ■ If approval has been sought from the ethics committee	Ethical standards were discussed. There was a clear explanation of informed consent and how confidentiality would be maintained. As the participants were in therapy, monitoring of the effects of participating in the study was addressed. Institutional review board approval from the researcher's university was sought and received.
Was the data analysis sufficiently rigorous?	Consider: ■ If there is an in-depth description of the analysis process ■ If thematic analysis is used. If so, is it clear how the categories/themes were derived from the data ■ Whether the researcher explains how the data presented were selected from the original sample to demonstrate the analysis process ■ If sufficient data are presented to support findings ■ To what extent contradictory data are taken into account ■ Whether the researchers critically examined their own role, potential bias, and influence during analysis and selection of data presentation	There was an in-depth discussion of the data analysis procedure. The data analysis method was appropriate for the research design. Through a 5-step process of data analysis, themes were identified. Through a systematic process of examining the participant's narratives it was clear how the themes were identified. Each was supported by participant narrative making the process and the choice of themes transparent. The researchers address minimization of bias through transparency. The researchers also did member checking by bringing their interpretations back to the participants.

(continues on page 136)

Table 10■4   **CASP Criteria** (continued)

Is there a clear statement of findings?	Consider: ■ If the findings are explicit ■ If there is adequate discussion of the evidence both for and against the researchers' arguments. ■ If the researchers have discussed the credibility of their findings (e.g., triangulation, respondent validation, more than one analyst) ■ If the findings are discussed in relation to the original research question	The findings were explicit and flowed from the themes and were supported by participant narrative. There were two researchers who agreed on the themes and finding. The findings were discussed in relation to the research question and provided relevance for clinical practice.
How valuable is the research?	Consider: ■ If the researcher discusses the contribution the study makes to existing knowledge or understanding (e.g., do they consider the findings in relation to current practice or policy or relevant research-based literature?) ■ If they identify new areas in which research is necessary ■ If the researchers have discussed whether or how the findings can be transferred to other populations ■ If the researchers considered other ways the research may be used	As there was not much research on this phenomenon, this study added to existing knowledge on this topic. The researchers identified the need for more research on this phenomenon.

From Public Health Resource Unit, UK. (2006). All rights reserved. Note: This appraisal is fabricated for illustrative purposes because no qualitative studies were found on AAT.

Making a Decision

Once you have appraised your evidence, how do you decide whether the study is of high enough quality to trust? Research is conducted in the real world and is therefore not always perfect. For a variety of reasons, research designs must adapt to certain problems in the process, and small compromises in quality are sometimes made. The question that drives the decision to use a study is whether the study is good enough or trustworthy enough to use in clinical decision making. This returns to the notion of best-available evidence. A study that does not meet any or few of the critical appraisal criteria would obviously be rejected, but if there are weaknesses found in some of the criteria and the researchers acknowledge the limitations, then the study might still be useful. An example is the study on AAT in the psychiatric setting that Kristen and Nicole appraised. During the appraisal process, they identified some severe limitations in the study. The fact that only 50 participants out of 230 completed the tools on both interventions surely reduces the validity and reliability of this study. However, the fact that the researchers acknowledged the limitations and their recommendations were appropriate for the study's limitations allowed for this study to still provide some useful information. An additional consideration is whether the findings of a particular research project will work in a particular context or setting. Are the recommendations feasible to carry out in your context? Are there resource limitations in your context? Finally, and most important, will it help your particular patient? To address these issues, clinical expertise and patient preference come into play. These can be difficult decisions for novice clinicians, but asking for advice and help is useful in gaining experience (Boxes 10■5 and 10■6).

BOX 10■5 Interdisciplinary Rounds

You would like to be able to receive some support when doing critical appraisal. You have read about journal clubs and think this is a good way for clinicians to improve their critical appraisal skills. How would you go about organizing such a group?

- Who could be involved?
- How often would you meet?
- What is involved in a journal club?
- How would you decide where and when to meet?
- What goals would you have for this journal club?
- How would the research be chosen?
- How would you choose your tools for appraisal?
- How would you know the journal club is meeting its goals

BOX 10■6 *Tools for Learning and Practice*

- Locate the Joanna Briggs Web site and find the *RAPid Assessment Handbook,* then locate and download the RAPid criteria.
- Locate the PHRU Web site and download the CASP tools.
- Locate the CINAHL Web site and search its database. Find one quantitative research report and one qualitative research report and find the correct RAPid00000000000000000000 or CASP tools. Try appraising each report. You might want to work with a partner or group at first.
- Write down the things that caused you the most difficulty when doing an appraisal. Discuss these with your instructor.

■ Summary

Critical appraisal is an important step in the evidence-based practice process. Clinicians need to maintain a skill set that allows them to critically appraise evidence to judge its ability to inform clinical decisions. A basic understanding of research language, methodologies, and methods is adequate to carry out a good critical appraisal. A good critical appraisal is also possible to do rapidly. Students and clinicians such as Kristin and Nicole can raise good clinical questions, search for the evidence, and appraise its quality. This leads to a clinician who is informed by the best available evidence and therefore making decisions that achieve better patient outcomes.

CHAPTER QUESTIONS

1. What started Kristin and Nicole on the search for more information?

2. How did they focus their search for evidence?

3. What skill sets do you need to carry out a good quantitative or qualitative critical appraisal?

4. What are the three main purposes of the critical appraisal process?

5. How would you explain rapid appraisal to a fellow student?

6. What does it mean when someone says that the critical appraisal tool must match the study design?

7. Compare reliability, external validity, and internal validity in quantitative paradigms to dependability, credibility, and transferability in qualitative paradigms?

References

Barker, S., & Dawson, K. (1998). The effects of animal-assisted therapy on anxiety rating of hospitalized psychiatric patients. *Psychiatric Services, 49*(6), 797–801.

Melnyk, B., & Fineout-Overholt, E. (2005). Rapid critical appraisal of randomized controlled trials (RCTs): An essential skill for evidence-based practice (EBP). *Pediatric Nursing, 31*(1), 50–53.

Joanna Briggs Institute. (2010). *RAPid appraisal users manual.* Retrieved from www.joannabriggs.edu.au/

Katrak, P., Bralocerkowski, A., Jassy-Westropp, N., et al. (2004). A systematic review of the content of critical appraisal tools. *BMC Med Research Methodology, 4*(22). doi:10.1186/1471-2288-4-22.

Lincoln, Y. S., & Gruba, E. G. (1985). *Naturalistic inquiry.* Beverly Hills, CA: Sage.

Public Health Research Unit. (2006). Critical appraisal skills program. Retrieved from http://www.phru.nhs.uk/pages/phd/resources.htm

CHAPTER 11

Appraise and Plan II
Pre-Appraised and Synthetic Sources of Evidence

Lisa Hopp

LEARNING OBJECTIVES

- Explain what an evidence hierarchy is and discuss different approaches to rating the quality and substance of an evidence source.

- Discuss the rigor of various evidence sources.

- Differentiate various types of pre-appraised sources of evidence according to their purpose, scope, and usefulness to busy clinicians.

- Discuss the advantages and disadvantages of using pre-appraised, digested sources of evidence.

- Assess a source of evidence for its transparency and rigor.

- Select and defend a pre-appraised source of evidence as best available evidence.

KEY TERMS

Case-controlled study
Cohort study
Digested evidence
Evidence hierarchies
Expert opinion

Grading of Recommendations Assessment, Development, and Evaluation (GRADE)
Working group
Homogeneity

(continues on page 140)

Levels of evidence
Levels (or grades) of recommendations
Meta-analysis
Narrow confidence intervals
Observational study
Pre-appraised evidence

Randomized controlled trial (RCT) with concealed randomization
Rigor
Synopses
Syntheses
Transparent

Clinical Story

When Jacob arrives at his medical-surgical unit one evening, his patient is a frail, elderly woman who has been on his unit for a week with dehydration caused by a urinary tract infection and subsequent septicemia. She needs frequent blood draws and IV medications. It has become increasingly difficult to obtain and maintain venous access. The resident physician decides to insert a multilumen central line to ensure access. Jacob is quite new to the unit and has not yet assisted with a central line insertion. However, he knows the unit has had a recent increase in bloodstream infections related to these catheters and that a multidisciplinary team revised the unit's policy relating to catheter insertion. He needs quick information that he can trust to make sure he knows key aspects of nursing care during the procedure. He wants a concise reference of the evidence to feel confident about his role and, in particular, the main interventions related to keeping the patient safe.

Jacob logs on to a computer in the central nurses' station and accesses the "evidence and policy resources" icon on the desktop; it takes him to a search page. He completes a basic search using the phrase "central venous line insertion" to find what he needs to know to assist with the procedure. He notes that the policy reflects the approval of a multidisciplinary panel (medical director, infectious disease team, quality improvement group, and nursing). He finds the policy has an embedded link to a brief evidence summary. The policy lists his responsibilities and the linked evidence provides the information he needs—a description of the type of evidence supporting the summary and key points to guide him just before he gathers the equipment he needs for the procedure. He also notices that a grade level (A, B, C or 1, 2, 3, 4) follows each recommendation. One of the recommendations that stands out is "maximum sterile barrier conditions and aseptic techniques are recommended in the procedure (grade A)." In addition, he reads that 2% chlorhexidine is superior to other skin-cleansing solutions (level 2) and that ultrasound-guided catheterization is recommended (grade A). The policy emphasizes that the assisting nurse can stop the procedure if these criteria cannot be met. Just minutes later, he heads to the room armed with the insertion kit and confidence in the knowledge he needs to keep the patient safe during the procedure.

Introduction

Critical appraisal is at the heart of evidence-based practice. That is, to properly employ the evidence-based practice process, you must be able to judge the strength and quality of the information you use to make decisions. In the previous chapter, you learned how to use specific tools to guide you in judging different types of research. You discovered that you need to use the right tool for the job. Although some appraisal questions are generic, others must match the design of the research to sensibly and fairly judge a particular study. These tools are very useful when you need to evaluate the quality of individual research reports. However, it may not be possible to appraise individual studies when you are making rapid decisions on the job. Even if you are an experienced expert, time constraints can affect your ability to be thorough in the middle of providing nursing care. A good solution for this dilemma is to use evidence sources in which someone else has already done the hard work of searching, appraising, and summarizing the evidence. Pre-appraised, digested sources of evidence are ideal for use at the point of care.

In this chapter, you will learn where to locate pre-appraised sources, how to judge their quality, and how evidence hierarchies can speed the process of appraising the strength of evidence that you can use during your busy clinical practice.

Pre-Appraised and Digested Sources of Evidence

Reader's Digest specializes in condensed material, giving you the most important points of an article concisely. In fact, maybe you have heard someone say, "Just give me the *Reader's Digest* version!" That means you want to get right to the heart of the issue and focus on the key points. When making simultaneous decisions in the midst of care, clinicians often need to use the *Reader's Digest* approach to find answers quickly and efficiently. However, they also need to be confident that the evidence that supports those answers is the best available evidence. **Pre-appraised evidence** is literature that an author or a group of experts has already reviewed and evaluated the evidence against quality indicators. **Digested evidence** is a source that an author or group of authors has carefully read, selected, and summarized; the most essential parts have been condensed into a shorter version so it is easier to read and understand quickly. **Synopses,** short abridged summaries of the evidence, can be very useful digests for busy clinicians who may only have a few moments to get to the heart of the matter. **Syntheses** refer to systematic reviews of quantitative or qualitative evidence that follow explicit methods of search, appraisal, and analysis of the evidence. Synopses of syntheses are particularly strong sources of evidence because they are brief, pre-appraised, and guided by rigorous methods.

You can recognize pre-appraised evidence by looking for a rating system and an explanation of the meaning of the rating. Many systems exist, so you need to look for a key to the ranking. Usually a rating of I, 1, or A is better than II, 2, or B; however, some systems are the opposite, meaning a IV may be better than a I. You can see how these different rating systems can be confusing, especially if you do not look at the key accompanying the evidence.

When evidence is packaged so that clinicians can more easily search and obtain a bottom-line recommendation, both physicians and nurses with advanced preparation are more likely to find the right answer to questions in the first 2 minutes of searching (Coiera, Westbrook, and Rogers, 2008). In some cases, 2 minutes may be the maximum amount of time you have. One observational study of resident physicians showed that many skipped searching for evidence for most questions they had, but if they did search, they spent only 2 minutes looking for answers. Most commonly, they asked another colleague for answers (Ramos, Linscheid, and Schafer, 2003). Other studies have shown that advanced practice nurses in primary care and nurses in hospitals are no different than their physician colleagues; they favor asking a colleague over searching an electronic database (Codgill, 2003; McCaughan, Thompson, Cullum, et al., 2005; Pravikoff, Tanner, and Pierce, 2005).

Clinicians consult other trusted colleagues because they believe one another, and it is a handy way to find an answer. But the quick consultation of a nearby coworker cannot be relied on for the validity of information in the same way that a published source of evidence can be. The ideal source is one that is as easy to access as a colleague but has already been judged for its quality (Box 11■1).

In this chapter's clinical story, Jacob consults a source of evidence on the desktop computer in his unit (i.e., the point of care) instead of asking a nearby colleague. He uses a simple search and quickly finds a brief summary of the evidence. In addition, he can quickly judge the quality of the best practice recommendations based on a simple A, B, or C rating or 1 to 4 level of evidence, although he needs to understand these rankings to determine how confident he can be in the evidence. Jacob soon discovers he needs know just how good the evidence is when he must defend the approach he thinks is right to protect the patient from possible adverse consequences of the central line insertion.

BOX 11■1   Significance of Pre-Appraised and Digested Evidence

- Most frequently, clinicians consult one another when they have a question about clinical practice; although convenient, it is difficult to know how trustworthy any one clinician's opinion or recommendation may be.
- Busy clinicians need access to brief summaries and synopses of evidence they can trust as high quality.
- When clinicians use a system that allows easy searching, they are more likely to find the best answer in the first 2 minutes of searching.
- Many evidence hierarchies exist; you need to understand the meaning of the hierarchy to know what an evidence rank means.
- Pre-appraised, digested evidence should be both transparent and rigorous to allow the clinician to know to trust the source.

Evidence Hierarchies

In the previous chapter, you learned that all evidence is not equally robust, credible, or trustworthy. Whether the best available evidence originates from quantitative or qualitative research, from local data, or from text and opinion, you need some method to rank your confidence and trust in the information you use to guide decisions. **Evidence hierarchies** are systems used to rank evidence statements according to certain criteria. They help you determine the amount of confidence you can have in a particular recommendation or source of evidence. However, many different hierarchies exist and it is easy to become confused. Some hierarchies rank the **level of the evidence** based on the design of individual studies or systematic reviews of several studies. In quantitative research, the level of evidence increases when the research design controls more extraneous variables. In qualitative research, the level of evidence increases when the credibility and dependability of the methods and the researcher's interpretations increase. Others combine the type of study with the magnitude of the effect or the degree of variability of results to determine rank. Still others are based on the quality of the information as well as the ease and feasibility of using the evidence.

Some hierarchies are based on the assumption that all evidence relates to the effectiveness of interventions, ignoring the idea that clinicians have a range of questions whose answers require different study designs. For example, if a hierarchy ranks a meta-analysis (a systematic review with a statistical summary of many individual studies) as the highest level of evidence, this system is not relevant for questions about the meaning of a symptom or experience in individuals with a certain condition. Questions of meaning need to be answered with study designs that produce narrative data, the words that people use to describe an experience.

Because there are many hierarchies, you need to locate the explanation of the hierarchy when you see a rating associated with a source of evidence or a particular recommendation. The following are three systems that you may encounter when you evaluate evidence-based guidelines or individual sources of evidence. Each system has a unique approach.

Grading of Recommendations Assessment, Development, and Evaluation Approach

The soundness of the research methods to answer any question is key to any rating system. However, an evidence rating system for effectiveness questions can include other factors as well. These factors include the relative importance of individual outcomes, the magnitude of effect, and the balance of harm and benefit (Guyatt, Oxman, Vist, et al., 2008). The **Grading of Recommendations Assessment, Development, and Evaluation (GRADE) Working Group** is an international group of evidence-based medicine experts who spent several years creating a rating system that takes all of these factors into consideration. They aim to provide a standard system that guideline developers can use to grade the quality of the evidence and the strength of recommendations that clinicians without strong backgrounds in critical appraisal can understand. Although this system stems from medicine, many disciplines have contributed to the debate and the system is used for multidisciplinary guidelines. The rankings for the quality of evidence in the GRADE approach are simply high, moderate, low, and very low (Table 11■1). However, a rigorous, transparent approach to appraisal of study designs and methods, consistency of results, directness of the measurement of results, potential for bias, precision and importance of outcomes, and size of the effect all influence the ultimate grade of evidence (Guyatt et al., 2008). You should have the greatest confidence in evidence with a "high" ranking because the source has the least possibility for bias, addresses the most important outcomes (e.g., mortality and highly morbid conditions), and has a large impact. Lower rankings can indicate a problem with some type of bias, inclusion of less important outcomes, or a smaller impact. Many international guideline groups have already adopted this approach, including the World Health Organization, Agency for Healthcare Research and Quality, the Scottish Intercollegiate Guidelines Network, and the European Respiratory Society, among many others (GRADE Working Group, n.d.).

Joanna Briggs Institute Levels of Evidence and Grades of Recommendations

The Joanna Briggs Institute (JBI) has developed a unique method to rank levels of evidence and recommendations. JBI embraces many types of evidence as both legitimate and important when answering questions relevant to enhancing global health. Therefore, it has created four parallel hierarchies for four different types of questions. The rating systems relate to questions of feasibility, appropriateness, meaningfulness, and effectiveness (Pearson, Wiechula, and Lockwood, 2005).

In Table 11■2, you see the top level of evidence for each category refers to a meta-synthesis or meta-analysis of the most trustworthy primary research. As in many other evidence hierarchies, JBI ranks a systematic review that nets a meta-synthesis or meta-analysis of the ideal findings or evidence as the most reliable and believable

Table 11■1   **GRADE Working Group Classification of the Quality of Effectiveness Evidence**

Quality Rating	Definition
High	Further research is very unlikely to change confidence in the estimate of effect
Moderate	Further research is likely to have an important impact on the confidence in the estimate of effect and may change the estimate
Low	Further research is very likely to have an important impact on the confidence in the estimate of effect and is likely to change the estimate
Very low	Any estimate of effect is very uncertain

Adapted from Guyatt et al. (2008).

Table 11■2 **Joanna Briggs Institute Levels of Evidence**

Level of Evidence	Feasibility	Appropriateness	Meaningfulness	Effectiveness
1	Meta-synthesis of research with unequivocal synthesized findings	Meta-synthesis of research with unequivocal synthesized findings	Meta-synthesis of research with unequivocal synthesized findings	Meta-analysis (with homogeneity) of experimental studies (e.g., RCT with concealed random assignment) OR one or more large experimental studies with narrow confidence intervals
2	Meta-synthesis of research with credible synthesized findings	Meta-synthesis of research with credible synthesized findings	Meta-synthesis of research with credible synthesized findings	One or more smaller RCTs with wider confidence intervals OR quasi-experimental studies (without random assignment)
3	a. Meta-synthesis of text/opinion with credible synthesized findings b. One or more single research studies of high quality	a. Meta-synthesis of text/opinion with credible synthesized findings b. One or more single research studies of high quality	a. Meta-synthesis of text/opinion with credible synthesized findings b. One or more single research studies of high quality c. Observational studies (without control group)	a. Cohort studies (with control group) b. Case-control studies
4	Expert opinion	Expert opinion	Expert opinion	Expert opinion, or physiology bench research or consensus opinion

RCT = randomized controlled trial

Adapted from Joanna Briggs Institute (2011b). Levels of evidence. Retrieved from http://www. joannabriggs.edu.au/About%20Us/JBI%20Approach/Levels%20of%20Evidence%20%20FAME source of evidence. Recall that *systematic review* is a general term, meta-syntheses are systematic reviews of qualitative evidence, and meta-analyses are systematic reviews that include statistical analyses of quantitative data. Systematic reviews rank highest because of their exhaustive, systematic search and rigorous appraisal, and the judicious selection of the evidence included in the systematic review (Joanna Briggs Institute, 2011b). Meta-syntheses and meta-analyses rely on methods that ensure rigor at multiple stages of the conduct of systematic reviews. Although a discussion of these techniques is beyond the scope of this book, there is good consensus among the many evidence hierarchies that this type of evidence ranks highest.

When you examine the JBI system of ranking levels of evidence, you will find that level 1 is the highest level and rankings decline to 4, the lowest level. For questions that are best answered with qualitative evidence (i.e., feasibility, appropriateness, and meaningfulness), meta-syntheses are still listed as level 2 and level 3a. However, for level 2, the trustworthiness of evidence contained in the meta-synthesis is not as high as level 1. Instead of being unequivocal, the evidence in a level 2 meta-synthesis is credible, meaning the findings are plausible but could be challenged. For level 3a, the meta-synthesis uses text and opinion rather than qualitative studies; this text and opinion may come from papers produced by scientific organizations or other non–research-based sources. Level 3b is a single qualitative research study of high quality (Joanna Briggs Institute, 2008). Finally, level 4 is evidence from expert opinion.

The evidence leveling for questions of effectiveness is similar to many other hierarchies. At level 1, two types of evidence rank highest: (1) a meta-analysis of randomized controlled trials (RCTs) with homogeneity of experimental studies, or (2) one or more large experimental studies with narrow confidence intervals. To understand why these types of evidence rank highest for questions of effectiveness, you need to understand more about these study designs.

A **meta-analysis** is a secondary research method that statistically pools data from multiple studies to produce a single statistic of effectiveness. Meta-analyses are highly regarded because they carry safeguards against bias, because they should only combine data from well-designed and well-conducted studies, and they follow a research protocol. In addition, they are more generalizable, and you can have greater confidence in the answers because the researcher combines data from more than one study. **Homogeneity** means that the results of each of the individual studies combined in the meta-analysis do not vary widely. Statistical methods can judge whether the results are homogeneous and the author should address this in the publication.

In an **RCT with concealed randomization,** participants are blindly assigned to a group (treatment or control). The RCT is stronger when those blinded include the person who allocates participants to the groups, the participants themselves, those who administer the treatment and collect data, and those who analyze the data. An example of a very rigorous approach to blinding is a study comparing two types of insulin administered by a subcutaneous injection. The control and experimental participants receive prefilled syringes that look identical, a computer program assigned the groups, the nurses providing the instructions do not know the group assignment, blood glucose data are gathered via computer associated only with a number, and the statistician who analyzes the data knows only which data belong to group A and B but is unaware of what each group means. Depending on the type of treatment, not all of those involved in the study can be blinded to group allocation.

Narrow confidence intervals is a statistical term that means how precisely the statistic estimates the true population value and to what degree of probability you can be sure of the estimate. In other words, it represents the "noise" around the estimate (Fig. 11■1). If the confidence interval is wide, the results are less precise and more noise exists in the study, meaning other known and unknown factors are making it difficult to determine the true result. Many factors can contribute to the size of the confidence interval, but the smaller the confidence interval, the more confident you can be in the result. Traditionally, most meta-analyses use a 95% confidence interval, meaning that you can be 95% confident that a true value is between the two ends of the interval. For example, in the RCT using two types of insulin, if the mean difference between glucose levels is 50 mg/dL with a 95% confidence interval of 45 to 55, then the average true difference in the effect of the two insulin treatments is 50 mg/dL. In addition, if you were to repeat the experiment again and again, 95% of the time the difference will fall between 45 and 55 mg/dL and 5% of the time the difference will be greater. If, instead, the 95% confidence interval was 49 to 51 mg/dL, the estimate was more precise and less noisy.

If you put all these factors together—a meta-analysis, homogeneity, concealed randomization, and a narrow confidence interval—you have the most powerful evidence of the effectiveness of an intervention. If you have only one study instead of a meta-analysis, you still have strong evidence, but your ability to generalize is lessened. Level 2 in the JBI hierarchy refers to one or more smaller RCTs with wider confidence intervals, meaning less precision and generalizability.

Three subcategories of single studies make up level 3. Each subcategory has the potential for more bias and less confidence in the results. However, many times these study types are the only feasible way to pursue an answer. **Cohort studies** with a control group are studies in which researchers follow an experimental cohort, or group of people, with something in common. They compare the cohort to another group whose members are otherwise similar, except for the factor that is being investigated. Researchers often use this design when they cannot feasibly or ethically manipulate

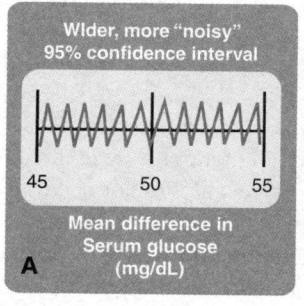
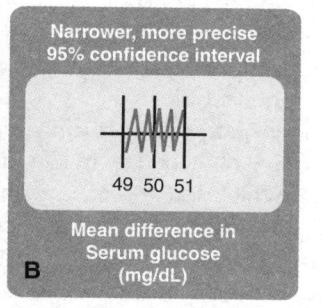

FIGURE 11■1 Confidence intervals and precision. **(A)** The wider confidence interval around the mean difference in glucose level means the estimate is less precise and more noisy (represented by the number of dots around the mean and the width of the interval). **(B)** The narrower confidence interval around the mean difference in glucose level means the estimate is more precise and less noisy (represented by fewer dots around the mean and the smaller interval).

the experimental conditions. For example, a cohort-controlled study might be a study of the effect of secondhand smoking on the incidence of asthma. The experimental cohort is a group of children who live in middle- to upper-class households with smokers who smoke one to two packs of cigarettes per day and expose the children to smoke at least 10 hours per day. The control group is children of the same age and similar socioeconomic status, but they live with nonsmokers. The researchers follow both groups from birth to 18 years of age and compare the number of children in each group who develop asthma. Obviously, it would not be ethical to randomly assign children to a smoking and nonsmoking family, but the question is important to the public health, and a cohort with control study allows researchers to obtain data and draw relevant conclusions in an ethical manner. However, there is greater risk of bias because the researchers have less control over other factors that may coincide with the children's smoking exposure status. Perhaps the families who do not smoke also have other healthy habits that could explain a difference in asthma rates. If the researchers could randomly assign children to smoking and nonsmoking families, they could assume other factors, like healthy eating or exercise habits, would occur at the same random rates in both the experimental and control groups. Without random assignment, researchers cannot assume similar rates in both the cohort and control groups. Despite this, they could strengthen the study design by measuring these healthy habits in both groups to see if there is a difference that contributes to the asthma outcome. Still, cohort-controlled designs rank lower because of the greater chance of bias.

In a **case-controlled study,** researchers select cases (those with a particular outcome) and the control group (those without a particular outcome) and compare the participants' history of exposure. In the asthma study example, the researchers are comparing 18-year-olds with asthma to those without asthma to see if there is a difference in family smoking habits since birth (DiCenso, Guyatt, and Ciliska, 2005).

Level 3c evidence concerns **observational studies** without a control group. These studies include different types of studies in which researchers simply observe what happens and take measurements. These studies can be fraught with bias because of lack of control over other variables that can influence outcomes. Conversely, sometimes an observational study may be the only feasible design, or it is a way to explore a relationship before using a more rigorous but expensive study design. For example, before doing a cohort-controlled study, researchers may have investigated the relationship between the incidence of asthma and secondhand smoke exposure by surveying households and counting how many children had asthma in smoking and nonsmoking households.

For all questions, **expert opinion** is ranked the lowest (level 4), but it does count as a legitimate source of evidence. In fact, not all hierarchies will include expert opinion in their rankings. When you are faced with no research evidence that ranks above expert opinion, you still need to make a decision. If expert opinion is the best available evidence, you need to use this type of evidence with caution. However, many nursing interventions have no stronger evidence than level 4 (expert opinion), yet we have incorporated these interventions into common practice. For example, there is no evidence beyond expert opinion that tells us how frequently we should turn patients who are unable to move themselves to prevent a pressure ulcer from forming.

However, expert opinion supports turning these patients at least every 2 hours and more frequently if signs of skin breakdown such as redness occur or they are high risk (Registered Nurses of Ontario, 2005). Of course, there are interventions that nurses can employ to prevent pressure ulcers in addition to turning patients. But if a highly controlled study is never conducted to compare turning frequencies, expert opinion may remain the best evidence that we will ever have to support the turning frequency of patients who are confined to their beds and unable to move themselves.

As do other organizations, JBI also has a system to rank recommendations. These **levels or grades of recommendations** incorporate the evidence that underpins the recommendations, as well as the appropriateness and relevance of the evidence to practice (Joanna Briggs Institute, 2011a). The grades of recommendations range from A to C, where A means that recommendation has strong support that merits application, B means moderate support that warrants consideration of application, and C means not supported.

In this chapter's clinical story, Jacob uses a policy with embedded evidence summaries much like the pre-appraised evidence summaries from the Joanna Briggs Institute collection called JBI COnNECT+. The summary includes a list of recommendations and associated grades. In addition, the evidence that supports the recommendations is ranked according to levels of evidence. Jacob's evidence summary is based on the highest level of recommendation—A (strong support and based on the highest level of evidence) and level II evidence (an evidence-based practice guideline) (Xue, 2010).

Keeping this information in mind, when Jacob opens the insertion kit, he is pleased to find chlorhexidine cleansing swabs. However, he finds only a small sterile barrier that will only partially cover the patient during insertion. In addition, there is no portable ultrasound machine in the room to help guide the insertion process. Jacob expresses his concerns to the physician about the lack of a full barrier and an ultrasound machine. The resident physician insists that they continue the procedure, as she is certain she can maintain a sterile field with the smaller barrier, and, considering her other responsibilities, she is unwilling to wait for a new, full-sized barrier and an ultrasound machine to be delivered to the unit. Jacob, knowing he has the support of medical and nursing leadership in his unit, informs the resident physician they must stop the procedure until these standards can be met. He further supports his decision by telling the physician that high-level evidence supports his stance. The resident physician interrupts the procedure, but Jacob can tell she is a bit impatient and not pleased about this turn of events.

The 6S Pyramid: Syntheses and Synopses

In addition to determining the quality and significance of evidence and recommendations, ease-of-use is an important practical determinant of whether clinicians will use an evidence source. DiCenso, Bayley, and Haynes (2009) proposed a hierarchy of pre-appraised evidence that ranks sources based on the degree of synthesis and summary. At the peak of the 6S pyramid is the ideal—a clinical decision support system in which evidence is filtered for quality, concisely summarized, and continually updated with emergent research and is linked to the electronic medical record (Figure 11■2). One example is a system that takes in all of the patient assessment data, uses algorithms to determine the patient's condition (e.g., risk for bloodstream infection related to a central line), and creates recommendations for interventions (e.g., full barrier precautions, aseptic technique, ultrasound guidance). This would happen at the point of care, seamlessly and automatically. Unfortunately, few systems such as this exist (DiCenso et al., 2009).

The next level in the 6S pyramid is summaries. These are summaries of evidence that are pre-appraised, filtered for excellence, and systematically developed and transparent; the authors explicitly detail the methods they used to ask, acquire, appraise, and synthesize the evidence. DiCenso et al. (2009) include clinical practice guidelines (CPGs) in this level of the pyramid. However, they emphasize the following: "A CPG should be based on comprehensive searches and appraisal of the literature (ideally current systematic reviews, if they exist), and each recommendation should be accompanied by levels of evidence" (p. 100). If the methods of the summaries are not clear, it is difficult to know if the source is truly based on the best available evidence. In this chapter's clinical story, Jacob uses an evidence summary from the JBI CONnECT+ system (Xue, 2010). This system falls in the category of summaries in the 6S pyramid because the methods of finding the summaries and the evidence that supports the recommendations are clear, and the summaries are regularly updated.

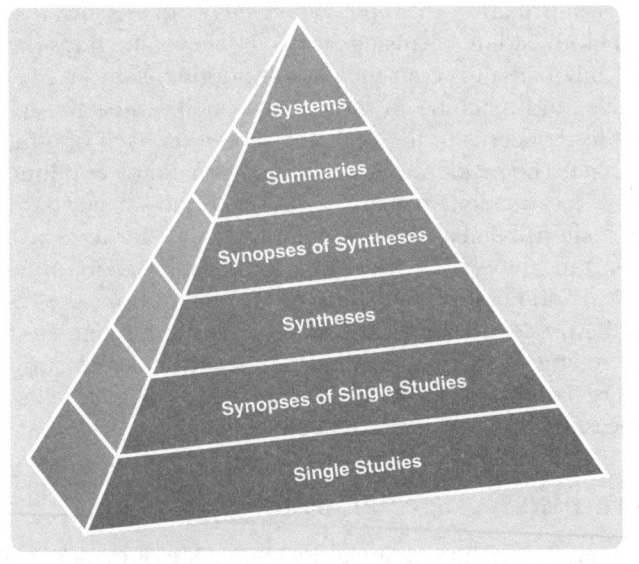

FIGURE 11■2　6S pyramid. DiCenso et al. (2009) adapted the 4S pyramid by adding two additional levels to the hierarchy. Systems = clinical decision support system, where evidence is filtered for quality, concisely summarized, and continually updated as new research emerges and is linked to the electronic medical record or clinical practice guidelines. Summaries = pre-appraised, filtered for excellence, and based on the systematically developed and transparent. Synopses of syntheses = brief summary of key elements of a synthesis such as a systematic review; synopses of single studies = brief summary of key elements of single study; single studies = original studies without filtering or pre-appraisal. (With permission from BMJ Publishing Group Ltd.)

The next level in the 6S pyramid is synopses of syntheses. These are brief summaries of systematic reviews. You can find synopses of syntheses in the Cochrane Nursing Care Field systematic review summaries published in journals such as the *International Journal of Nursing Practice, AORN Journal, Clinical Nurse Specialist Journal and Neonatal, Paediatric & Child Health Nursing,* and many others. You will also find summaries of both systematic reviews and single studies at McMaster University's *Nursing+, Best Evidence for Nursing Care,* which is a free, pre-appraised synopsis online service. In addition, there are abstracting journals that publish synopses of syntheses, such as *Evidence-Based Nursing.* If you need more detail than a synopsis of a synthesis or no synopses exists, you can find the actual systematic reviews published in general literature or in libraries of systematic reviews such as the Cochrane and Campbell Libraries and the Joanna Briggs Institute Library of Systematic Reviews. Finally, if no syntheses exist, you can seek synopses of individual studies found in the same abstracting journals that publish synopses of syntheses, or individual reports of original studies that have not been pre-appraised. Remember, you must use caution when using this pyramid; make sure you find evidence that has undergone a rigorous and transparent filtering and appraisal process to be certain you can trust the source (DiCenso et al., 2009).

Judging the Quality of Pre-Appraised Sources

The advantage of using pre-appraised sources is that you can more quickly determine a source's quality and strength, which helps you decide if you should use the evidence and the appropriate level of confidence you can have in the source (Box 11■2). However, you must still evaluate whether the pre-appraised source can be trusted. Once you have established that the methods of the pre-appraised sources are solid, you can quickly screen content for its quality (see Box 11■3 for tips and best bet sources).

You have seen the word *transparent* several times in this chapter as well as other chapters. This is a key concept to quality evidence. When an evidence source is **transparent**, the authors provide details about its purpose and methods. For example, they need to specify the goals of the guideline, synthesis, synopsis, or summary in the form of a statement or question. They need to explain their search process including where they searched (e.g., databases, organizations) and how they searched. The following statement is an example of good transparency of the search strategies and inclusion criteria used for one summary of a systematic review in the Cochrane Library:

> We searched the Cochrane Central Register of Controlled Trials, MEDLINE, CINAHL, EMBASE (from inception to December 2006), reference lists of identified trials, and bibliographies of published reviews. We also contacted researchers in the field. There were no language restrictions....We included randomized controlled trials comparing central venous catheter insertion routes. (Hamilton and Foxcraft, 2008, Abstract, para. 4–5)

This is typical of a systematic review. Other sources may only discuss the overall methods for a resource somewhere on their Web site or in upfront materials. This

---

BOX 11■2 Interdisciplinary Rounds

- All health-care disciplines need evidence in a form that is easy to use and trustworthy.
- Search for high-quality synopses and summaries of syntheses in any discipline that relates to your clinical problem or question.
- Regardless of the disciplinary source, make sure you understand the ranking system or hierarchy for the evidence you consider using.
- Some systems of evidence are created for many disciplines and others are aimed at more singular audiences.
- Ask colleagues from other disciplines what pre-appraised and digested evidence sources they use.
- Be ready to support your decisions when other professionals challenge your position; understanding the level of evidence and degree of confidence in the evidence may affect how vigorously you argue the point.
- Having ready access to evidence at the point of care that is pre-appraised and summarized may foster a culture of evidence-based decision making among all disciplines.

BOX 11■3 Tools for Learning and Practice

Free Pre-Appraised, Digested Evidence Sources

- http://www.tripdatabase.com/—The Turning Research Into Practice (TRIP) is an easy-to-use, free tool to search across several databases. It uses a color-coded method of identifying the quality of evidence and you can filter evidence to find summaries of systematic reviews or clinical practice guidelines. The search process is not exhaustive but it is somewhat transparent. The focus is on both medical and nursing decisions.
- http://www.rnao.org—Registered Nurses of Ontario Nursing Best Practice Guidelines Are based on transparent methods and a rigorous approach, using tools to help with implementation. Each guideline has a short summary with grades of evidence for each recommendation.
- http://www.joannabriggs.edu.au. Brief synopses of systematic reviews called "Best Practice Information Sheets" are freely available after 6 months of publication date.
- http://plus.mcmaster.ca/NP/Default.aspx—A unique service of pre-filtered evidence based on quality indicators and rated for relevance and interest by an international group of nurses. It is searchable and customizable to areas of interest within nursing; e-mail alerts are available.
- http://www.guideline.gov—Includes summaries of clinical practice guidelines for nursing and other healthcare disciplines. Use the Compare tool to quickly look for quality indicators. Appraise these guidelines for their rigor and transparency.

BOX 11■3 **Tools for Learning and Practice** (continued)

Subscription-Based Pre-Appraised, Digested Evidence Sources

- http://connect.jbiconnectplus.org/—A subscription-based service of nursing and health-care disciplines. Evidence sources include summaries as well as systematic reviews of evidence of effectiveness as well as feasibility, appropriateness, and meaningfulness. Systematic reviews are highly transparent.
- http://clinicalevidence.bmj.com—Clinical Evidence is a product of the *British Medical Journal* publication that uses an explicit approach to searching and the GRADE evidence rating system. The majority of evidence relates to medical rather than nursing decisions.
- http://www.ebscohost.com/dynamed—Dynamed uses an explicit and comprehensive approach to the search and appraisal of evidence with regular, ongoing updates. It is more heavily oriented toward medical practice but nursing-relevant content can be found. It can be linked to the electronic health record and can be used with a portable digital assistant.
- http://www.uptodate.com/index—Like Dynamed, this source is aimed primarily at medical practice. Its methods are somewhat transparent but not easily found. It can be used with a personal digital assistant, contains brief summaries of many types of evidence, and is updated regularly.

makes the source less transparent and more difficult to judge when you must hunt for the methods. You should use caution if a source lacks any description of the method of the search, how exhaustive the search was (i.e., the breadth and number of databases), and what criteria were used to include studies or information in a source.

In addition to transparent methods, look for how the authors ensured **rigor,** meaning the way in which the authors appraise the evidence (look for appraisal checklists and levels of evidence or grades of recommendations) and if more than one person validates the appraisal (if it is a clinical practice guideline or systematic review). For example, in the same systematic review from the Cochrane Library above, Hamilton and Foxcraft (2008) wrote, "Two authors assessed potentially relevant studies. We resolved disagreements by discussion. Relevant outcomes were: venous thrombosis, venous stenosis, infection related to CVA devices, mechanical complications" (Abstract, para. 6). Generally, you will see this degree of transparency and rigor only with syntheses, such as systematic reviews.

Defending Your Evidence-Based Position

Once you have selected the best pre-appraised evidence from a synthesized or other digested source, you need to be ready to defend your choice. Not all health-care workers will be familiar with evidence hierarchies, and they may even be skeptical of evidence-based practice itself. You may need to go beyond a plain, uninformative statement such as "My information and reasons are evidence based." Instead, be ready to briefly discuss where your evidence came from, its quality, and a quick summary of the results.

In the clinical story, Jacob discovers the physician is reluctant to wait for a full drape to cover the patient and an ultrasound machine that would help the physician know if a vein was patent (i.e., had good circulation and blood flow). Jacob is ready to support his stance. He explains to the physician that the reason he asks her to stop the procedure is that strong evidence from systematic reviews supports full barrier precautions and ultrasound guidance. He says that he used the Joanna Briggs Institute evidence summaries, which are based on Cochrane Library systematic reviews. In addition, he mentions that he understands her urgency, but the unit standard of practice is consistent with this evidence, and he must stop the procedure to ensure the patient's safety. Once Jacob is able to find the correct equipment, he and the physician start the procedure again.

Increasingly, nursing staff members are empowered to interrupt medical procedures when those involved deviate from the recommended practices (Institute for Healthcare Improvement, ND). Jacob is confident in his decision to interrupt the procedure because of the high-quality evidence. Having the evidence in hand enhances the nurse's position, even in a situation of conflict with the physician.

■ Summary

In this chapter, you learned about the value of pre-appraised and summarized evidence. In the clinical story, Jacob was able to quickly locate a pre-appraised evidence summary that provided him with important knowledge to maintain the patient's safety. Busy clinicians need systems of evidence they can trust and access quickly at the point of care. You need to understand evidence hierarchies and what they mean in terms of your confidence in the evidence. To this end, evidence ratings can help you quickly assess the trustworthiness of any source and help you defend your clinical decisions. As with any evidence source, pre-appraised sources must be evaluated for their transparency and rigor, but they can be a valuable asset in a busy healthcare environment.

CHAPTER QUESTIONS

1. In this chapter's clinical story, what type of evidence source did Jacob rely on? What did it mean that some recommendations were level A and other pieces of evidence were level 2? What is the difference between the level of evidence and level or grade of recommendation?

2. What factors contribute to the rigor of the evidence? What is meant by *transparency*?

3. What are the main similarities and differences among the GRADE Working Group, Joanna Briggs Institute, and the 6S approaches to ranking evidence?

4. What is a meta-analysis? Is it considered a type of systematic review?

5. Why do most hierarchies rank systematic reviews and meta-analyses as the most ideal evidence?

6. Why does random assignment and concealment of group assignment strengthen a study?

7. How do cohort control, case control, and observational study designs compare? Provide an example of each. How do they compare in their ability to control the research conditions?

8. Go to http://www.guidelines.gov. Search the term "smoking cessation." Select two guidelines from the list and use the Compare tool. Which guideline is more transparent and rigorous? Support your answer.

9. Consider this chapter's clinical story. Do you think that it was right for Jacob to stop the procedure? How would you approach a similar situation?

References

Codgill, K. W. (2003). Information needs and information seeking in primary care: A study of nurse practitioners. *Journal of Medical Library Association, 9,* 203–215.

Coiera, Westbrook, & Rogers (2008). Clinical decision velocity is increased when meta-search filters enhance an evidence retrieval system. *Journal of American Medical Informatics Association, 15,* 638–646. doi:10.1197/jamia.M2765

DiCenso, A., Bayley, L., & Haynes, R. B. (2009). Accessing pre-appraised evidence: Fine-tuning the 5S model into a 6S model [Editorial]. *Evidence-based nursing, 12*(4), 99–101. doi:10.1136/ebn.12.4.99-b

DiCenso, A., Guyatt, G., & Ciliska, D. (2005). *Evidence-based nursing: A guide to clinical practice.* St. Louis, MO: Elsevier Mosby.

GRADE Working Group. (n.d.). Organizations that have endorsed or that are using GRADE. Retrieved from http://www.gradeworkinggroup.org/society/index.htm

Guyatt, G. H., Oxman, A. D., Vist, G. E., et al. (2008). GRADE: An emerging consensus on rating quality of evidence and strength of recommendations. *British Medical Journal, 336,* 924–926.

Hamilton, H. C., & Foxcroft, D. (2007). Central venous access sites for the prevention of venous thrombosis, stenosis and infection in patients requiring long-term intravenous therapy. *Cochrane Database of Systematic Reviews, 3.* doi:10.1002/14651858.CD004084.pub2

Institute for Healthcare Improvement. (n.d.). Central line insertion checklist. Retrieved from http://www.ihi.org/IHI/Topics/CriticalCare/IntensiveCare/Tools/CentralLineInsertionChecklist.htm

Joanna Briggs Institute. (2008). *Joanna Briggs Institute reviewer's manual 2008 edition.* Retrieved from http://www.joannabriggs.edu.au/Documents/JBIReviewManual_CiP11449.pdf

Joanna Briggs Institute. (2011a). Grades of recommendation. Retrieved from http://www.joannabriggs.edu.au/About%20Us/About%20Us/JBI%20Approach/Grades%20of%20Recommendation

Joanna Briggs Institute. (2011b). Levels of evidence. Retrieved from http://www.joannabriggs.edu.au/About%20Us/JBI%20Approach/Levels%20of%20Evidence%20%20FAME

McCaughan, D., Thompson, C., Cullum, N., et al. (2005). Nurse practitioner and practice nurses' use of research information in clinical decision making: Findings from an exploratory study. *Family Practice, 22,* 490–497. doi:10.1093/fampra/cmi042

Pearson, A., Wiechula, R., & Lockwood, C. (2005). The JBI model of evidence-based healthcare. *International Journal of Evidence Based Healthcare, 3,* 207–215.

Pravikoff, D. S., Tanner, A., & Pierce, S. T. (2005). Readiness of U.S. nurses for evidence-based practice. *American Journal of Nursing, 105*(9), 40–51.

Ramos, K., Linscheid, R., & Schafer, S. (2003). Real-time information-seeking behavior of residency physicians. *Family Medicine, 35,* 257-260.

Registered Nurses of Ontario (2005). Risk assessment & prevention of pressure ulcers. Retrieved from http://www.rnao.org/Page.asp?PageID=924&ContentID=816

Xue, Y. (2010). Evidence summary: Central venous access device (CVAD) insertion. *JBI COnNECT+.* Retrieved from http://connect.jbiconnectplus.org/ViewDocument.aspx?0=1854

CHAPTER 12

Apply and Implement I

Decision Making and Integrating Preference and Clinical Expertise

Leslie Rittenmeyer

LEARNING OBJECTIVES

- Discuss the concept of patient-preference and its relationship to evidence-based practice.

- Explain shared decision making (SDM).

- Summarize the responsibilities of the clinician in SDM.

- Discuss the role of clinical expertise in clinical decision making.

KEY TERMS

Clinical decision making
Clinical expertise
Local context

Meaning
Patient preference
Shared decision making

Clinical Story

Pat, a newly graduated nurse practitioner, is working at a clinic in a rural farming community. The people who work and live in this community are known for their independent thinking and willingness to communicate their ideas and opinions. Pat views these traits as positive, generally leading to an effective, joint decision-making process between patient and clinician, one that moves beyond the research evidence to include patient preferences, values, and clinical expertise. Pat knows this is the most desirable model for evidence-based practice clinical decision making but admits to her evidence-based practice mentor that it is difficult for her when patients express a preference that she disagrees with. Pat provides an example from her current caseload: a patient who refuses prescribed antihypertensive medication for his high blood pressure. The patient, a 55-year-old farmer who works extremely hard and is exposed to the daily stressors common to the occupation of farming, communicates that the last time he was on this type of medication, his sexual functioning was affected to the point that he prefers not to take them again. At this point in time he seems adamant about his decision. Pat wonders what should drive her next actions.

Introduction

It has often been said that knowledge is power. In nursing, knowledge is derived from many sources, such as systematic reviews, primary research, pre-appraised sources, clinical guidelines, and expert opinion. However, Pravikoff, Tanner, and Pierce (2005) surveyed 3000 nurses across the United States and found that although nurses needed information to make clinical decisions, they often relied more on peers, colleagues, and the Internet than they did on bibliographic databases, such as the Cumulative Index to Nursing and Allied Health Literature (CINAHL) and PubMed, to obtain it. The study results showed there was more of a reliance on human sources of knowledge and the study participants felt generally unprepared to do the things necessary to practice evidence-based nursing. In evidence-based practice, knowledge holds a prominent place because its purpose is to inform clinical decision making with the best available evidence. As a nurse, you need to understand how to access knowledge and use it to inform your clinical decisions.

However, this is not the complete story. In clinical decision making, the research evidence alone is not necessarily justification for action. There are other considerations such as **patient preference, clinical expertise,** and **local context.**

- Patient preference is the right of an individual to be involved in the planning of his or her own care and ultimately having the final say about which interventions he or she chooses to accept or not accept.
- Clinical expertise is the accumulated knowledge of the professional and how it influences clinical decisions.
- Local context is the circumstances particular to a situation.

All of these considerations together give you the ability to make clinical decisions more clear or, conversely, muddy them. This chapter will address the issues relevant to clinical decision making.

Evidence-Based Clinical Decision Making

Haynes, Devereaux, and Guyatt (2002) define evidence based decision making as the integration of the best available research evidence with clinical expertise and patient values. Clinical decisions are made by balancing four equally important constructs: the clinical circumstance, patient preferences, research evidence, and clinical expertise. Pearson, Wiechula, Court, et al. (2005) describes **clinical decision making** within the perspective of giving equal weight to the best available evidence, the context in which the care is given, client preference, and the professional judgment of the health-care professional. The equal weighting of these factors means that research evidence cannot eliminate the wishes of the patient or the clinical expertise of the professional. This fact dispels the belief that evidence-based practice is "cook-book" nursing, making nursing care too prescriptive and removing all creativity. This would be true if clinical decisions were based solely on the research evidence, but that is not the case in actual evidence-based practice. When the research evidence, preferences of the patient, and the clinical expertise of the professional are in agreement, and there are no contextual issues, the course of action is clear. However, the process gets murky when the research evidence points to one intervention, and the preference of the patient is in opposition. When this happens, it is often the expertise of the clinician that influences the situation.

Pat, the nurse in this chapter's clinical story, understands what should influence clinical decision making but has a hard time accepting patient preference when she feels it is counter to what is medically sound practice. The evidence and her clinical expertise are in accord, but the preference of her patient is not. She asks herself what she should do and what her responsibility is. The answers to these questions should become clear as this chapter progresses.

What Does Patient Preference Really Mean?

There are two ways in which patients and their values and preferences are considered in evidence-based practice. The first is to what extent patients are involved in shared decision making, and the second is the right of patients to choose or reject an intervention.

Shared Decision Making

Shared decision making (SDM) is a key part of evidence-based practice because it brings together clinical expertise and patient preference. In reviewing the literature, Makoul and Clayman (2006) found that there was great variation in the definitions of shared decision making. The two ideas that appeared most often in the literature were "patient preferences" and "options." Legare, Elwyn, Fishbein, et al. (2008) define SDM as decision-making process jointly shared by patients and their health-care provider, whereas Thistlethwaite, Evans, Tie, et al. (2006) describe SDM as a patient-centered consultation in which the patient and clinician discuss disease management and come to mutual decisions. In addition, Towle and Goldolphin (1999) explain that SDM is based on the best evidence of the risks and benefits of all the alternatives. This means that for any clinical decision there are alternatives; you and your patient must weigh the potential harm and potential benefit of any intervention.

Silow-Carroll, Alteras, and Stepnick (2006) state that "the U.S. health care system is experiencing a slow and subtle shift from a professionally driven approach toward one that is 'patient centered' or 'consumer centered.' This stems from a growing recognition that incorporating an individual patient's perspective and greater involvement in his/her care result in better health outcomes and satisfaction" (p. 4). Using an iterative process of reviewing the existing literature and research, the authors identified the following eight core components as a comprehensive patient-centered care approach, especially when caring for vulnerable populations:

1. Welcoming environment
2. Respect for patients' values, and expressed needs
3. Patient empowerment and activation
4. Sociocultural competence
5. Coordination and integration of care
6. Comfort and support
7. Access and navigation skills
8. Community outreach

Pat is proud of the fact that her clinic embraces the patient-centered approach to care. She and her colleagues place value on treating their patents within a holistic perspective. She feels that this approach is vital to setting the stage for SDM. Davis, Schoenbaum, and Audet (2005) refer to patient-centered primary care as a system that allows individuals access to a form of health care that works for them, and the Institute of Medicine (IOM) has identified patient-centered care as one of its six aims of quality. This statement illustrates an obvious trend away from the paternalistic view that the health care provider knows best; however, Legare et al. (2008) contend that data exist that suggests that SDM has not been broadly adopted in reality. Despite those claims, Clark, Nelson, Valero, et al. (2009) cite a large amount of existing literature that suggests SDM is at least being widely discussed in health care.

SDM is not without it controversies. Studies indicate that many patients wish to have active participation in their care (Deber, Kraetschmer, Urowitz, et al., 2007; Funk, 2004; Gilbar and Gilbar, 2009; Heesen, Segal, Kopke, et al., 2004). Conversely, some patients prefer that their health-care provider make decisions for them. Vogel, Helmes, and Hasenburg (2008), found that 40.2% of the breast cancer patients in their study preferred that their physician make decisions for them. In another study that examined decision-making preferences of 150 women with breast cancer (Beaver, Luker, Owens, et al., 1996), researchers found that 20% of the study participants wanted an active role in decision making, 28% wanted to make a joint decision, and 52% wanted their surgeon to decide for them. In a related follow-up study (Beaver, Bogg, and Luker, 1999), researchers compared the preferences of breast cancer patients (n = 150) against patients with colorectal cancer (n = 48). Results showed that 78% of the colorectal cancer patients preferred to play a passive role in decision making in contrast to 52% of the breast cancer patients.

What does this confusing and sometimes contradictory evidence mean? The answer is not easy, because you cannot assume that you and your patients have the same values. Patient values are as diverse as patients themselves. The important lesson is always to be aware of the differing preferences and values and to communicate respect for your patients. After an exhaustive search of the literature, Clark et al. (2009) conclude that preferences for SDM might be age related and possibly a generational phenomenon. The authors posit that younger patients seem to have a preference for patient–provider interaction in health care, possibly because of higher expectations for participation and communication, whereas older individuals seem to be more comfortable with leaving the health-care decisions in the hands of the provider. It is up to the clinician to explore how much or how little involvement the patient wants.

Strategies to Encourage SDM

Ford, Schofield, and Hope (2003) researched the characteristics of a successful evidence-based patient choice consultation. Interviews were done with general practitioners, hospital doctors, practice nurses, academics, and lay people. Six themes emerged from the data:

1. Research evidence/medical information
2. The doctor-patient relationship
3. Patient perspective
4. Decision-making processes
5. Time issues
6. Establishing the patient problem

Box 12■1 summarizes some of their findings into practical information. Fraenkel and McGraw (2007) also looked at the essential elements to enable participation in medical decision making. They identified five key elements. Box 12■2 summarizes these elements.

It should be clear from the research evidence that SDM does not happen spontaneously. Implementation of an SDM process is a must for patient-centered environments. There needs to be system investment and acceptance from all staff. Elwyn, Laitner, Coulter, et al. (2010) identify three major forces that must be present to make SDM part of mainstream clinical practice: (1) access to evidence-based knowledge about treatment options, (2) help in weighing the pros and cons of the various options, and (3) a culture that facilitates patient engagement.

Patient Choice

As previously discussed, patients come to the health-care setting with many different perspectives and values. As Hope (1996) observes, patients differ both in what they value and their tendency to accept risk. In this chapter's clinical story, Pat's patient

BOX 12■1   **Skills Required for Evidence-Based SDM**

- Communicating complex information using nontechnical language
- Tailoring the amount and pace of the information to the patient needs/preferences
- Drawing diagrams to aid patient comprehension
- Checking patient understanding
- Weighing medical evidence about treatment options while considering patient values
- Conveying objective, nondirective information regarding possible options
- Explaining probability of harm and risk for each option
- Using facilitative skills to encourage patient involvement
- Evaluating Internet information that patients might bring with them
- Creating an environment in which patients feel able to ask questions.
- Negotiating skills

Summarized from Ford, S., Schofield, T., & Hope, T. (2003). What are the ingredients for a successful evidence-based patient choice consultation? A qualitative study. *Social Science & Medicine, 56,* 589–602.

BOX 12■2   **Elements That Enable Patient Participation in Medical Decision Making**

- Patient knowledge: Patients being adequately informed is absolutely essential for them to participate in the decision-making process.
- Explicit encouragement of patient participation: Aside from clarifying information, clinicians should facilitate patient participation in decision making by encouraging patients to ask questions.
- Appreciation of the patient's responsibility/rights to play an active role in decision making: Patiens should feel that they have a reasonability to actively participate in decisions involving their care.
- Awareness of choice: To participate in decision making, patients must first be aware of the uncertainty in medicine. Patients should realize the importance of participation, particularly when decisions are value based.
- Time: The lack of time spent with patients has been identified as a barrier. Limited time has been seen as a barrier to becoming informed.

Summarized from Fraenkel, L., & McGraw, S. (2007). What are the essential elements to enable patient participation in medical decision-making? *Journal of General Internal Medicine, 22*(5), 614–619.

is choosing to reject the treatment recommendation. She acknowledges his right to do so but admits it upsets her that he is making that decision. In this case, the patient seems to value his sexual function more than he values treating his hypertension.

The right of a patient to choose health-care options has existed for some time. When talking and writing about patient-centered care, nurses have long recognized patient autonomy. Ford et al. (2003) describe patient choice as originating from the doctrine of informed consent. They state that in English and U.S. law, a competent individual has a legal right to refuse even lifesaving treatment. Patient choice from an evidence-based practice context goes beyond just informed consent; it actively involves the patient in the decision-making process. Knowledge is given to patients with the explicit purpose of giving them choice. This is more than respect for patient autonomy but instead full recognition of individual preferences (Hope, 1996).

In the clinical story, Pat might speculate about why her patient values his sexual function more than he values his health, but in trying to understand his decision she should consider the **meaning** both have for him. Until Pat is able to discover this information, she will probably have difficulty engaging in SDM with him. *Meaning* is the subjective interpretation an individual places on something. To glean the meaning of something, you have to attempt to understand your patient's story. Nurses should ask, "Help me understand how you came to this decision," so the patient can provide insight into his or her decision-making process. Although it is sometimes difficult, it is always better to bring a nonjudgmental attitude to the nurse-patient relationship. If you are to be given the privilege of hearing the patient's story, then the patient has to feel comfortable sharing it with you.

Another way in which you might get in touch with the meaning of particular phenomena is by searching for research evidence or synthesized evidence that will give you more information. For example, Pat decides to explore the evidence for anything that will provide her with a greater understanding of her patient's decision. Realizing that systematic reviews are a higher level of evidence, she first goes to the CINAHL and MEDLINE databases and searches for any systematic reviews (in the form of a meta-synthesis or meta-aggregation) on the meaning of "sexual dysfunction as a result of taking hypertensive medication." She does not find a systematic review but is excited to find a primary qualitative research study in which Volis, Sandelowski, Dahm, et al. (2008) explored the adherence to antihypertensive medications as a patient-driven means to preserving sexual potency. Pat first critically appraises the study and determines that it is of high quality. After reading this study, she thinks she better understands her patient's decision. Box 12■3 summarizes what Pat learned from this study that helped her to better understand the context of her patient's preferences.

After reading this meaningfulness study, Pat believes she has a better understanding of the factors that are influencing her patient's decision. Next, she needs to search for the best available evidence that will assist her in identifying alternative forms of hypertensive treatment that might target the diagnosis but not have the same side effects. Armed with some new insights and information, Pat now plans to engage her patient on the next office visit to further explore his perspective. She wishes to discuss if he has considered how this decision will affect his relationships with

BOX 12■3 **Findings on Preserving Sexual Potency While on Hypertensive Medication**

■ The male patients felt that sexual activity reduced stress caused by high blood pressure.
■ The male patients felt that sex lowers your blood pressure and the lack of it is unnatural.
■ "Sexual intercourse is part of your make-up. Part of your spiritual make-up, part of your mental make-up and you need to get some."
■ Patients felt the antihypertensive medications interfered with their desire and ability to have sexual intercourse causing them to pursue strategies to preserve sexual function
■ Some reported selecting adhering to the medication, stopping when a romantic time was planned.
■ Spouses thought the sexual dysfunction took low priority to health.

Findings summarized from Volis, C., Sandelowski, M., Dahm, P., et al. (2008). Selective adherence to antihypertensive medications as a patient-driven means to preserving sexual potency. *Patient Preference and Adherence, 2,* 201–206.

significant others and if he has shared his preference with significant others. If he is firm in his decision, then Pat wants to discuss potential risks and offer him some alternative treatment options.

Whatever the patient's final decision, Pat has researched and answered her own questions about her responsibility when a patient's preference is different from the evidence-based recommended intervention. She realizes she must (1) struggle to understand the meaning of the patient's decision; (2) search for the best available evidence of alternative treatments that will minimize the patient's perception of risk but still target the diagnosis; (3) empower the patient with the necessary knowledge to make the decision; (4) enter into a shared decision-making dialogue; and (5) ultimately accept the patient preference.

The Role of Clinical Expertise

What is the role of clinical expertise in evidence-based health care? Does clinical expertise hold more weight than other factors, such as research evidence or patient preference? As previously mentioned in this chapter, clinical expertise should be weighed equally with research evidence and patient preference. Although the research evidence is of utmost importance as a starting place, an expert clinician will address an array of other considerations like sociocultural factors, access to transportation, insurance converge, and ethical concerns before making decisions. Pat, the nurse in our clinical story, used her expertise to diagnose her patient's hypertension and suggest evidence-based treatment. When her patient declined the treatment, she then used her expertise to better understand his decision and to look for alternatives that would decrease his perception of risk.

Within the evidence-based practice movement it is expected that expert clinicians will inform their practice with the best available evidence (Boxes 12■4 and 12■5). As Haynes et al. (2002) state, "Application of current best evidence from healthcare research is now an expected adjunct to clinical acumen" (p. 36). In that context, clinical expertise is a union of knowledge of the best available evidence, competent clinical skills, and clinical experience. In an evidence-based practice setting, the clinician will use his or her clinical expertise to balance relevant research evidence, the patient's clinical state and circumstances, and the patient's preference and values before determining action. See Figure 2■1 for an illustration of how the role of clinical expertise relates to the patient's clinical state and circumstance, the patient's' preferences, and the research evidence.

■ Summary

Clinical decision making is a process that includes more than the application of the best available research evidence to a clinical situation. This alone is not sufficient to justify any action on the part of the health-care provider. Consideration of other factors such as preferences and values of patients, the context or circumstances that influence the situation, and the available resources is warranted. Patient preference is valued through shared decision-making models and respect for patients' autonomy in accepting or refusing a treatment.

BOX 12■4 Interdisciplinary Rounds

You would liked to find out how experienced clinicians implement a shared decision-making model in their evidence-based practice. You talk to some colleagues from different disciplines and organize a brown bag lunch once a month to discuss shared their perspectives on patient preference and shared decision making.

BOX 12■5 Tools for Learning and Practice

■ Read Haynes, R. B., Devereaux, P. J., and Guyatt, G. H. (2002). Clinical expertise in the era of evidence-based medicine and patient choice. *Evidence-Based Medicine, 7,* 36–38, and summarize the article's six most salient points.
■ Ask three people in your family how involved would they like to be in making clinical decisions in conjunction with their health-care practitioner.
■ Conduct an Internet search for the term "patient-centered care" and compare the characteristics with evidence-based clinical decision making.

Clinical decision making is not always an unambiguous process because patients sometimes choose not to accept a suggested treatment. It is during this time that clinicians need to explore the meaning of the patient's decision to better understand it and to search for acceptable alternatives. The expertise of the clinician is what drives this process. Combining knowledge of the best available research evidence with competent clinical skills and clinical experiences while respecting the preference and values of patients within the context or circumstance of the situation, influence the achievement of good clinical outcomes. Including patient preference and clinical expertise into the clinical decision-making process is essential for maintaining the theoretical underpinning of holistic nursing practice.

CHAPTER QUESTIONS

1. Why do you think Pat in the clinical story felt concerned about her patient's decision?

2. What steps would you take if this happened to you?

3. How much weight do you feel should be given to patient preferences?

4. What role does meaning have when considering patient preferences?

5. What are the most important elements to consider in SDM?

6. Explain the role of clinical expertise in clinical decision making.

References

Bensing, J. (2000). Bridging the gap: The separate worlds of evidence-based medicine and patient centered medicine. *Patient Education and Counseling, 39*(1), 17–25.

Beaver, K., Bogg, J., & Luker, K. A. (1999). Decision making role preferences and information needs: A comparison of colorectal and breast cancer. *Health Expectations 2,* 266–268.

Beaver, K., Luker, K. A., Owens, R. G., et al. (1996). Treatment decision making in women newly diagnosed with breast cancer. *Cancer Nursing, 19*(1), 8–19.

Clark, M., Nelson, B., Valero, M., et al. (2009). Consideration of shared decision making in nursing: A review of clinician's perceptions and interventions. *The Open Journal of Nursing, 3,* 65–75.

Davis, K., Schoenbaum, C., & Audet, A. (2005). A 2020 vision of patient-centered primary care. *Journal of Internal General Medicine, 2*(10), 953–957.

Deber, R. B., Kraetschmer, N., Urowitz, S., et al. (2007). Do people want to be Autonomous patients? Preferred roles in treatment decision making in several patient populations. *Journal of Public Participation in Health Care and Health Policy, 10*(3), 248–258.

Elyn, G., Laitner, S., Coulter, A., et al. (2010). Implementing shared decision making in the NHS. *BMJ: British Medical Association, 341,* c5146

Ford, S., Schofield, T., & Hope, T. (2003). What are the ingredients for a successful evidence-based patient choice consultation? A qualitative study. *Social Science & Medicine, 56,* 589–602.

Fraenkel, L., & McGraw, S. (2007). What are the essential elements to enable patient participation in medical decision-making? *Journal of General Internal Medicine, 22*(5), 614–619.

Funk, L. M. (2004). Who wants to be involved? Decision making preferences among residents of long-term care facilities. *Canadian Journal of Aging, 23*(1), 47–58.

Gilbar, R., and Gilbar, O. (2007). The medical decision making process and the family: The case of breast cancer patients and their husbands. *Bioethics, 23*(3), 183–192.

Haynes, R. B., Devereaux, P. J., & Guyatt, G. H. (2002). Clinical expertise in the era of evidence-based medicine and patient choice. *Evidence-Based Medicine, 7,* 36–38.

Heesen, C., Segal, J., Kopke, S., et al. (2004). Decisional roles preference, risk knowledge, and information interests in patients with multiple sclerosis. *Multiple Sclerosis, 10*(6), 643–650.

Hope, T. (1996). *Evidence based patient choice.* London: Kings Fund.

Legare, F., Elwyn, G., Fishbein, M., et al. (2008). Translating decision-making into healthcare clinical practices: Proof of concepts. *Implementation Science, 3*(2). doi:10.11866/1748-5908-3-2

Makoul, G., & Claymom, M. L. (2006). An integrative model of shared decision making in medical encounters. *Patient Education and Counseling, 60*(3), 301–312.

Pearson, A., Wiechula, R., Court, A., et al. (2005). The JBI model of evidence-based healthcare. *Inernational Journal of Evidence-Based Healthcare, 3,* 207–215.

Pravikoff, D. S., Tanner, A. B., & Pierce, S. T. (2005). Readiness of U.S. nurses for evidence-based practice. *American Journal of Nursing, 105,* 40–45.

Silow-Carrol, S., Alteras, T., & Stepnick, L. (2006). *Patient-centered care for underserved populations: Definition and best practices.* Washington, DC: Economic and Social Research Institute.

Thistlewaite, J., Evans, R., Tie, R., et al. (2006). Shared decision making and decision aids—a literature review. *Australian Family Physician, 35*(7), 537–540

Towle, A., & Goldolphin, W. (1999). Framework for teaching and learning informed shared decision making. *British Medical Journal, 319,* 766–771.

Vogel, B., Helms, A. W., & Hasenburg, A. (2008). Information and decision making: Patients needs and experiences in the course of breast cancer treatment. *Patient Education and Counseling, 71*(1), 79–85.

Volis, C., Sandelowski, M., Dahm, P., et al. (2008). Selective adherence to antihypertensive medications as a patient-driven means to preserving sexual potency. *Patient Preference and Adherence, 2,* 201–206.

CHAPTER 13

Apply and Implement II
Individual Nurse Implementation

Lisa Hopp

LEARNING OBJECTIVES

- Given a clinical scenario, identify the problem that is amenable to using evidence to inform an individual nurse's decision to intervene.

- Discuss common barriers and nurses' characteristics that relate to their use of research.

- Explore the concept of knowledge translation and how it relates to using evidence in nursing practice.

- Considering common barriers and facilitators for using evidence in individual nurse's daily practice, develop a plan to overcome these barriers.

- List evidence-based strategies related to improving how nurses implement evidence.

KEY WORDS

Academic detailing
Audit and feedback
Conceptual research utilization
Context
Implementation science
Instrumental research utilization

Knowledge translation (KT)
Opinion leaders
Patient-mediated strategies
Persuasive research utilization
Reminders

Clinical Story

The first sign of trouble in Ms. B's breathing is the telltale wheeze that Rory could hear without a stethoscope. When she sees Ms. B. in the emergency department's (ED) triage area at 3 a.m., Rory knows that she needs to move the patient to the back for treatment immediately. Ms. B. is 20 years old and her family physician diagnosed her asthma just a few days prior to her visit to the ED. When she arrives, Ms. B. has a difficult time speaking because of her shortness of breath. Her respiratory rate is 22 breaths per minute. She is sitting upright and working hard to breath. Rory listens to her chest and hears distant breath sounds and expiratory wheezes. The ED physician immediately orders a nebulizer treatment with a fast-acting bronchodilator. Within about 15 minutes of the treatment, Ms. B. begins to feel better; her respiratory rate decreases and she can talk more easily. She tells Rory she has been taking inhaled medicines since her physician prescribed them but she wasn't sure if she was using the inhaler correctly. She says she recognized her symptoms but then began to panic as her wheezing and chest tightness seemed to worsen. She tells Rory she just didn't know what to do.

In her years as a nurse, Rory has seen many patients in the ED who cannot recognize and care for their early asthma symptoms. She knows that a patient needs to use the right technique for the inhaled medications to reach the bronchioles. She also knows that if patients wait until they have audible wheezing and chest tightness, they may have waited too long for the rescue inhaler to work. Rory wants to use the best evidence to teach her young patient how to control her asthma as much as possible to avoid future hospital visits and the fear associated with severe shortness of breath. Ms. B. will be discharged from the ED in about an hour, so Rory needs to find the best evidence and tools for teaching quickly.

To start her search, Rory thinks about the issues facing Ms. B. that she can feasibly address, and she prioritizes these issues. Rory is highly motivated to find the right answers to help Ms. B. because she has seen patients newly diagnosed with asthma return to the emergency room in distress many times. Even though she has only a short amount of time to work with patients once their attack is controlled, she knows can make an impact when they have recovered from the severe symptoms but can to focus on some "just-in-time" teaching. To help Ms. B. and future patients, Rory wants to provide the best resources and information that she can. ∎

Introduction

Clinical reasoning and decision making are at the center of nursing care. Individual nurses decide how and when to assess patients; they identify problems and make diagnoses; they select, implement, and evaluate their interventions. At each step, they need to use information to make the best decisions. The evidence-based practice movement calls for this information to be based on the best available evidence from research. In the last chapter, you learned that evidence is rarely the only factor to consider. Patient preferences, clinician expertise, and available resources also play roles in the decision-making process. In addition to using evidence to inform their decisions, nurses do not make decisions in a vacuum. They are part of the clinician–patient/family relationship and members of a patient care unit, a multidisciplinary team, a health-care organization, and a public health context. In this chapter, you will learn how to use evidence in your everyday decision making as an individual practitioner. Although you make autonomous decisions for which you are accountable, you make these decisions in the midst of many influences in your practice setting (Box 13■1).

Nurses and Research Utilization

Research utilization is one aspect of the evidence-based practice process. Nurse researchers have studied how nurses use research for several decades, yet a research-practice gap remains. Uptake of research is not fast or consistent enough, so patients do not consistently benefit from the investment in research and may even be harmed because of slow uptake (Squires, Estabrooks, Gustavsson, et al., 2011). A number of researchers have studied how nurses perceive how they use research. Squires, Hutchinson, Bostrom, et al. (2011) conducted a systematic review to identify and analyze how nurses use evidence in their practice. They searched the international literature, including English and Scandinavian languages. They retrieved 133 articles from an initial list of 12,418 titles, with the most recent titles published in March 2008. After using standard tools to appraise all of the articles

---

BOX 13■1 **Significance of Individual Implementation of Evidence in Nursing Practice**

- When nurses do not use the evidence from research and other sources, uptake is slow and patient outcomes may be affected.
- Research use may take the form of influencing others, changing thinking or actual practices.
- The characteristics of the evidence, setting, and nurse affect how individual nurses use evidence.
- Clinical context including organizational culture, leadership, and evaluation practices can positively and negatively affect how bedside nurses use evidence.
- Individual characteristics that are more likely associated with research utilization are holding an advanced practice degree, being in a leadership roles, practicing in a specialty area (e.g., critical care, diabetes care), and being satisfied in the job.

they retrieved, they ultimately included 55 studies of varying research designs. They found researchers used several different tools to measure nurses' research use, and they summarized the level of research use with a simple "low to high" research use scale. The studies represented nurses from North America (71%), Europe (22%), Asia (5%), and Oceania (2%). The trend showed more studies were conducted after 1995 and nurses reported increasingly higher levels of research use since 1995. Overall, nurses classified their research use in the moderate-high level (the second highest level) (Squires, Hutchison, et al., 2011). The authors of this systematic review are cautious about the validity of the research and recommended further research to measure research use more directly.

The manner in which nurses use research is important and varies depending on the person, the evidence, and the situation. Some researchers differentiate instrumental, conceptual, and persuasive ways of using research. In **instrumental research utilization,** you apply the research in some concrete way. For example, if a systematic review indicates a pressure-reducing bed surface is best for preventing pressure ulcers in at-risk adults and this causes nurses to change from a standard mattress to a specialized bed surface for certain patient, then they would be using research in an instrumental manner. In **conceptual research utilization,** you think differently after understanding research but do not change your behavior. Consider the following example. Nurses read about pregnant women's experience of being confined to bed because of the threat of premature labor, and they consider this research the next time they work with a pregnant woman who has been put on bedrest. However, they ultimately do not use the evidence to make a decision about counseling the patient on her activity. In **persuasive research utilization,** you use research to influence the others. For example, nurses might use evidence related to the effectiveness of bed rest in premature labor to persuade midwives when they make recommendations (Squires, Hutchinson, et al., 2011).

The evidence-based practice movement has changed the way nurses think about using research. Now, they focus on finding the best available evidence instead of just any piece of research. The goal is to use evidence in concrete, instrumental ways to improve patient outcomes. Moreover, the definition of evidence-based practice includes clinical expertise and patient preferences in the decision-making process.

Barriers to Evidence Utilization

Moving evidence into practice is the responsibility of both individual nurses and the organizational context in which they work. This means you, as an individual nurse, are accountable for using the best available evidence. However, you work within an organization, whether it is an acute care hospital, a community health agency, a long-term care setting, or some other type of health-care facility. Organizations, their leaders, and systems of care greatly affect how individual nurses use evidence; they share the responsibility for providing nursing care based on the best available evidence. Any individual nurse will find it difficult to use evidence if elements of the organization pose too many barriers. Similarly, organizations can create a positive context, making it easier for individual nurses to act and advance evidence uptake (Estabrooks, Scott, Squires, et al., 2008; McCormack, Kitson, Harvey, et al., 2002).

A great deal of literature exists related to barriers to evidence implementation. You need to be aware of these barriers so that you are able to anticipate common challenges you may face and to understand the complex process of moving evidence into practice. Barriers tend to cluster around the following themes: the nature of the evidence (e.g., amount, novelty, presentation of evidence, quality, accessibility), the setting (e.g., time, resources, support, leadership), or characteristics of the individual nurse (e.g., knowledge, time, attitude) (Kajermo, Bostrom, Thompson, et al., 2010; Kent, Hutchinson, and Fineout-Overholt, 2009).

In the next chapter, you will learn more about these barriers and how important the organizational culture and systems are to the success of evidence implementation. This chapter explores what individual nurse characteristics are most important to successful implementation of evidence.

Individual Nurse Characteristics That Pose Barriers to or Aid Evidence Implementation

In a systematic review of barriers related to nurse characteristics, Kajermo et al. (2010) found the top three hurdles to using research in practice were (1) nurses being unaware of research, (2) nurses not feeling capable of evaluating the quality of research, and (3) nurses being isolated from knowledgeable colleagues with whom they could discuss research. Closely related to these nurse characteristics were barriers related to organizational setting: insufficient time on the job to implement new ideas, insufficient time to read research, lack of authority for patient care procedures, unsupportive staff, and uncooperative physicians.

Pravikoff, Tanner, and Pierce (2005) surveyed a broad spectrum of practicing nurses in the United States. They found the most frequent individual barriers to using research in practice were the following: lack of value for research in practice, lack of skills for using or accessing electronic information and databases, and difficulty understanding research. These individual attributes can change if nurses are willing to learn the information management skills, are open to using evidence, and are willing to learn more about judging the quality of evidence. Appraisal checklists that are brief and include hints about what to look for in the research are very helpful to help the novice as well as the experienced appraiser (see Chapter 10). Nurses can build confidence in their appraisal skills by joining a journal club on their unit. In addition, clinical and academic educators can provide opportunities for nurses to acquire the appropriate skills and knowledge.

Researchers have studied what conditions aid or slow the use of evidence in nursing practice. In a recent systematic review, Squires, Estabrooks et al. (2011) found the following individual nurse characteristics were more commonly associated with the use of research-based evidence:

- Having a positive attitude toward research
- Being engaged in research activities
- Having a greater tendency to seek information

- Holding a graduate degree
- Having certain professional characteristics.

According to the review, nurses were more likely to use evidence if they held advanced practice degrees or leadership roles, practiced in a specialty area (e.g., critical care or diabetes care), or were satisfied in their jobs. Years of experience did not relate to evidence use (Squires, Estabrooks, et al., 2011). This evidence reinforces the need to remain curious, inquisitive, and interested in continuously searching for evidence that helps you provide the right intervention to the right patients in the right way at the right time.

Knowledge Translation—Part of the Implementation Puzzle

Although individual nurses are responsible and accountable for using the best available evidence to make clinical decisions, you still need to learn how to accomplish that goal. The next phase in the evidence-based practice movement begins with investigators focusing on how best to translate knowledge from research and other sources into everyday practice. Some refer to this process as **knowledge translation (KT).** Many countries, including Canada, the United States, the United Kingdom, and Australia, have developed programs to enhance the uptake of evidence. For example, the Canadian Institutes of Health Research has committed resources and devotes a branch of the institutes to knowledge translation. It defines KT as "a dynamic and iterative process that includes synthesis, dissemination, exchange and ethically sound application of knowledge to improve the health of Canadians, provide more effective health services and products and strengthen the health care system" (Canadian Institutes of Health Research, 2010, Knowledge Translation—Definition, para. 1). This means that moving knowledge from research to practice does not happen in a linear fashion via a lone practitioner, and it is not context free. The implementation process requires the knowledge creators and the users to interact, reflect, revise, and reflect again on practice changes within their own environments. The tools and mechanisms of KT involve synthesizing multiple sources of knowledge (i.e., more than one study as well as other sources of knowledge such as local data, patient experiences, and clinician expertise) and novel, innovative ways of getting the information to the knowledge users (clinicians and patients).

Exchange is another important characteristic of effective KT. This step may be as simple as engaging patients and their families in the discussion and shared decision-making process about their care. It can be as complex as national and international networks of patients, researchers, and clinicians working together for evidence-based solutions.

You can become a part of future KT efforts by volunteering to take part in research or evidence-implementation projects. Some KT models indicate that you could be involved from the very inception of the research project by helping researchers identify important questions to your nursing practice and the health needs of your patients. If you become a part of the research process itself, you can help ensure the relevance of the findings and use the evidence in your practice to contribute to the advancement of the profession.

Context of Care

Although this chapter focuses on what the individual nurse can do to implement evidence in practice, it is important to recognize that this always occurs within a context which influences how and if change can happen. Context is a very broad concept with many definitions. For individual nurses making evidence-based decisions, the most relevant definition comes from Promoting Action on Research Implementation in Health Services (PARIHS), which defines **context** as "the environment or setting in which the proposed change is to be implemented" (Kitson, Harvey, and McCormack, 1998). According to PARIHS, context includes the subelements of organizational culture (e.g., values, beliefs, regard for individuals, how learning happens, teamwork), leadership (style, structures, roles, methods of teaching), and evaluation (feedback mechanisms, sources and methods of measurement) (McCormack et al., 2002). Other evidence-based practice models (see Chapter 5) also take context into consideration in some manner. However, although there is broad recognition that context and organizational cultures affect the implementation of evidence, a systematic review of strategies for change in organizational culture indicates evidence is lacking about how to effectively change cultures (Parmelli, Flodgren, Beyer, et al., 2011).

Kent and McCormack (2010) note that the emphasis on quality, safety, and effectiveness in health care has caused organizational cultures to shift away from paternalistic, provider-centered care toward more patient-centered care. To work in this culture, practitioners need to change how they approach care, and nurses need to be reflective, critical thinking, "knowledge-based doers" (p. 11).

In this chapter's clinical story, Rory is always pressed for time in the busy emergency department. Despite the rapidly changing conditions of the environment, she is open to using evidence to make a difference in the many patients she sees with acute exacerbations of asthma, but she must be able to trust the information she uses to advise her patients. She needs the skills to find the information quickly, to judge the quality of the information rapidly, and to use the tools to intervene within a short window of opportunity with her patient. Rory values the evidence from research and she has good searching skills so she can quickly find evidence from the databases immediately available on the computers in the patient-care bays and at the nurses' station. She must also understand she has the authority to make these decisions about using evidence in patient care; her manager and the organizational leaders not only support her but expect that she will use the evidence in collaboration with her patient.

Not all nurses in the United States and in other countries experience these ideal conditions. In this chapter's clinical story, Rory has an inquisitive mind, knowledge, and resources, which lead to her use of evidence. She did not have to overcome barriers such as no access to electronic databases, lack of skill or confidence to search and evaluate the evidence, or inadequate autonomy to pursue the issue. If she had to face these barriers, she may have discharged the patient without an evidence-based solution to address the patient's need to understand and manage her asthma symptoms.

From Question to Evidence

In previous chapters, you studied how to ask, acquire, and appraise the evidence to decide how to apply the evidence in a particular context while also considering the patient's values and preferences. Just as Rory did when she first assessed Ms. B, you can form a mental checklist to help you quickly move from messy, poorly structured problems to focused questions that will lead to the right evidence. For example, ask: What is at the center of the patient's condition that you can change? What are the nursing interventions that relate to the patient problem? If you keep the focus on the patient's needs, you will stay centered on the higher priority questions.

In the clinical story, Rory identifies that the patient needs to understand how to self-manage her asthma. This problem could generate many questions such as: What is the effectiveness of asthma self-care action plans (intervention) versus brief oral instruction (comparison) on frequency of asthma exacerbations (outcome) in newly diagnosed adult asthma patients (population)? Rory is time pressured and needs to find a brief summary of the evidence to help her counsel the patient. She searches "asthma self-care" in the Joanna Briggs Institute's evidence database, which is available in the emergency room. She immediately finds two evidence summaries that fit the patient's problem—one on self-management and another on effective inhaler techniques. This type of evidence is ideal for point-of-care use. The summaries are short yet transparent, meaning Rory can immediately determine the level of evidence supporting each recommendation. In fact, she can see the original sources cited along with a summary of the type of evidence underpinning the recommendations (Schultz, 2010).

If Rory did not have access to this type of evidence source, she could have generated several questions (see Chapter 8 for more information on questioning) from her mental checklist such as the following:

- What is the effect of a written self-management action plan that includes self-adjusting medications versus regular visits with a primary care provider on the number of return emergency room visits for acute exacerbations in patients with new diagnosis of asthma?
- What is the effect of regularly using a peak-flow meter (a handheld device that measures airflow) versus no self-monitoring to identify worsening symptoms in patients with asthma?
- What is the effect of time of day on the occurrence of wheezing, chest tightness, and cough in patients with asthma?
- What are effective ways to manage allergy-related triggers of bronchospasm and an asthma attack?

The experience of an acute exacerbation merits exploration as well. Rory could ask the following meaningfulness questions:

- What is the experience of dyspnea (shortness of breath) in patients in the midst of an acute exacerbation?
- What is the meaning of receiving a diagnosis of asthma?
- What is the meaning of avoiding allergic triggers and its impact on quality of life of people with asthma?

Implementing the Evidence

You have read about several conceptual frameworks and models to guide the evidence-based practice process. Once you have worked through the question, evidence search, and appraisal process, the next step is to apply the evidence. The model or framework that you choose will influence how you apply the evidence. In addition to theory, there is a growing body of research that supports how to improve the uptake or application of evidence. This evidence comes from KT and implementation science work. **Implementation science** means the "scientific study of methods to promote the systematic uptake of clinical research findings and other evidence-based practices into routine practice, and hence to improve the quality and effectiveness of health care. It includes the study of influences on healthcare professional and organizational behavior" (Eccles and Mittman, 2006, para. 2). Just as you use the evidence to determine the right intervention, you need to consider what works to apply evidence.

Several systematic reviews have already been conducted of implementation methods but they reveal this is an emerging science and much remains to be learned. In addition, most of the completed studies relate to physician uptake of evidence-based guidelines (Table 13■1). Thompson, Estabrooks, Scott-Findley, et al. (2007) reviewed the evidence related to enhancing research use in nursing practice. Despite screening over 8000 titles in their initial search of multiple databases, only 4 studies met their quality criteria. The most frequent intervention to enhance research uptake was an educational meeting of some sort, but no study showed an increase in evidence uptake. Educational meetings with a local opinion leaders and multidisciplinary committees

Table 13■1   **Strategies and Examples That May Promote Evidence Uptake**

Strategy	Potential Application
[1]Audit and feedback	Observations and chart review to monitor adherence to evidence-based interventions for central-line infections with monthly feedback to the nursing care unit
[2]Reminders	Colored patient wrist bands indicating allergies, risks for falls or pressure ulcers
[3]Opinion leaders	Well-respected staff nurses give a demonstration of an evidence-based procedure and work one-on-one with other nurses to coach them through the procedure
[4]Patient-mediated interventions	When orienting patients and families to the hospital, inform them that everyone who enters the room should wash their hands or use the alcohol scrub before working with the patient
[5]Academic detailing	A nursing instructor from the local university works with the nursing staff to develop evidence-based interventions

[1]Jamtvedt, Young, Kristoffersen, et al., 2006; [2]Shojania, Jennings, Mayhew, et al., 2009; [3]Flodgren, Parmelli, Doumit, et al., 2007; [4]Fraenkel & McGraw, 2007; [5]O'Brien, rogers, Jamtvedt et al., 2007.

showed more promise, but the authors concluded that current evidence has not produced much guidance on effective strategies (Box 13■2). This somewhat dismal picture reflects that practitioners are just beginning to uptake evidence. This is a complex problem, and new ways are needed to intervene and study the effectiveness of these efforts.

In the clinical story, Rory is ready to use the evidence in the short time she has to work with the Ms. B. Although she recognizes that asthma self-management can be complicated for patients, she has just a brief opportunity to intervene and that shapes how she uses the evidence. After reading the one-page summary on asthma self-care, she focuses on three key goals for her intervention:

1. The patient will be able to demonstrate how to use a peak expiratory flow meter and record her measurement in a diary.
2. The patient will be able to demonstrate how to use a rescue inhaler.
3. The patient will be able to state what to ask her primary care provider to help her manage her asthma.

The evidence related to strategies to achieve these outcomes is ranked level I, the most trustworthy type, which is based on systematic reviews of randomized controlled trials, with grade A recommendations (strong support for application) (Schultz, 2010). Rory gathers the equipment she needs (a peak expiratory flow meter and diary to record the reading, date, and time that accompanies the meter), a metered-dose inhaler with the appropriate medication (a handheld "puffer" device

---

BOX 13■2 **Interdisciplinary Rounds**

- Consider evidence from multiple disciplines when searching for the best evidence to make well-informed decisions.
- Join an interdisciplinary journal club to review research related to a topic of common interest.
- More systematic reviews of research exist related to strategies to promote individual physician adoption of evidence-based decisions. Brainstorm with other nurses how this research does or does not translate to nurse behaviors.
- Collaborate with other disciplines to build consensus around evidence-based patient care to increase the chance that practitioners use evidence.
- With physicians, physiotherapists, occupational therapists, and other professionals, discuss the use of patient-mediated interventions that result in empowering patients to urge their health-care providers to use evidence. What are their concerns and ideas about this strategy?
- Become a part of an interdisciplinary team to improve a patient outcome through the implementation of an evidence-based practice. How might you use audit and feedback, reminders, and prompts? For each discipline involved in the project, consider who would be the most effect opinion leader. Would an outside expert influence the adoption of the evidence?

and short-acting bronchodilator to relax the airways), and a simple patient instruction pamphlet with brief instructions about using the meter and inhaler as well as a reminder to schedule a visit with her primary care provider and a prompt for questions to ask her provider.

Engaging Patients in the Evidence That Affects Their Care

Nurses have long valued the idea that patients should be partners in their care. Recall that the definition of evidence-based practice includes patient preferences and values. But evidence related to the role of patients in shared evidence-based decision making is still emerging. In the previous chapter, you learned about the evidence that currently exists. Some of the key recommendations from this work (Buzza, Williams, Vander Weg, et al., 2010; Ford, Schofied, and Hope, 2002; Fraenkel and McGraw, 2007) include the following:

- Use plain language for explanations to ensure that patients understand their options.
- Explicitly encourage their participation.
- Provide an unhurried atmosphere of listening.
- Encourage patients to ask about the evidence-based approaches to care (activating the patient to encourage their providers to use evidence-based strategies).
- Use decision aids to help patients understand their alternatives.

In the clinical story, Rory closes the drapes so she can remain focused on what the patient says. Rory then sits down so she can maintain level eye contact, and she listens to her patient's main concerns about being able to manage her asthma. Ms. B. says she was very frightened by her attack, and she worries that it will happen again. She states she wants to take care of herself. Rory focuses her interventions on these issues. Rory tells Ms B. there is good evidence that patients can manage their asthma with the help of a written action plan (Schultz, 2010) and by working with their primary care provider. In addition, by using a peak flow meter, patients can better detect when their asthma is flaring so they can give themselves the right medicine to prevent worsening symptoms. Ms. B. is relieved and asks for more information. Rory teaches her how to perform a good measurement with the peak expiratory flow meter by blowing out as hard and fast as she can through the mouthpiece. In just a few tries, Ms. B. is able to reproduce her best measurement. Because her medicine has not completely opened her airway yet, the meter registers a decreased measurement. Rory discusses the result with Ms. B. and asks her to record the measurement, her current shortness of breath, and the time of day in the diary (4 a.m.). Rory emphasizes that patients often experience more bronchospasm and coughing during the nighttime than during the daytime. Next, Rory shows Ms. B. how to use the inhaler, emphasizing the need to coordinate activation of the inhaler by taking a deep breath in and then holding it as long as she can. Ms. B. practices first without activating the medicine and then demonstrates the technique with the medication as she still has some airflow limitation (the key breathing problem in asthma). Rory congratulates her on her good technique and again encourages her to record taking the medication in the diary.

After about 15 minutes, Rory returns to Ms. B. and asks her to repeat her peak flow measurement and to write it down. They are both happy to see that the measurement has improved. Rory assesses Ms. B.'s chest sounds one last time and is pleased to hear very few wheezes. Finally, Rory provides Ms. B. with the written pamphlet of the techniques they discussed and asks Ms. B. to make sure she contacts her primary care provider the next day to schedule a return visit. Rory sits with her for 5 more minutes to generate the following questions that Ms. B writes down to ask her primary provider:

1. How often and when shall I measure my expiratory peak flow?
2. What medicine should I use and in what sequence should I use them when my expiratory flow decreases?
3. What is the written plan that I will use to take care of my asthma?
4. When should I call my primary care physician?
5. Under what circumstances should I go to the emergency room?

These are the top five questions based on Rory and Ms. B.'s shared concerns about Ms. B.'s condition and ability to manage her asthma. Ms. B. leaves the ED breathing better and armed with the information that Rory is confident reflects the best available evidence, represents the desires and preferences of the patient, and will help Ms. B. manage her asthma.

■ Summary

Bedside clinicians rarely make decisions in isolation or out of context. Rather, they are part of a larger system and environment that influence how they use evidence and make decisions. Barriers and facilitators of knowledge translation can arise from the individual practitioner, the evidence itself, or the context of the evidence implementation. Strategies to help individuals translate knowledge into practice include **audit and feedback, reminders, opinion leaders, patient-mediated interventions, academic detailing** and combinations of these strategies (Box 13■1). When nurses engage patients in the process of knowledge translation, the patient preferences are honored, and the gap between research and practice narrows.

BOX 13■3 Tools for Learning and Practice

- Use brief, trustworthy pre-appraised evidence summaries when making individual decisions on the fly.
- Checklists, prompts, and reminders can be good memory aids and help all bedside practitioners use evidence in their everyday practice.

(continues on page 180)

BOX 13■3   **Tools for Learning and Practice** (continued)

■ Seek feedback from clinical audits to check your own adherence to evidence-based practices.
■ Work with advanced practice nurses to uncover the best available evidence to create pre-appraised evidence sources about the high-frequency, high-impact nursing care interventions if no existing summaries are available.
■ Provide patients and their families with information and resources that help them ask the right questions and engage in shared decision making, including the following:
  ■ Joint Commission Speak Up Program: http://www.jointcommission.org/speakup.aspx
  ■ Agency for Healthcare Quality and Research consumer and patient information: http://www.ahrq.gov/consumer/
  ■ Agency for Healthcare Quality and Research Health Tips: http://healthcare411.ahrq.gov/
  ■ United Kingdom National Health Services Choices for consumers: http://www.nhs.uk/Pages/HomePage.aspx
  ■ Explore Canadian Institutes of Health Research's Café Scientifique idea for developing a local consumer discussion or to take part in an online discussion: http://www.cihr-irsc.gc.ca/e/34951.html

CHAPTER QUESTIONS

1. Think about a time when you were unsure about what to do in a certain clinical situation. What could be on your mental checklist to help you formulate a question that enables to you isolate the main questions and locate evidence?

2. Consider this scenario: You are searching for new employment as a bedside nurse. You are passionate about using evidence in your nursing practice. You want to determine if the organization is an environment that would enable you to use evidence in your everyday practice. What are some questions that you would ask during your interview with the human resources representative, the nursing leader of the unit you are considering, and a staff nurse who currently works on the unit?

3. What are common individual barriers to using evidence that nurses commonly identify? How might you overcome those barriers to enhance how you and your colleagues use evidence?

4. Using a common search engine such as Google, search the term "knowledge translation." How are different organizations and national groups defining "knowledge translation" and supporting knowledge translation efforts? Do you think that knowledge translation is important to everyday nursing practice?

5. Think about a routine nursing practice. How do you know that the practice is right? Have you questioned a nursing procedure or intervention in the past? Have you noticed any clinical reminders, prompts, or cues in your practice setting? How well have they worked? Did they represent an evidence-based practice? Does the effect of these strategies change over time?

6. Consider this situation: You are a staff nurse caring for a patient in a critical care unit. The unit policy limits visitors to 10 minutes on the even hours. You find yourself needing to frequently bend the rules because some families and their critically ill loved ones want to spend more time together and they want more flexibility to visit. How might you investigate whether this practice reflects the best available evidence? How might patients' and families' wishes be better incorporated to change the practice?

References

Buzza, C. D., Williams, M. B., Vander Weg, M. W., et al. (2010). Part II, provider perspectives: Should patients be activated to request evidence-based medicine? A qualitative study of the VA project to implement diuretics (VAPID). *Implementation Science, 5*(24). doi:10.1186/1748-5908-5-24

Canadian Institutes of Health Research. (2010). More about knowledge translation at CIHR. Retrieved from http://www.cihr-irsc.gc.ca/e/29418.html

Eccles, M. P., & Mittman, B. S. (2006). Welcome to *Implementation Science*. *Implementation Science, 1*(1). doi:10.1186/1748-5908-1-1

Estabrooks, C. A., Scott, S., Squires, J. E., et al. (2008). Patterns of research utilization on patient care units. *Implementation Science, 3*(31). doi:10.1186/1748-5908-3-31

Flodgren, G., Parmelli, E., Doumit, G., et al, M. P. (2007). Local opinion leaders: Effects on professional practice and health care outcomes. *Cochrane Database of Systematic Reviews, 1.* Art. No.: CD000125. doi:10.1002/14651858.CD000125.pub3

Ford, S., Schofield, T., & Hope, T. (2002). Barriers to the evidence-based patient choice (EBPC) consultation. *Patient Education and Counseling, 47,* 179–185.

Fraenkel, L., & McGraw, S. (2007). What are the essential elements to enable patient participation in medical decision making? *Journal of Internal Medicine, 22,* 6114–6119.

Jamtvedt, G., Young, J. M., Kristoffersen, D. T., et al. (2006). Audit and feedback: Effects on professional practice and health care outcomes. *Cochrane Database of Systematic Reviews, 2.* Art. No.: CD000259. doi:10.1002/14651858.CD000259.pub2

Kajermo, K. N., Bostrom, A. M., Thompson, D. S., et al. (2010). The BARRIERS scale—the barriers to research utilization scale: A systematic review. *Implementation Science, 5*(32). doi:10.1186/1748-5908-5-32

Kent, B., Hutchinson, A. M., & Fineout-Overholt, E. (2009). Getting evidence into practice—understanding knowledge translation to achieve practice change. *Worldviews on Evidence-Based Nursing, 6,* 183–185. doi:10.1111/j.1741-6787.2009.00165.x

Kent, B., & McCormack, B. (2010). Context: Overview and application. In B. Kent & B. McCormack (eds.)., *Clinical context for evidence-based nursing practice.* West Sussex, UK: Wiley-Blackwell.

Kitson, A., Harvey, G., & McCormack, B. (1998). Enabling the implementation of evidence-based practice: A conceptual framework. *Quality and Safety in Health Care, 7,* 149–158.

McCormack, B., Kitson, A., Harvey, G., et al. (2002). Getting evidence into practice: The meaning of "context." *Journal of Advanced Nursing, 38*(1), 94–104.

O'Brien, M. A., Rogers, S., Jamtvedt, G., et al. (2007). Educational outreach visits: Effects on professional practice and health care outcomes. *Cochrane Database of Systematic Reviews, 4.* Art. No.: CD000409. doi:10.1002/14651858.CD000409.pub2

Parmelli, E., Flodgren, G., Beyer, F., et al. (2011). The effectiveness of strategies to change organisational culture to improve healthcare performance: A systematic review. *Implementation Science, 6*(33). doi:10.1186/1748-5908-6-33

Pravikoff, D. S., Tanner, A. B., & Pierce, S. T. (2005). Readiness of U.S. nurses for evidence-based practice. *The American Journal of Nursing, 105*(9), 40–51.

Schultz, T. (2010). Evidence summary: Asthma self-management education. *JBI Connect+.* Retrieved from http://connect.jbiconnectplus.org/ViewPdf.aspx?0=4120&1=2)

Shojania, K. G., Jennings, A., Mayhew, A., et al. (2009). The effects of on-screen, point of care computer reminders on processes and outcomes of care. *Cochrane Database of Systematic Reviews, 3.* Art. No.: CD001096. doi: 10.1002/14651858.CD001096.pub2.

Squires, J. E., Estabrooks, C. A., Gustavsson, P., et al. (2011). Individual determinants of research utilization by nurses: A systematic review update. *Implementation Science, 6*(1). doi:10.1186/1748-5908-6-1

Squires, J. E., Hutchinson, A. M., Bostrom, A-M, et al. (2011). To what extent do nurses use research in clinical practice? A systematic review. *Implementation Science, 6*(21). doi:10.1186/1748-5908-6-21

Thompson, D. S., Estabrooks, C. A., Scott-Findlay, S., et al. (2007). Interventions aimed at increasing research use in nursing: A systematic review. *Implementation Science, 2*(15). doi:10.1186/1748-5908-2-15

CHAPTER 14

Apply and Implement III
Nursing Systems of Evidence Implementation

Beth Vottero

LEARNING OBJECTIVES

- Distinguish among organizational, setting, and individual barriers to evidence implementation.

- Describe how the organizational culture affects evidence implementation.

- Explain how knowledge of system barriers can facilitate evidence implementation.

- Develop a planning process to minimize system barriers while maximizing system facilitators.

- Examine your own individual barriers and facilitators for evidence implementation.

KEY TERMS

Accountability
Ad hoc committees
ANCC Magnet Recognition
    Program®
Authority to change practice
Barriers
Chief nursing officer/chief
    nursing executive
Embedded evidence
Empirical quality outcome

Enculturation
Facilitators
Forces of magnetism
Journal clubs
Levels of administration
Magnet model
Organizational culture
Shared governance
Structural supports
Unit practice councilst

Clinical Story

Ann is the quality representative on a critical care unit. As part of her responsibilities, she monitors data from catheter-associated urinary tract infections (CAUTI). Over the past two quarters she notices an increase in the number of CAUTIs on her unit. As a nurse-sensitive indicator, CAUTIs reflect the quality of care provided for catheterized patients. Ann is determined to make a change. As a start, she reviews the current policies and protocols on the care of patients with an indwelling catheter to see if she can find discrepancies between care provided and current protocols. Ann believes that she could make a change but is unsure about how to go about it.

Introduction

The success of any evidence implementation project is directly associated with **organizational culture.** The culture of an organization is the bedrock for germinating new ideas and innovations. Why is organizational culture important? Similar to creating a garden, where starting with the right soil mix and fertilizer ensures healthier plants, organizational culture can foster opportunities and sustain integration of evidence implementation. The culture reflects the values of the organization, from the bedside nurse to the highest levels of administration.

You may have noticed that different organizations have different cultures, manifested in part through nurse-sensitive outcomes and nurse satisfaction, autonomy, and accountability over nursing practice as well as patient outcomes. Health-care organizations that nurture a culture of evidence demonstrate higher nursing satisfaction and lower turnover rates while maintaining positive patient outcomes (Kramer, Schmalenberg, and Maguire, 2010). However, the creation of such a culture is a multifaceted and complex endeavor, requiring the inclusion of nurses from the bedside to the boardroom. This leads us to the question: what are the **barriers** and **facilitators** to creating an effective culture for evidence implementation?

To understand barriers and facilitators, it helps to organize them in terms of organizational, setting, and individual. Organizational barriers consist of management/administration priorities involve evidence-based practice processes, communication channels, organizational culture, and resources for skill development. Examples of setting barriers include policies and procedures, design and type of unit, and the workload constraints that affect implementation of evidence-based practice. Finally, individual barriers consist of nurse competence in evidence-based practice procedures, presence or lack of skills, and ability to apply research to practice.

Organizational Barriers and Facilitators

In the clinical story, Ann is positioned to affect a change in practice. As a first step, Ann approaches her director about her analysis of the data and redesigning care related to indwelling catheters. She believes that the current protocols should be reviewed against the most current evidence to support care, but is unsure about how to begin. The director recognizes an opportunity to meet the organizational goals of providing evidence-based care as well as aligning the **chief nursing officer**'s (CNO) or **chief nursing executive**'s (CNE) vision with nursing practice on the unit level. The CNO or CNE is the most senior nursing leader in the organization who is administratively responsible for all aspects of the nursing care including budget, patient care services, and the like. Sometimes the CNO or CNE carries the title of vice-president. The director encourages Ann to enlist other nurse's involvement during the next unit meeting.

Organizational Priorities

Although much of the duty for evidence-based practice falls on clinical nurses, the actuality is that evidence-based practice is a complicated undertaking requiring organizational dedication to embrace an evidence-based practice culture (Box 14■1). Organizational barriers strongly affect the ability of nurses to implement evidence. In the overall leadership structure, it is essential to have a CNO or CNE with a voice and vote to represent nursing and evidence-based practice at the highest levels of the organization's **administration.** The administration includes all of the executive leaders in the organization who make critical financial, strategic, and patient care decisions on behalf of all aspects of the agency. Embedding a value for evidence-based practice at the administrative level ensures that leadership of the entire organization shares the same goals. Subsequently, evidence-based practice becomes an essential part of the strategic plan for the organization. Direct care nurses need an advocate at the highest levels to obtain resources in finance, human resource, operations,

---

BOX 14■1 Significance of Nursing Systems in Implementing Evidence

- Organizations that foster a culture of evidence have higher nurse satisfaction, a more stable workforce, and positive patient outcomes (Kramer, Schmalenberg, and Maguire, 2010).
- Leaders set the tone and expectations for the members of the organization.
- Systems that enhance evidence uptake include effective communication channels; shared, decentralized governance structures; resource allocation; access to evidence; coaches; and mentors.
- Evaluation systems that enhance evidence uptake provide meaningful, accessible data and feedback mechanisms that are timely, individualized, and focused.

technology, quality information, and procurement as well as from other departments in the facility. The CNO/CNE is positioned to initiate critical conversations on evidence-based practice with an opportunity to provide a clear vision for the entire organization.

Similarly, the CNO/CNE's ability to understand and support evidence implementation reflects down the hierarchy to middle management's appreciation for evidence-based nursing practice. Unit managers/directors must have explicit expectations to grow a climate that values and supports evidence-based practice. The CNO/CNE functions as a catalyst, bringing together the appropriate high-level administrative entities and the middle management layer to ensure that the direct care nurse has the necessary resources to implement evidence into practice. The ability of middle management to cultivate interest and opportunities for EB initiatives is the beginning of culture development. In the clinical story, the director recognizes how Ann's project is aligned with the organization's values.

Organizational Culture

Enculturation—the process of being socialized to a culture—of evidence-based practice as an organizational value has a strong impact on frontline nursing. To understand the true barriers to evidence-based practice implementation, one must be aware of nurse-identified management issues. Such barriers include a lack of interest, motivation, leadership, vision, strategy, and direction (DiCenso, 2003). To counteract such barriers, organizations have initiated ongoing leadership development, communication training, and education on evidence-based practice and coaching and mentoring skills. Some facilities use outside consultants, whereas others work with professional organizations such as the American Organization of Nurse Executives (AONE) or the American Nurses Credentialing Center (ANCC) to offer preparation courses for certification as a nurse executive. The ANA's certification requires that candidates are well versed in the body of knowledge, consisting of leadership and management styles, theoretical underpinnings of management, culture development, and strategic planning. These skills are essential for progressing an organizational culture and philosophy that is founded on evidence-based practice.

The CNO/CNE can instill **accountability** for evidence-based practice implementation into performance evaluations for middle nursing management. This includes setting explicit expectations for developing evidence-based practice opportunities. Middle managers are charged with the task of creating an environment supportive of practice innovations, and assume direct responsibility for setting the stage for evidence-based nursing practice. When looking at the clinical story, it is clear that Ann's manager supported her initiative and promoted involvement of other nurses. Identifying potential facilitators, supporting time to work on the project, bringing key stakeholders to the table, and acquiring access to databases for literature reviews make up some actions that middle management take to support nurse-driven initiatives. Managers also must learn how to gather and watch how data are trending regarding the effectiveness of evidence-based practice initiatives. Supportive documentation exposes the degree of enculturation for evidence implementation projects, including the significance for enhancing patient outcomes.

Adding an evidence-based practice component to the nurse's position description, leveled for educational preparation, can support commitment to evidence-based practice. Clearly detailing expectations for evidence-based practice increases nurse awareness and responsibility for providing evidence-based care. In 2003, the Institute of Medicine (IOM) initiated discussion on the need to include evidence-based practice processes in the education of health-care workers through their publication, *Health Professions Education—A Bridge to Quality.* The IOM proposed that all health-care professionals be educated to deliver patient-centered care as members of an interdisciplinary team, emphasizing evidence-based practice, quality improvement approaches, and informatics (IOM, 2003). For direct care nurses, the expectation could include identifying practice issues, using organizational resources to develop an EB project, creating a PICO question, participating in an evidence-based project, becoming a member of the research committee, or attending educational offerings that increase awareness of research and evidence-based nursing practice. When the position description includes evidence-based practice processes, there must be coexisting structural supports to help nurses achieve expected performance levels.

Communication

A key to successful implementation of evidence-based practice organization-wide is having clear channels of communication. This is important when working on evidence-based practice projects on a unit within a larger organization. Communication allows a sharing of ideas, thoughts, practices, challenges, and promotes collaboration among various units and disciplines (Box 14■2). For example, if another unit revises its CAUTI care practices, the sharing of their experience and knowledge could help Ann with her project. In addition, communication is significant for enhancing collaboration between disciplines (Agency for Healthcare Research and Quality, 2008). An essential piece of any nursing care project is the input from other disciplines. If Ann were to work on her project without the input from other areas such as laboratory personnel, physicians, or infection control staff, she might lose out on some wonderful opportunities to bring in various elements needed for a successful project. Laboratory information affects turnaround time for urinalysis results. Physician collaboration assists by creating orders responsive to the patient's need and nurse's judgment for catheter removal. Infection control's participation includes bringing data from CAUTI rates to the table and determining effective practice changes.

One method for enhancing communication is a **shared governance** structure. Ideally, when a functional shared governance structure is in place, nurses are given the power, autonomy, and authority to control nursing practice. "Shared governance is a structural configuration of councils and committees that provide formal mechanisms that ensure nurses' responsibility, right, and power to make decisions and to control nursing practice" (Kramer et al., 2009). Organizations with strong shared governance structures are shown to demonstrate sustained evidence-based practice integration (Rycroft-Malone, 2008). One of the **forces of magnetism** (American Nurses Credentialing Center, 2008) is decentralized decision making, whereby nurses throughout an organization are engaged in self-governance and

BOX 14■2   **Interdisciplinary Rounds**

- All disciplines contribute to the organizational culture, including the chief executives of various disciplines such as nursing, medicine, and information services.
- Most problems affect other disciplines. For example, preventing CAUTIs requires collaboration and cooperation among nurses, nursing care technicians, physicians, infectious disease professionals, quality and safety officers, purchasing and supply chain managers, clinical educators, advanced practice nurses, finance officers, and risk managers.
- Some disciplines like nurses affect how evidence informs practice directly because they are at the point of care. Other disciplines, such as purchasing and supply chain managers, affect how the organization uses evidence indirectly because they influence the structures important to evidence uptake. For example, those who make decisions about what urinary catheter to buy must understand the evidence related to the effectiveness of one catheter type over another.
- Magnet-recognized facilities promote interdisciplinary engagement by creating structures for nurses to participate in diverse teams and work groups.
- Depending on the problem you approach, the departmental leaders can facilitate or pose barriers to evidence implementation.
- Effective and respectful interdisciplinary communication helps move evidence into practice and creates a positive organizational culture.

forums to address practice issues. A variety of shared governance structures are found in the literature, the most common being the council format. In this model, councils are created based on functions (quality, research, evidence-based practice, education, advocacy, retention/recruitment, etc.) and include nursing representation (Fig. 14■1). The different councils work toward improving patient care and the patient/family experience. With the patient/family at the center, the model ensures that all issues keep a focus on the patient and family. Unit-based councils focus on specific unit practice issues being the only council that includes direct care nurses on each specific unit. All other councils have a representation and a voice to promote communication of issues.

Establishing a formal communication configuration allows the sharing of ideas among all areas. For example, **ad hoc committees** can develop from the original group, allowing key stakeholders to work with nurses to support implementation of evidence-based practice innovations. Ad hoc committees are formed by the owner of the project to address short-term issues. Composition of the committee includes experts in the area, those directly affected by the practice, and both managers and direct care nurses. The committee works solely on the identified issue, then disbands after completion of the project.

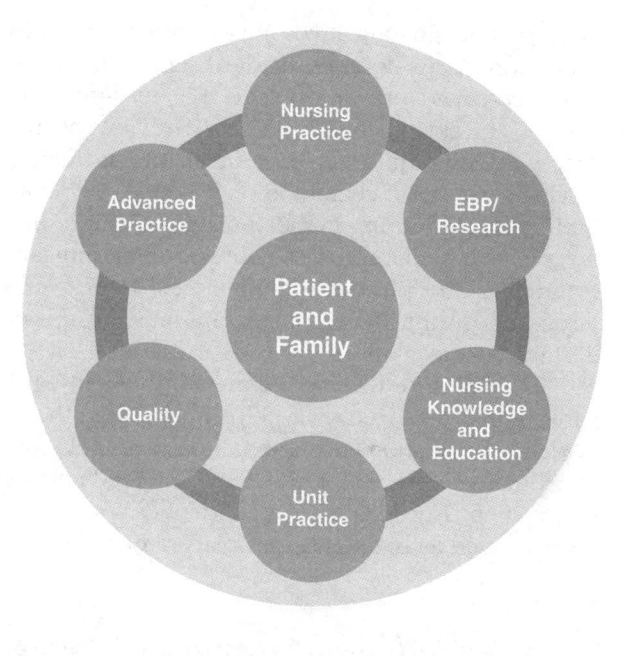

FIGURE 14■1 Example of a shared governance council structure.

In the clinical story at the beginning of the chapter, Ann presented her project at the unit practice council meeting. Two other nurses expressed an interest in working with Ann on the project. Ann also communicated her ideas to the evidence-based practice council as a project proposal. To help Ann and her team, the committee suggested working with a mentor who could help work through the process of an evidence-based practice project with the team. The evidence-based practice council works in concert with the other councils to establish a roster of nurses who possess training and experience in evidence-based practice processes. From this roster, an appropriate mentor is contacted and agrees to work with Ann and her team.

Resources at the Organizational Level

Organizational support for evidence-based practice is critical, especially in organizations where nurses think they lack the authority, autonomy, or power to implement a change in patient care practices (Brown, Wickline, Ecoff, et al., 2009). Such barriers relate to the critical need for leadership styles that promote a patient-centered environment in which nurses believe they are valued and incorporate a learning culture that encourages evidence-based practice. To counteract the barriers, some organizations create evidence-based practice councils, teams, mentors, interdisciplinary councils, and evidence-based practice-focused education, all designed to support nurse participation in evidence-based practice. Such tools and resources can effectively promote evidence-based practice when used in conjunction with leadership empowerment for nurse participation.

A critical need exists for collaboration with physicians on evidence-based practice initiatives from a big picture perspective. Having a physician champion does not mean that nursing initiatives must transform into medical projects. Rather, a physician champion opens doors to medical staff committees that might have a piece of your evidence-based practice puzzle. For instance, in the clinical story Ann wants to change current practice based on a review of the evidence for CAUTIs. The new protocol may require changes in treatment, including pharmacology management. Having a physician champion on board at the beginning of discussions can minimize problems later during implementation. During the stages of protocol development, the physician champion becomes a communication conduit between the CAUTI committee and physician committees. Issues, problems, concerns, and ideas are discussed during development, minimizing the chance that opposition will arise during implementation.

To appreciate the big picture of potential barriers and **facilitators** from an organizational perspective, it helps to see how the structure and resources can affect evidence integration (Box 14■3). It is clear that consideration of organizational issues affecting evidence integration is widespread and varied. Having a basic understanding of such issues can help you identify your own organization's potential problem areas as well as highlight exemplary processes.

BOX 14■3 Tools for Learning and Practice

- Ask for an organizational chart to understand the reporting structure in your organization.
- Find out if your organization has an evidence-based practice council and determine if you are eligible to participate on the council or find out who your representative is.
- When planning a unit-level or systemwide evidence-based change, use tools to assess the organizational culture, context, and stakeholders:
  - Use the *Context Assessment Index (related to PARIHS model) to determine the strengths of leadership, evaluation methods and organizational culture.
  - Use the Guideline Implementation Toolbox available from the Registered Nurses' Association of Ontario to analyze a system's readiness for change, stakeholders, and to plan implementation strategies, available at http://www.rnao.org/Storage/12/668_BPG_Toolkit.pdf
  - Systematically identify barriers and promoters of change.
- Work with an advanced practice nurse to help you find, appraise, and plan change.
- Engage your information technology team to create quick links to excellent evidence-based sources available through one-click on your unit's desktops.
- Support and get involved with policy committees to make evidence transparent and embedded in the policy.
- Participate in journal clubs and encourage peers to join.

Setting Barriers and Facilitators

Organizations with successful evidence integration have something in common; each embeds evidence into policies, procedures, clinical pathways, standards, protocols, and documentation systems (Agency for Healthcare Research and Quality, 2008). These actions build strong structural supports that externalize the internal cultural value for evidence-based nursing practice. When providing care for a specific patient population and diagnosis, such as asthmatic children or adults with heart failure, pathways or protocols prescribe nursing interventions. When based on evidence, the pathway or protocol can increase the likelihood of achieving desired patient outcomes.

Ann's team has worked diligently for over a month on the new protocol. During one meeting, a team member tells the group that besides her normal 40-hour work-week, she has put in at least 20 hours per week of her own time on the project. The other team members agree that project is time-consuming, provides no reimbursement, and is beginning to affect their family life. The team members also discuss difficulties accessing databases, not knowing how to search effectively, and needing help to find articles. Ann can feel the group's enthusiasm starting to decline and decides to speak to the director about the new issues.

Time Constraints

Nurses very commonly perceive that insufficient time poses a primary setting barrier to being able to implement new practices (Carlson and Plonczynski, 2008; Koehn and Lehman, 2008; Pravikoff, Tanner, and Pierce, 2005). These time constraints include short-staffing, lack of time for patient care, too much work, and high patient acuity. In addition, nurses may believe that time constraints extended to personal time (Brown et al., 2009). All are valid and pertinent points. You may have considered the amount of time needed for developing and instituting an evidence-based practice project and wondered how you will incorporate it into your nursing practice. Strategies to overcome the time barrier require an organizational commitment to evidence-based nursing practice. For example, the CNO/CNE can develop and support a policy allowing paid time off for working on research or evidence-based practice that directly relates to the area of nursing. In addition, the unit director or manager may allow time off to work on initiatives that improve the quality of care. In both cases, the key issue is that nurses need dedicated time away from direct care responsibilities to work on evidence implementation.

Ann speaks to her director about the concerns of the group. The director acknowledges the validity of the concerns and to bring it up to the CNO/CNE. During the meeting, both identify the need to support direct care nurses engaged in evidence-based practice initiatives and brainstorm on creative ways to meet the need for time release. A unique feature of their organization is the presence of a highly functioning and nurse-dedicated foundation. The foundation agrees to fund half a nurse's salary for 1 month while working on an evidence-based practice project and promises to expand the program up to a total of five nurses per year. The program allows Ann's team to split the time off and continue with the project.

Resource Availability

Another organizational characteristic involves resources available to nurses. In the clinical story, Ann's team quickly identified the need to access databases to review the literature on catheterized patients. When you encounter a practice issue, you will need to have accessible and reliable databases for reviewing the literature. Professional literature is essential for developing a change in practice that is consistent with best evidence (Pravikoff et al., 2005). This step requires a dedicated budget for purchasing appropriate library resources. The economics of health-care makes it important to have a champion at the administrative level that values knowledge generation and defends the need for budget allocations. Imagine if Ann and her team did not have access to the necessary literature; the entire project would have been compromised.

Having accessible databases demonstrates the dedication of the organization for knowledge growth. In addition, an experienced on-staff librarian can help immensely when locating appropriate and reliable literature. Some smaller organizations employ a librarian for use by both physicians and nurses, whereas others have dedicated staff for each department. The function and title of a hospital-based librarian varies in each facility. Some may combine several duties together, whereas other facilities maintain a pure librarian position. However it is handled in your organization, you should be familiar with the structure and position of the librarian as he or she will become an invaluable resource to you.

Even with database resources, the logistics of accessing information can still be a barrier. Having Internet access on computers throughout the units with the ability to acquire full-text articles or guidelines on the nursing unit is significant to linking evidence to the point of care. Minimizing the steps nurses must perform to get the evidence into practice facilitates the process. Some of the more technologically advanced health-care organizations have **embedded evidence** into their charting systems by linking policies, protocols, and pathways to specific nursing care instances. For example, while caring for a patient with ventilator-acquired pneumonia (VAP), the nurse is prompted to perform certain care when entering information into the patient's medical record. A link to the protocol allows the nurse to access the evidence-based care interventions at the point of care.

Some organizations, recognizing the need to provide strong **structural supports** for evidence-based practice have created dedicated nursing education departments. These departments go beyond teaching; they can also include primary responsibility for purchasing and maintaining resources such as databases and memberships for the organization. Education departments identify the learning needs of the organization and develop or bring in experts to meet such needs. The departments also help make connections between those desiring to work on an evidence-based project and those experienced in the processes. For example, Kaiser Permanente, a large health-care organization in California, wanted to expand its nursing workforce's knowledge of research and evidence-based practice. The organization's Nursing Education Department developed a Nursing Pathways Web site devoted to knowledge generation and dissemination (http://nursingpathways.kp.org/national/research/index. html). This action allows nurses to expand their understanding of evidence-based practice and share initiatives throughout the organization.

Dedicated mentors, well versed in evidence-based practice processes, can provide a support mechanism for initiating and sustaining evidence-based practice initiatives. Having someone knowledgeable in the process of crafting a question from a practice issue, experienced in searching the literature, and familiar with the organizational policies for putting evidence into practice is vital for constructing an evidence-based practice culture. Some larger organizations employ a dedicated nurse researcher. Smaller organizations may have nurse mentors who are practicing nurses experienced in evidence-based practice processes. Regardless of how the process is handled, having available mentors demonstrates organizational commitment toward initiating and sustaining an environment for evidence-based practice.

Even with available time for evidence-based practice, adequate database resources, a mentor to assist in the process, support from management, and Internet access, other unexpected issues can still arise. The key is that with the aforementioned support mechanisms, most of the other barriers can be overcome or minimized to increase an organization-wide culture for evidence-based practice.

Individual Barriers and Facilitators

Ann's team completes the project and is ready to present their protocol and supportive evidence to the unit's practice council. While preparing for the meeting, Ann begins to think that she might not be able to affect changes in practice, even though she knows that the team developed a valid process and is confident in the project findings.

Individual barriers consist of both intrinsic and extrinsic factors such as lack of knowledge and skills, uncertainty about how to proceed with a project or formulate a question, belief that the goal of implementing evidence-based practice is unattainable, heavy workloads, lack of resources, and minimal support (Fineout-Overholt and Johnston, 2006). Research shows that there are six individual determinants that affect evidence implementation at the individual level; beliefs and attitudes, education, and involvement in research activities (Estabrooks, Floyd, Scott-Findlay, et al., 2005). Education about evidence-based practice processes is fundamental to building the foundation for an evidence-based practice culture but is most effective when lack of knowledge is identified as a primary barrier. A multifaceted approach includes seminars and workshops. The education is most effective when it is highly interactive, the content is highly relevant and nursing leaders indicate that attendance is important. Education by itself will probably not change complex behaviors (Forsetlund, Bjorndal, Rashidian, et al., 2009). (Health-care opinion leaders providing educational outreach are successful in reducing bias.)

Beliefs and Attitudes

A frequently cited individual barrier to evidence implementation is the nurses' perception that they did not feel they had the **authority to change practice** (Brown et al., 2009). This brings up an interesting question: If nurses do not have control over their practice, then who does? Contrary to what some nurses may believe, nurses absolutely have authority to change practice and should take control of the process. The bigger issue is the reason that nurses feel this way and what can be done to counteract it. This feeling can be related to the culture of the organization as well as an understanding of the professional nursing concepts of accountability and autonomy.

Continuity of care is another means of supporting nurses in applying evidence-based practice. When nurses have the same assigned patients (i.e., a caseload), they not only develop relationships with their patients, but they also have the opportunity to learn about their patients' preferences. When nurses' patient assignments change each day, they cannot easily identify subtle changes in their patients' status. They will need more time to understand trends, to apply interventions for the specific patient's care needs, and to see outcomes from interventions when the patient load varies.

It helps when there is a structure in place for nurses to bring practice issues forward. **Unit practice councils** or similar formal venues allow nurses to voice their concerns and be involved in making practice changes. Councils, made up of direct care nurses, allow exploration of practice issues and create opportunities for supporting evidence-based practice. Such formats encourage all nurses to take an active role in deciding how nursing care will be provided. Consider in the clinical story how Ann was part of a unit practice council with a direct link to larger, hospital-wide nursing councils. The larger nursing councils also had a direct link to various committees made up of management. How would the progression and sustainability of the initiative change if this chain of support and communication were not present?

Education

Knowledge of research, including how to read, understand, and assimilate findings, can be a barrier to evidence-based initiatives. It is estimated that 40% of direct care nurses possess an Associate's level degree (HRSA, 2004). Because of this, research knowledge and skills cannot be expected from nurses who have not had formal education on this topic. To counteract this, many facilities have initiated RN-BSN or RN-MSN program affiliations with academic partners. Such partnerships bring a twofold benefit to the organization. First, the partnership supports the continuation of professional development for nurses by encouraging formal education for the nursing staff. Second, it links academic resources to the organization. For some organizations this partnership has helped to formalize research committees and journal clubs, and provided research opportunities for educators.

Other organizations have turned to advanced practice nurses (APNs) to help support evidence-based initiatives. In particular, **clinical nurse specialists** (CNSs) are APNs with master's or doctoral degrees and they are prepared with a specialty focus and are able to lead practice change a multiple levels including influencing individual nurses, unit and systemwide change (National Association of Clinical Nurse Specialists [NACNS], 2004). Having access to APNs such as CNSs is essential to the enculturation and sustainability of evidence-based initiatives. Depending on the organization and role delineation for APNs, such nurses can provide mentorship, guidance, facilitation, and dissemination for evidence-based nursing practice (Rycroft-Malone, 2008).

In the clinical story, the mentor for the CAUTI project is Mary, who is an MSN. Mary is the medical-surgical CNS who volunteers to work with Ann and the team on their project. She begins by helping them develop a PICO question and provides guidance on available resources for searching the literature. Mary also is available to answer questions and help develop an understanding of evidence-based practice. She helps the team to develop a protocol for catheterized patients and provides assistance with various committee approvals by attending meetings and supporting their project.

The clinical story demonstrates how an APN was accessible and supportive of the evidence-based initiative. Her ability to guide Ann through the processes helped move the project forward. If Ann did not have a mentor, guide, facilitator, and support system, she would have expended a large amount of time learning before doing, which could lead to frustration and discouragement, and to dropping the project. Of course a project can be completed, and done well, without an APN; if the team is lacking knowledge of processes involved with evidence-based practice, an APN can provide needed mentorship. Research knowledge and mentoring support is an effective facilitator for evidence-based practice, especially when an APN is involved (Nutley et al., 2003; Thompson, McCaughan, Cullum, et al., 2001; Rycroft-Malone, 2008).

Recall that the PARIHS model suggests that you will more likely be able to implement evidence when the organizational culture, leadership, and evaluation processes are strong and facilitators such as CNSs have excellent skills, and clear roles and purposes (Kitson, Rycroft-Malone, Harvey, et al., 2008). Until evidence-based practice processes are integrated and standardized into academic nursing curriculums, having a mentor who is knowledgeable and experienced in evidence-based practice is essential to the success of a project.

Involvement in Research Activities

Journal clubs have gained popularity in recent years. Such clubs are based on the premise that reading, reviewing, and discussing research, systematic reviews, and evidence-based practice protocols can generate an awareness of evidence-based practice. Although there is varied research on the success of journal clubs to increase the number of new research studies, understanding of how research affects nursing care by those attending is still a viable outcome. Members must attend regularly scheduled meetings and discuss the research using a standardized evaluation method in a nonthreatening and learning environment (Fineout-Overholt and Johnston, 2006). A twist on the journal club is to hold open forums via a learning management system, e-mail subscriber list, or blog. Similar to e-learning, participants discuss the topic online as an interactive activity. This method allows participation at the nurse's convenience.

Information Seeking

Information seeking is an attribute of those nurses who question their clinical practice and actively seek out answers in the professional literature. Similar to the characteristic of the setting, the availability of databases can enhance information-seeking behaviors. The significance to the individual is the immediacy of information at the point of care, satisfying the internal need for appropriate clinical information, and encouragement for nurses to read available literature. For example, while caring for a patient you might question an intervention or practice. Possessing the characteristic of information seeking means you might consult reliable databases or repositories of information to actively seek out answers to your question. In addition, reviewing peer-reviewed journals from your professional organization can provide insights into how others addressed the same or similar issues specific to your area of nursing.

Individual barriers are just that; they arise from the value and worth placed on evidence-based practice by the individual. Such issues vary with the type of organization, educational level of nurses, and support structures available. The culture of an organization strongly affects the willingness of the nurse to participate in evidence-based initiatives. Whether addressing organizational, setting, or individual barriers to implementing evidence, adopting multifaceted and targeted methods for the variety of barriers is more effective than any single intervention (Farquhar, Stryer, and Slutsky, 2002; Glasgow, Lichtenstein, and Marcus, 2003; Pearson, 2004).

Sustaining Change

Once system barriers are minimized and facilitators are supported, the need to sustain change emerges. It is easy to fall back into the routine of what was always done. The challenge is to integrate changes into our everyday routine. This holds true for evidence-based practice initiatives as well. Once we make the change, how do we sustain it?

Having a dedicated person or team responsible for auditing the evidence-based practice protocol outcomes provides information on how well the initiative is working. Assigning this task ensures that data reflecting the outcomes are routinely gathered and analyzed. If the task is not clearly assigned, then who is actually monitoring the outcomes becomes muddled, with each person thinking the other is completing the task. It makes sense that the committee or nurse who initiated the evidence-based practice change also assumes the responsibility for gathering data. The team must also plan how they will feed the data back so that it is timely, does not punish, and is targeted and specific.

Piloting the evidence-based practice protocol with a small population is generally done to identify such issues prior to implementing on a larger scale (Fineout-Overholt and Johnston, 2006). At this point, feedback from nurses is essential to identify potential problems and rework or retool the process you will use to make the practice change. The owner of the evidence-based practice project is typically the one to gather such information, make necessary changes, and reevaluate the process. This cyclical process is done prior to larger scale implementation to identify and rectify potential problems. When you plan a practice change you will want to find issues before they become problems. A small-scale pilot run allows you to fix issues that you might not have known existed before you start the large-scale implementation.

Another essential feature for sustaining change is the need for feedback to those who are implementing the protocol or practice change as well as to the organizational committees. Feedback to nurses using the evidence-based practice protocol on data shows how the care influenced patient outcomes. Enabling nurses to see how their participation in the application of the evidence-based practice affected the outcomes of care received. Many times nurses are asked to change their practice but are not told why or given information about how it affected their care outcomes. You can imagine the frustration you would feel if you were left out of the communication process. Consistently bringing data back to nurses reflecting care provided encourages engagement and commitment to the practice issue and EB protocol.

Evidence indicates that certain feedback techniques are more powerful than others to help start and sustain change and adherence to EB guidelines. When the audit team feeds the data back in a way that is individualized, nonpunitive, and timely, those who are trying to change their behavior are more likely to adhere to the EB guideline (Hysong, Best, and Pugh, 2006). In addition, the feedback may be most effective for those who were used the EB practices before the change. In addition, the intensity and individualization and higher intensity of feedback works better (Jamvedt, Young, Kristoffersen, et al., 2009). Expert facilitators can help you craft the feedback message so that it does not place blame but is specific about where adherence is low and needs to improve and happens as close to the time of the data collection as possible.

Bringing audit data to the larger organizational committees demonstrates the impact of evidence-based practice on patient outcomes. Connecting the various layers to the direct care of patients helps bring the focus back to patient care outcomes. Different departments can begin to understand the importance of their role in nursing care. For example, in the clinical story, Ann brought the data back to a committee composed of department managers and directors. This action provided information on how the various non-nursing departments influenced the patient care outcomes. In addition, the process of disseminating data from initiatives links the strategic plan back to the direct care of patients.

The Impact of Magnet Recognition Program®

The American Nurses Credentialing Center (ANCC) developed and revised the **ANCC Magnet Recognition Program.®** This program is based on the Magnet model. Those organizations seeking Magnet recognition (or redesignation) find ways to overcome barriers to evidence implementation. The **Magnet model** requires organizations to demonstrate transformational leadership; structural empowerment; exemplary professional practice; and new knowledge, innovations, and improvements. Each piece is essential to achieving empirical quality outcomes, the central focus of the model. An **empirical quality outcome** is a measurement of a patient-centered and organizational health outcome and is the result of organizational commitment to excellence in nursing care. It is within the process of working toward Magnet recognition that an organization identifies areas of opportunity and develops structures to support nursing practice. Table 14■1 describes select forces and the impact on evidence-based practice implementation.

Table 14■1   **Forces of Magnetism and Impact on Evidence-Based Practice Integration**

Force of Magnetism	Types of Evidence	Impact on Evidence Integration
Transformational leadership	Strategic planning	Represent nursing's mission, vision, values at the organizational strategic plan level
	Advocating for resources	Meeting nurses' needs for evidence-based practice such as databases, time, mentors, etc.
	Visibility, accessibility, and communication	Maintains lines of communication with direct care nurses to identify and support practice changes
Structural empowerment	Professional engagement	Nurse involvement in decision-making entities through shared governance
	Professional development	Educational activities that develop nursing knowledge of evidence-based practice processes.
Exemplary professional practice	Interdisciplinary care	Nurse inclusion and leadership on interdisciplinary committees Interdisciplinary collaboration on quality improvement initiatives All levels of nurses involved in developing policies and standards of care
	Accountability, competence, and autonomy	Autonomous practice supported by access, routine use, current literature, and professional standards Nurse involvement in annual goal settings including participation in evidence-based practice initiatives Support for nursing involvement in practice decision making and autonomy Nurse accountability for clinical practice
	Culture of safety	Nurse-sensitive indicator data the mean of the national benchmarks used. Nurses participate in initiatives to reduce or eliminate barriers to safe patient care.

Force of Magnetism	Types of Evidence	Impact on Evidence Integration
	Quality monitoring and improvement	Nurse responsibility for coordinating care among disciplines Trending care outcomes against national benchmarks to identify nursing practice issues Patient satisfaction is addressed using interdisciplinary methods with nurse involvement
New knowledge, innovations, and improvements	Research	Evaluating and using research findings in nursing practice Nurse participation on the Institutional Review Board for research studies Dissemination of knowledge from research studies
	Evidence-based practice	Structure and processes in place to allow the evaluation of current practice Clearly defined method for translating new knowledge into nursing practice Evaluation of how the translation of new knowledge affects patient outcomes

Adapted from American Nurses Credentialing Center. (2008). *Magnet Application Manual.*

■ Summary

In the clinical story, the group works for several months to implement the new protocol. They look at the number of CAUTIs during the next two quarters and are delighted to find that the number of CAUTIs fell to zero during a 6-month period. The CNO publicly thanked Ann and her group for taking the initiative to work on the problem. The unit director encourages the group to submit their protocol as a paper presentation to a nursing conference. Ann felt good about improving patient care outcomes and reflected on the experience, knowing that she received support and encouragement throughout the process.

The organizational culture depends on the type of leadership, available resources, enculturation of value for evidence-based practice, expectations of nurses, and the individual nurse. The culture, values, and norms of an organization all affect evidence implementation. As you develop an understanding of an organization, you will recognize both barriers and facilitators for evidence-based practice implementation at the organizational, setting, and individual levels. Such knowledge will prepare you to successfully navigate and direct an evidence implementation project.

CHAPTER QUESTIONS

1. Identify frequently encountered barriers found at the organizational, setting, and individual levels.

2. Describe facilitators that could counteract barriers found in the organizational, setting, and individual levels.

3. Explain how knowledge of setting barriers can facilitate evidence implementation.

4. Describe a plan for overcoming the following barriers:
   a. You identify a clinical practice issue. You ask another nurse what he thinks about investigating the problem further and receive the following response: "Only doctors can make changes to clinical practice."
   b. While caring for a patient on a ventilator, you wonder if your interventions are current and based on evidence. What resources could increase access to appropriate information?
   c. This is your fourth shift in a row with a different team of patients assigned to you.
   d. You want to join the research committee but the meetings always occur during your scheduled time to work.

5. Think about one of your clinical experiences to answer the following questions:
   a. What formal structure was in place to facilitate the generation and movement of clinical issues?
   b. How did the nurses use evidence to direct bedside care?
   c. What databases were available to the nurses for accessing systematic reviews?
   d. Do you know if the patient care policies were based on evidence? Why or why not?

6. Reflect on your clinical experiences to answer the following questions.
   a. Based on the barriers discussed in the chapter and your own experiences in the clinical setting, do you think they are valid? Why?
   b. Would you have had time to incorporate evidence into your care of patients during your clinical experience?
   c. In your experience, what facilitation method would have helped you integrate evidence into your clinical practice?

7. If you are interviewing for a new position and you want to determine if the organization has a culture of evidence based practice, what questions would you ask during your interview?

References

Agency for Healthcare Research and Quality. (2008). *Patient safety and quality: An evidence-based handbook for nurses* (AHRQ Publication No. 08-0043). Retrieved from http://www.ahrq.gov/qual/nurseshdbk/

American Nurses Credentialing Center. (2008). *Magnet recognition program: Application manual.* Silver Springs, MD: Author.

Brown, C. E., Wickline, M. A., Ecoff, L., et al. (2009). Nursing practice, knowledge, attitudes and perceived barriers to evidence-based practice at an academic medical center. *Journal of Advanced Nursing, 65,* 371–381.

Carlson, C. L., & Plonczynski, D. J. (2008). Has the BARRIERS scale changed nursing practice? An integrative review. *Journal of Advanced Nursing, 63,* 322–333. doi:10.1111/j.1365-2648.2008.04705.x

Estabrooks, C. A., Floyd, J. A., Scott-Findlay, S., et al. (2003). Individual determinants of research utilization: A systematic review. *Journal of Advanced Nursing, 43,* 506–520.

Farquhar, C. M., Stryer, D., & Slutsky, J. (2002). Translating research into practice: The future ahead. *International Journal for Quality in Health Care, 14,* 233–249.

Fineout-Overholt, E., & Johnston, L. (2006, 4th Quarter). Implementation of evidence: Moving from evidence to action. *Worldviews on Evidence-Based Nursing,* 194–200.

Forsetlund, L., Bjorndal, A., Rashidian, A., et al. (2009). Continuing education meetings and workshops: Effects on professional practice and health care outcomes. *Cochrane Database of Systematic Reviews, 2*All of your cases can be related or each different fro each other. Art. No.: CD003030. doi: 10.1002/14651858.CD003030.pub2

Glasgow, R. E., Lichtenstein, E., & Marcus, A. C. (2003, August). Why don't we see more translation of health promotion research to practice? Rethinking the efficacy to effectiveness transition. *American Journal of Public Health, 93,* 1261–1267.

Hysong, S. J., Best, R. G., & Pugh, J. (2006). Audit and feedback and clinical practice guideline adherence: Making feedback actionable. *Implementation Science 1,* 9

HRSA. (2004). The registered nurse population: Findings from the National Sample Survey of Registered Nurses. Retrieved from http://bhpr.hrsa.gov/healthworkforce/reports/nursing/samplesurvey00/chapter2.htm

Institute of Medicine. (2003). *The education of healthcare professionals: A bridge to quality.* Washington, DC: National Academies Press.

Jamvedt, G., Young, J. M., Kristoffersen, D. T., et al. (2006). Audit and feedback: effects on professional practice and healthcare outcomes. *Cochrane Database of Systematic Reviews, 2.* Art. No.: CD000259. doi: 10.1002/14651858.CD000259.pub2

Kitson, A., Rycroft-Malone, J., Harvey, G., et al. (2008). Evaluating the successful implementation of evidence into practice using the PARiHS framework: Theoretical and practical challenges. *Implementation Science, 3.* doi:10.1186/1748-5908-3-1

Koehn, M. L., & Lehman, K. (2008). Nurses' perceptions of evidence-based nursing practice. *Journal of Advanced Nursing, 62,* 209–215.

Kramer, M., Schmalenburg, K., & Maguire, P. (2010). Nine structures and leadership practices essential for a magnetic (healthy) work environment. *Nursing Administration Quarterly, 34,* 4–17.

Kramer, M., Schmalenberg, C., Maguire, P., et al. (2009, June). Walk the talk: Promoting control of nursing practice and a patient-centered culture. *Critical Care Nurse, 29*(3), 77–93.

National Association of Clinical Nurse Specialists. (2004). *Statement on clinical nurse specialist practice and education* (2nd ed.). Harrisburg, PA: Author.

Pearson, A. (2004). Getting research into practice. *International Journal of Nursing Practice, 10,* 197–198.

Pravikoff, D. S., Tanner, A. B., & Pierce, S. T. (2005). Readiness of U.S. nurses for evidence-based practice. *American Journal of Nursing, 105*(9), 40–51.

Rycroft-Malone, J. (2008). Evidence-informed practice: From individual to context. *Journal of Nursing Management, 16,* 404–408.

Thompson, C., McCaughan, D., Cullum, N., et al. (2001). Research information in nurses' clinical decision-making: What is useful? *Journal of Advanced Nursing, 36,* 376–388.

Yano, E. M. (2008). The role of organizational research in implementing evidence-based practice: QUERI series. *Implementation Science, 3*(29). Retrieved from http://www.implementationscience.com/content/3/1/29.

CHAPTER 15

Apply and Implement IV
National and International Systems of Evidence Implementation

Leslie Rittenmeyer

LEARNING OBJECTIVES

- Discuss the basic concepts of health-care policy.
- Explore health-care policy in the context of evidence-based practice.
- Describe how individual nurse decision making is influenced by larger systems.
- Discuss how evidence-based practice innovations can be driven by governmental policy.

KEY TERMS

Agency for Healthcare Research and Quality (AHRQ)
American Health Quality Association
Beveridge model
Bismark model
Centers for Disease Control and Prevention (CDC)
Centers for Medicare & Medicaid Services (CMS)
Core measures
Cost sharing
Deductible

Department of Health and Human Services (HHS)
Evidence-based health care
Health Care Commission
Hospital-acquired conditions (HACs)
Indian Health Services (IHS)
Institute for Healthcare Improvement (IHI)
Joint Commission (JC)
Joint Commission Patient Safety Goals (NPSGs)
Lobbyists

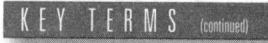

Clinical Story

Winnifred is in her last semester of a BSN program. She is currently enrolled in a health-care policy course. Her final assignment is a project that will require her to integrate a multitude of concepts from the course. The grading rubric for this project indicates that Winnifred should address the following objectives:

- Describe the basic concepts of public policy and health-care policy.
- Describe the steps of how policy is made.
- Compare the different models of health-care delivery and provide some national and international examples.
- Compare the concept of regulatory responsibility in the United States to that in the United Kingdom.
- Describe how public policy influences quality, safety, and practice and explain why government would be interested in evidence-based health care.
- Choose a practice problem that is targeted by a governmental or accreditation policy that also has reimbursement or accreditation ramifications. Describe why an agency would target this problem.
- Explain how the policy has implications for practice change and the steps that might be taken to address the problem at the institutional level. ■

Introduction

Most health-care professionals would claim they want to provide their patients the best-quality health care possible. But what does *best quality* really mean in the context of health care? Who defines *best quality,* and how do you know if you are providing it? Is *best quality* framed differently from the practitioner's perspective than from a management perspective? Does best quality always mean the care you are providing is evidence based and flows directly from the best available evidence? Can you provide best-quality health care and make good health-care decisions without being aware of the best available evidence? Is best-quality care based on rigorous and scientific guidelines and standards generated with transparent methods? Does best-quality care mean safe health care?

Governmental and accrediting entities continue to develop health-care policy that affects how nurses practice. From a governmental perspective, the purpose of an evidence-based practice is to provide care that is less variable and more standardized, with emphasis on patient safety, better patient outcomes, continuing quality monitoring, and improvement. This chapter begins by explaining the dimensions of public policy, with a focus on health-care policy. A discussion of who influences the making of public policy follows. Health-care delivery models in both the United States and internationally are then compared and regulatory responsibilities discussed. This discussion leads to an exploration of the influence of public policy on health-care quality, safety, and practice. The chapter ends with an example of the implementation process for an evidence–based program that addresses a clinical problem that has safety and reimbursement ramifications.

What Are the Dimensions of Public Policy?

Winnifred starts her project by reviewing her notes and readings for the various definitions of public policy and health-care policy. She begins her paper with some basic definitions and explains the public policy process, including how it is influenced by different groups.

Dye (1995) defines **public policy** as whatever governments choose to do or choose not to do. He points out that a lack of a policy is a policy statement in itself. Kilpatrick (2000) describes public policy as a system of laws, regulations, courses of action, and funding priorities in the context of a given issue promulgated by a governmental entity or its representative.

The role of public policy in the health-care context is complex because it addresses issues such as health-care coverage, health-care cost, health-care philosophy, and health-care quality. These issues are emotionally charged, and the role of government in health-care policy is often debated along the lines of political ideology. Buse, Mays, and Watt state that health policy is "assumed to embrace courses of action (and inaction) that affect the set of institutions, organizations, services and funding arrangements of the health system" (2005, p. 6).

How Is Policy Made and Influenced?

Public policy is generated by laws and enforced by governmental entities. Elected politicians set the agenda and the regulatory framework. Health-care policy falls under the heading of **social policy** (policies that address things such as welfare, crime, education, and health care). Remember, governments also make economic and foreign policy. The development of any type of policy usually starts with the identification of a problem. Sometimes the government identifies the problem or sometimes other stakeholders identify it. Once the problem has been defined, the next step is debate between conflicting interest groups. These groups vary but can consist of stakeholders, politicians, consumers, and special interest groups. An example of a special interest group is the insurance industry. Special interest groups are represented by political activists and **lobbyists** (persons who attempt to influence legislation on behalf of special interests). Walt (1994) contends that health-care policy is about process, power, and influence at play when policy is being made. Kilpatrick (2000) believes advocacy in the context of public policy is an attempt to influence policy through education, lobbying, or political pressure. Advocacy groups not only attempt to influence policy makers but the general public as well. An example of such a group is the American Nurses Association, which lobbies Congress and regulatory agencies on health-care issues. Another example is the **American Health Quality Association,** whose mission is to advance quality of care and patients safety nationwide. Box 15■1 is a representative sample of issues related to health policy associations.

A study from the Center for Responsive Politics (CRP), Northwestern University, and the *Chicago Tribune,* reported that lobbyists spent $862 million between 2008 and 2009 to influence senators and congressional representatives involved in the debate over health-care restructuring legislation (Martin, 2009). In addition, the drug industry spent $199 million on lobbying over a 9-month period, making the industry the second biggest spender next to the insurance companies. Unfortunately, conflicting agendas and competing interests can significantly slow the process of reaching consensus on a health-care reform or public policy.

If a policy is finally formulated at the end of the debate, legislators vote on it; if it passes the vote, the policy is enacted into law. Following the vote, the law is then signed or vetoed by the president, and it is then decided which governmental entity will enforce the policy.

BOX 15■1   **Representative Sample of Health Policy Associations**

- Alliance for Health Reform
- Alliance to Improve Medicare
- American Association for Health Care Risk Management
- American Association of Retired Persons
- American Hospital Association
- American Pharmaceutical Association
- Citizen Advocacy Center (CAC)
- Henry J. Kaiser Family Foundation\
- Institute for Health Policy Solutions
- National Rural Health Association

The Role of Government in Health Care From a National and International Perspective: A Comparison

National Health-Care Policy (United States)

To understand the role of government in our national health-care system, it is necessary to understand how health care is structured in the United States. Simply put, the financing of health care in this country is shared by two entities, private insurance and the government, and the United States is considered to have a **multipayer system.** In the private sector, employer-sponsored group insurance is the most common. Individuals who do not have employer-sponsored insurance are free to purchase private, nongroup insurance. This means these individuals pay out-of-pocket premiums. These premiums are usually very expensive and difficult for most people to afford, so that there are so many uninsured and underinsured in this country. More recently, because of the prohibitive cost of health care, it is not unusual for employers to ask employees to pay a portion of their health-care premium. This is called **cost sharing.** There is even some cost sharing in the federal programs (e.g., Medicare) in the form of **deductibles,** the amount of money an individual pays each year before his or her benefits begin.

Government Funded Health Care in the United States: What Is It and Who Uses It?

The primary government funded health-care programs in the United States are **Medicare, Medicaid, State Children's Health Insurance Program (SCHIP), TRICARE, Veterans Health Administration (VA),** and the **Indian Health Service (HIS).** Box 15■2 summarizes the function of each of these entities.

The Kaiser Commission on Medicaid and the Uninsured/Urban Institute Analysis (2010) report provides statistics on health-care coverage in the United States. Box 15■3 provides a summary of the distribution of health insurance coverage in the United States for 2009.

Kaiser (2010) also presents some additional interesting facts about the portion of the U.S. population that is uninsured:

1. The majority of uninsured are working families (6 in 10 have at least one full-time worker, and 16% have only part-time workers).
2. 80% of the uninsured are legal U.S. residents.
3. Uninsured workers are more likely to have low-wage and blue-collar jobs.
4. More than half of uninsured adults have no education beyond high school, making it difficult for them to find jobs that pay for health-care benefits.
5. 40% of the uninsured have family incomes below the federal poverty level ($22,050 a year for a family of four).
6. Nine in ten uninsured have family incomes below 400% of the federal poverty level and would be eligible to receive Medicaid or subsidized coverage under the new health-care reform bill.

BOX 15■2   **Functions of Federal and State Funded Health-Care Programs**

- **Indian Health Service (IHS)** is an operating division within the Department of Health and Human Services and provides medical and public health services to members of federally recognized Native American tribes and Alaskan tribes.
- **Medicaid** is a funded by both the federal government and the states. It is administered at the state level. It covers low-income children and their families.
- **Medicare** is a federally funded program that insures persons 65 years and older and some individuals with disabilities. Part A pays for hospital care, Part B, for physician services, and Part D, for prescription benefits.
- **State Children's Health Insurance Program** (SCHIP) is funded by both the federal government and the states to provide health care to children whose families earn too much income to qualify for Medicaid but do not have enough money to pay for private insurance.
- **TRICARE** is a program that provides health coverage to all military retirees, their spouses, survivors, and other qualified dependants.
- **Veterans Health Administration** (VA) is a federally funded and administered program for veterans. Health care is delivered in government-run health-care facilities.

BOX 15■3   **Distribution of Health Insurance Coverage in the United States (2009)**

- Employee-sponsored insurance: 49%
- Medicare and other public forms of insurance: 17%
- Medicare: 12%
- Private nongroup insurance: 5%
- Uninsured: 17%

Total population: 303.3 million

Data from Kaiser Commission on Medicaid and the Uninsured/Urban Institute Analysis of March 2010. CPS.

Health-Care Reform

The recently enacted **Patient Protection and Affordable Care Act (PPACA)** (2010) (Pub. L. No. 111-148) is a large bill with many provisions that are likely to change over time. Some of the noteworthy provisions in the bill include the following:

- Federally mandated health insurance will be implemented, with the government covering legal residents whose incomes are below 400% of the federal poverty level.

- Adults with pre-existing conditions are eligible to join a high-risk pool and will be able to obtain health insurance at the same published rate, no matter what their health status, by 2014.
- It will be illegal for health insurers to deny coverage, raise premiums, or cancel policies.

This law is currently being challenged in the courts, and it is difficult to predict what will be the final outcome.

Regulatory Responsibility

The agency with primary responsibility for protecting the health of Americans and providing essential human services, especially for the most needy, is the **Department of Health and Human Services (HHS).** HHS represents close to a quarter of all federal outlay of funds and administers more grant dollars than all other federal agencies combined. The Medicare program, managed by HHS, is the nation's largest health insurer, handling more than a billion claims a year. HHS works closely with state and local governments, and many HHS-funded programs are provided at the local level by state or county agencies or through private sector grantees. The programs are administered through 11 operating divisions, which include 8 agencies in the U.S. Public Health Service and 3 human services agencies (http://www.hhs.gov). Box 15■4 includes the agencies that comprise the HHS.

Although describing all of the sub-agencies of HHS is beyond the scope of this chapter, A description of three of the subagencies of HHS is important to the focus of the chapter:

- The **Agency for Healthcare Research and Quality's (AHRQ)** supports research that helps people make more informed decisions and improves the

---

BOX 15■4 Structure of the Department of Health and Human Services

- Administration for Children and Families (ACF)
- Administration for Children, Youth and Families (ACYF)
- Administration on Aging (AoA)
- Agency for Healthcare Research and Quality (AHRQ)
- Agency for Toxic Substances and Disease Registry (ATSDR)
- Centers for Disease Control and Prevention (CDC)
- Centers for Medicare & Medicaid Services (CMS)
- Food and Drug Administration (FDA)
- Health Resources and Services Administration (HRSA)
- Indian Health Service (HIS)
- National Institutes of Health (NIH)
- National Cancer Institute (NCI)
- Office of the Inspector General (OIG)
- Substance Abuse and Mental Health Services Administration (SAMHSA)

quality of health-care services. AHRQ was formerly known as the Agency for Health Care Policy and Research (http://www.ahrq.gov).

- The **Centers for Medicare & Medicaid Services (CMS)** administers the Medicare program, providing health-care security and choice for aged and disabled people. Jointly with the state governments, CMS administers the Medicaid program and the **State Children's Health Insurance Program (SCHIP)**. CMS is the largest purchaser of health care in the United States—its programs account for more than one-third of the dollars spent on health care in the U.S. economy. In 2001, CMS programs provided health-care coverage for 70 million people—nearly 1 out of every 4 Americans (http://ASPE.hhs.gov).

- The **Centers for Disease Control and Prevention (CDC)** collaborates to create the expertise, information, and tools that people and communities need to protect their health through health promotion; prevention of disease, injury, and disability; and preparedness for new health threats. The CDC seeks to accomplish its mission by working with partners throughout the nation and the world to monitor health, detect and investigate health problems, conduct research to enhance prevention, develop and advocate sound public health policies, implement prevention strategies, promote healthy behaviors, and foster safe and healthful environments (http://www.cdc.gov).

The health-care system is the United States is very complicated. Dialogue concerning health disparities, health access, efficiency, patient safety, value, and quality to some extent raises more questions than it provides answers to and certainly keeps the health-care reform debate alive. The next section provides a comparison of U.S. health-care policy with international health-care policy.

International Health-Care Policy

According to the Institute of Medicine of the National Academy of Sciences (2004), the United States is the only industrialized nation that does not offer universal medical insurance coverage for its citizens. Despite that fact, the United States spends more on health care than does any other country. Table 15∎1 illustrates comparisons of health-care expenditures among industrialized nations.

In his book on international health care, Reid (2010) states that health-care systems tend to follow patterns, creating four basic systems throughout the world. The first system he describes is called the **Beveridge model,** named for William Beveridge, the designer of National Health Service (NHS) in the United Kingdom. It is also called a **single-payer system**—only a single entity pays the bill. In this system, health care is provided and financed by the government (the single payer) through a system of tax payments. In Britain, citizens never receive a bill for health-care services. Countries that adopt this model tend to have low costs per capita, because the government, as a sole payer, controls what doctors can do and can charge. Examples of nations using the Beveridge model are the United Kingdom and almost all of the Scandinavian countries.

The second system is called the **Bismark model**. This model is more like segments of the U.S. system in that it uses an insurance system jointly financed by employers and employees. However, insurance companies in Bismark-type health

Table 15■1 Comparisons of Health-care Expenditures Among Industrialized Nations

Country	Life Expectancy	Infant Mortality Rate	Physicians per 1000 People	Nurses per 1000 People	Per Capita Expenditure on Health (USD)	Health-care Costs as a Percentage of GDP	Government Revenue Spent on Health (%)	Health Costs Paid by Government (%)
Australia	81.4	4.2	2.8	9.7	3137	8.7	17.7	67.7
Canada	80.7	5.0	2.2	9.0	3895	10.1	16.7	69.8
France	81.0	4.0	3.4	7.7	3601	11.0	14.2	79.0
Germany	79.8	3.8	3.5	9.9	3588	10.4	17.6	76.9
Japan	82.6	2.6	2.1	9.4	2581	8.1	16.8	81.3
Norway	80.0	3.0	3.8	16.2	5910	9.0	17.9	83.6
Sweden	81.0	2.5	3.6	10.8	3323	9.2	13.6	81.7
United Kingdom	79.1	4.8	2.5	10.0	2992	8.4	15.8	81.7
United States	78.1	6.7	2.4	10.6	7290	16.0	18.5	

Source: Davis, K., Schoen, C., Schoenbaum, S., et al. (2007). Mirror mirror on the wall: An international update on the comparative performance of American health care. The Commonwealth Fund.

insurance plans are mandated to cover all citizens, and they do not make a profit. Although this is a multipayer system, tight regulations give government as much cost control clout as in the single-payer system. Germany, Japan, and Spain are three prominent nations that have adopted this model.

The third model is the **national health insurance model.** This model, Reid contends, has elements of both the Beveridge and Bismark models. It uses private sector providers, but reimbursement comes from a government-run insurance company that is funded by all residents. Because there are no marketing costs, no financial motives to deny claims, and no profit to be made, these universal programs tend to be cheaper and simpler to manage. In addition, the single-payer system has more power to negotiate for lower prices, which can include the cost of prescription drugs. National health insurance plans also cut costs by limiting the amount or type of medical services they will pay for or making patients wait for treatment. Canada has this type of system.

The last system Reid describes is the **out-of-pocket model.** He suggests most nations are too poor to have any formalized health care. In these countries, rich citizens can pay out of pocket for health care, whereas the poor citizens cannot afford care and usually stay sick or die. He provides examples of people in rural Africa, China, and India who have never seen a doctor in their entire lives.

Comparison of the U.S Health-Care System and International Systems

According to Reid (2010), America's health-care system is unique; the system is fragmented and has elements of all the models explained above. He compares our VA system (which is a single-payer system) to the Beveridge model employed by the United Kingdom and Cuba. For those Americans over the age of 65, he compares the Medicare system to the national health insurance model employed in Canada and Taiwan. He compares employer-paid health insurance to the Bismarck model practiced in Germany, France, and Japan (even though those countries have strong government regulations controlling quality and cost). Finally, he compares the 15% of Americans who have no insurance and no ability to pay out of pocket to parts of Africa, China, and India. He believes the United States is unlike any other country because it maintains separate systems for separate classes of people. Other countries have settled on one model for everyone, which he believes is fairer and cheaper.

Despite differences in health-care delivery systems, Gray (2009) believes many of the problems and potential solutions to those problems are similar. His opinion is based on the belief that across the globe, despite the differences in the way health-care services are paid for and delivered, many of the major problems are the same. He cites some of the following as examples:

- Increasing cost
- Lack of capacity of any country to pay for the totality of health-care services
- Provision of inappropriate care
- Aging population
- Technological advances
- Rising professional and patient expectations

In addition to the macro problems listed above, Gray identifies the following eight problems that can be found in any health-care service:

1. Errors and mistakes
2. Poor-quality health care
3. Waste of resources
4. Variation in policy and practice
5. Patients' poor experience with health care
6. Overenthusiastic adoption of interventions of low value
7. Failure to find evidence and to put new interventions of high value into practice
8. Failure to manage ignorance and uncertainty (pp. 1–2)

He goes on to state, "In order to meet these powerful challenges, the principles of **evidence-based health care** can be applied to great effect, regardless of whether a health service is organized nationally (as in the United Kingdom [UK]), or by province (as in Canada) whether it is tax-based or insurance based (as in Japan), or whether the main source of funding is public or private (as in the USA)" (p. 3). Gray suggests the practice of evidence-based health care can have a great impact on some of the aforementioned challenges in any health-care delivery system.

The next section addresses how governmental policy influences health-care quality, safety, and practice, and the relationship to evidence-based health care.

Returning to this chapter's clinical story, Winnifred believes she understands the definition of *public policy* and its relationship to health care. She thinks she can give a good elemental description of the health-care delivery system in the United States and compare it to at least two international health-care systems. She also understands the structure of regulatory responsibility and now feels ready to tackle what she sees as the influence of government policy on quality, safety, and practice. She is beginning to see how larger systems and government policy can affect individual nurse practice.

The Influence of Governmental Policy on Health-Care Quality, Safety, and Practice: Why Evidence-Based Health Care?

There is great interest in evidence-based health care from both the private and public sectors because there is increasing concern about high cost, poor quality, and waste of resources. The imperative for evidence-based health care is more formalized and more embedded into public health-care policy in some countries than it is in others. For instance, the United Kingdom has taken a systematic approach to quality improvement in the National Health Service (NHS). Through formal public policy, the boards of NHS organizations have a duty to ensure the quality of health care is improved. To reach this goal, it has created new organizations such as the **National Institute for Health and Clinical Excellence (NICE), National Service Framework (NSF),** and the **Health Care Commission** (Craig & Smith, 2007). Box 15■5 summarizes the NHF quality assurance structure.

> BOX 15▪5 **The Roles of the Organizations That Make Up the United Kingdom's Quality Structure**
>
> ▪ **National Institute for Health and Clinical Excellence (NICE)** is an independent organization responsible for providing national guidance on promoting good health and preventing and treating ill health. NICE develops and defines the standards of health care that people can expect to receive. These standards will indicate when a clinical treatment (or set of clinical procedures) is considered highly effective, cost effective, and safe as well as being viewed as a positive experience by patients. (http://www.nice.org.uk)
>
> ▪ **National Service frameworks (NSFs)** and strategies set clear quality requirements for care. These are based on the best available evidence of what treatments and services work most effectively for patients. (htt://www.nhs.uk/nhsengland/nsf/)
>
> ▪ **Health Care Commission** regulates care provided by the NHS, local authorities, private companies, and voluntary organizations. It aims to make sure better care is provided for everyone—in hospitals, care centers, and private homes. It seeks to protect the interests of people whose rights are restricted under the Mental Health Act. (http//www.cqc.org.uk)

In the United States, there are several agencies that recognize the value of evidence-based practice in improving health-care quality and safety. The **Agency for Healthcare Research and Quality (AHRQ)** is one of the subdivisions of HHS, and its mission is to improve the quality, safety, efficiency, and effectiveness of health care for all Americans. AHRQ launched an initiative to promote evidence-based practice in everyday care through the establishment of 12 evidence-based practice centers (EPCs). The EPCs develop evidence reports and technology assessments on topics relevant to clinical, social science/behavioral, and economic areas, as well as other health-care organization and delivery issues—specifically issues that are common, expensive, and/or significant for the Medicare and Medicaid populations. With this program, AHRQ became a "science partner" of private and public organizations in an effort "to improve the quality, effectiveness, and appropriateness of health care" by synthesizing the evidence and facilitating the translation of evidence-based research findings (http://www.ahrq.gov/).

In an attempt to improve patient safety and control cost, the **Centers for Medicare & Medicaid Services (CMS)** recently implemented policies that attached reimbursement ramifications for facilities when patients experience certain secondary **hospital-acquired conditions (HACs).** Medicare does not want to pay for medical complications that are the result of errors. Section 5001(c) of the Deficit Reduction Act of 2005 required the secretary of the Department of Health and Human Services to identify conditions that are (a) high-cost or high-volume or both, (b) result in the assignment of a case to a drug-related group that has a higher payment when present as a secondary diagnosis, and (c) could reasonably have been prevented through the application of evidence-based guidelines.

On July 31, 2008, in the *Inpatient Prospective Payment System (IPPS) 2009, Final Rule*, CMS included 10 categories of conditions that were selected for the hospital acquired conditions (HAC) payment provision (http://www.cms.gov/HospitalAcqCond/06_Hospital-Acquired_Conditions.asp#To). See Box 15■6 for the current list of hospital-acquired conditions.

BOX 15■6   Current CMS List of Hospital-Acquired Conditions

1. Foreign Object Retained After Surgery
2. Air Embolism
3. Blood Incompatibility
4. Stage III and IV Pressure Ulcers
5. Falls and Trauma
   - Fractures
   - Dislocations
   - Intracranial Injuries
   - Crushing Injuries
   - Burns
   - Electric Shock
6. Manifestations of Poor Glycemic Control
   - Diabetic Ketoacidosis
   - Nonketotic Hyperosmolar Coma
   - Hypoglycemic Coma
   - Secondary Diabetes with Ketoacidosis
   - Secondary Diabetes with Hyperosmolarity
7. Catheter-Associated Urinary Tract Infection (UTI)
8. Vascular Catheter-Associated Infection
9. Surgical Site Infection Following:
   - Coronary Artery Bypass Graft (CABG) - Mediastinitis
   - Bariatric Surgery
     - Laparoscopic Gastric Bypass
     - Gastroenterostomy
     - Laparoscopic Gastric Restrictive Surgery
   - Orthopedic Procedures
     - Spine
     - Neck
     - Shoulder
     - Elbow
10. Deep Vein Thrombosis (DVT)/Pulmonary Embolism (PE)
    - Total Knee Replacement

Source: U.S. Department of Health and Human Services, Centers for Medicare and Medicaid Services, *Hospital-Acquired Conditions,* http://www.cms.gov/HospitalAcqCond/06_Hospital-Acquired_Conditions.asp#Top

Never events are extremely serious, preventable patient safety incidents that should not occur if the relevant evidence-based practice measures are in place. The **National Quality Forum (NQF)** has identified 28 incidents that qualify as never events; these are listed in Box 15■7. These incidents are very serious and costly from both a personal and fiscal perspective because people can and often do die from them. In 2007 (enacted October 2008), the CMS announced it would not reimburse the extra costs for complications caused by serious error. This is another example in which governmental policy influences clinical decision making and practice.

The Role of Accrediting Agencies

Accreditation of health-care organizations is technically voluntary. However, reimbursement by some entities, such as Medicare and Medicaid, requires organizations

---

BOX 15■7 Current List of Centers for Medicare & Medicare Services Never Events

1. Wrong site surgery (existing)
2. Wrong implant/prosthesis (new)
3. Retained foreign object post-operation (existing)
4. Wrongly prepared high-risk injectable medication (new)
5. Maladministration of potassium-containing solutions (modified)
6. Wrong route administration of chemotherapy (existing)
7. Wrong route administration of oral/enteral treatment (new)
8. Intravenous administration of epidural medication (new)
9. Maladministration of insulin (new)
10. Overdose of midazolam during conscious sedation (new)
11. Opioid overdose of an opioid-naïve patient (new)
12. Inappropriate administration of daily oral methotrexate (new)
13. Suicide using non-collapsible rails (existing)
14. Escape of a transferred prisoner (existing)
15. Falls from unrestricted windows (new)
16. Entrapment in bedrails (new)
17. Transfusion of ABO-incompatible blood components (new)
18. Transplantation of ABO or HLA-incompatible organs (new)
19. Misplaced naso- or oro-gastric tubes (modified)
20. Wrong gas administered (new)
21. Failure to monitor and respond to oxygen saturation (new)
22. Air embolism (new)
23. Misidentification of patients (new)
24. Severe scalding of patients (new)
25. Maternal death due to postpartum hemorrhage after elective caesarean section (modified)

Source: National Quality Forum (http://www.qualityforum.org) and U.S. Department of Health and Human Services, Agency for Healthcare Research and Quality (AHRQ) (http://www.ahrq.gov/)

to be accredited. Therefore, if an organization wishes to be paid by Medicare and Medicaid, it must seek accreditation. Accrediting agencies set certain standards and then evaluate the organization through a process of review to determine if the organization meets those standards. Although not the only accreditation organization, the **Joint Commission (JC)** is the agency of this chapter's focus. The Joint Commission is an independent, not-for-profit organization that accredits and certifies more than 18,000 health-care organizations and programs in the United States. An accreditation or certification from the Joint Commission represents quality health care and recognition of the organization's commitment to meeting certain performance standards. Its mission, in collaboration with other stakeholders, is to continuously improve health care for the public by evaluating health-care organizations and inspiring them to excel in providing safe and effective care of the highest quality and value. (http://www.jointcommission.org/)

Each year the JC releases the **Joint Commission Patient Safety Goals (NPSGs).** The 2011 NPSGs are readily found on the JC Web site and include the following categories:

- Ambulatory health care
- Behavioral health care
- Critical access hospital
- Home care
- Hospital care
- Laboratory services
- Long-term care
- Medicare and Medicaid
- Office-based surgery

NPSGs are discussed later in the chapter.

The JC also developed a set of care processes called the **core measures.** The core measures were developed from a set of quality indicators defined by the CMS. The purpose of the core measures is to help institutions improve quality of patient care by focusing on outcomes. Although the core measures tend to be medically centered as opposed to nurse sensitive, the job of monitoring the measure often falls to nurses.

The role of government influence in health-care quality, safety, and practice is somewhat of a "carrot and stick" story. Public governmental policy can be influential in the use of an evidence-based practice model across a large spectrum of health-care agencies by using the "stick" of denied reimbursement and the "carrot" of incentives. The threat of delivering care that will not be reimbursed causes many organizations to pay attention, and the incentives keep that attention. Conversely, when there is not a "stick" and only a few "carrots" to go around, the influence of policy on practice diminishes. This means that some policies, even if based on solid evidence, are sometimes slow to trickle down or be embraced by the practice community.

In the clinical story, the last part of Winnifred's paper must provide an example of a potential clinical problem targeted by government policy that has safety and cost implications. She needs to explain the significance of the problem and also how she is going to use evidence-based knowledge to address it. She begins by looking at the CMS Web site to see the current list of HACs. She easily finds the list, and after some consideration, she chooses "surgical site infections, post orthopedic surgery," as her clinical problem (see Box 15■6 for a review of HACs). The rationale for her choice is both personal and academic; her grandmother suffered a surgical site infection after hip replacement surgery in which the cost in pain and suffering was high and she knows hospital acquired infections should be preventable. Most important, she wants to know how she can ensure that her own nursing actions are based on the best available evidence and safe.

To learn more about the prevention of surgical site infection, Winifred decides to search the Web sites of the governmental and accrediting agencies that address this safety problem. She already knows that the CMS has identified surgical site infection after orthopedic procedures as a HAC. She also knows this condition has reimbursement ramifications because of that HAC designation. In looking at the NPSGs for 2011 from the Joint Commission, Winnifred notes that "prevention of hospital infection" is one of its safety goals as well. However, the JC safety goals address hospital acquired infections in general, whereas the CMS addresses surgical site infection specifically. She decides to stick with surgical site infection and theorizes how she would approach this problem in an actual clinical situation.

After reading the clinical guidelines for prevention of surgical site infection, she realizes she will not be able to address all of the recommendations found in the CDC guideline because they are extensive. For this particular project, she decides to narrow her scope to just one of the recommendations. She feels she can adequately illustrate how a government regulation can influence individual practice by following through with this one recommendation. She chooses recommendation 3b: Postoperative Incision Care. This recommendation states, "Wash hands before and after changing dressings and any contact with the surgical site" (CDC, 1999).

When you decide to address a clinical problem, you must first define the dimensions of the problems, as Winnifred's situation illustrates. For example, if you are concerned there is poor compliance to the hand hygiene policy or if there is a high rate of surgical site infections in your unit, you might decide to launch a hand hygiene and glove compliance intervention program. How would you do that? A good place to start would be the **Institute for Healthcare Improvement (IHI).** This organization offers a publication, "How-To Guide: Improving Hand Hygiene" (2002). This guide was developed in conjunction with the CDC, the Society of Healthcare Epidemiology of America, and the Association for Professionals in Infection Control and Epidemiology, and it provides a tool kit to implement such a program. Box 15■8 summarizes some of the recommendations. (The full program is part of the public domain and readily available at the IHI Web site.)

A part of any program (such as the one from the IHI) is data collection and analysis. Data are gathered to assess the extent of the problem and to measure improvement after implementation. Data are also gathered from the stakeholders as the program is being implemented, to assess the process. Once you have analyzed the various types of data, you can search the literature to see if there are clinical guidelines based on the best available evidence that could inform you on the best way to frame a plan for implementing quality improvement measures and ultimately monitoring improvements.

BOX 15■8   **Approaches to Developing a Hand Hygiene and Glove Intervention Program**

- Give a diverse group of personnel a stake in the process, gather a multidisciplinary team, including physicians and administrators who can help remove barriers to implementation.
- Assess current practice and compliance.
- Perform a survey to determine hand hygiene and glove compliance rates. Determine how these rates compare to those in the literature.
- Set clear aims and time-specific improvement targets. Set the bar high.
- Allocate adequate resources and personnel to achieve target levels.
- Establish measures that will indicate whether changes are leading to improvement.
- Organize an educational program that teaches the core principles and hand hygiene and glove practice to clinical staff throughout the hospital.
- Assess satisfaction with current hand hygiene products.
- If alcohol-based hand products are not used by the hospital, have a select group of nurses and physicians test two or three products. Poorly functioning dispensers do not improve compliance.
- Introduce program to entire staff and have team members visit the units to answer questions.
- Provide a patient safety tip sheet for staff and families.
- Use measurement tools to monitor compliance.

Institute for Healthcare Improvement (http://www.IHI.org).

In the case of hand hygiene compliance, the CDC and **World Health Organization (WHO)** have well-established, evidence-based guidelines on hand hygiene. Box 15■9 provides the links to both the CDC and WHO hand hygiene recommendtions, with explanations about the levels of evidence that informed the guidelines.

The best available evidence should guide the implementation and evaluation of any program meant to improve hand hygiene compliance in hospital staff

BOX 15■9   **Links to the Centers for Disease Control and Prevention and World Health Organization Hand Hygiene Recommendations**

WHO I The evidence for clean hands
http://www.who.int/gpsc/country_work/en/
CDC I Guideline for Hand Hygiene in Health-Care Settings
http://www.cdc.gov/mmwr/pdf/rr/rr5116.pdf
CDC I Hand Hygiene in Healthcare Settings
http://www.cdc.gov/handhygiene/

(Box 15■10). The IHI program was developed in part from the recommendations of the CDC. However, other considerations will enter into your decision making. Factors such as context, available resources, personal knowledge of the institution, facility limitations, and geographic location all must be considered in your planning.

■ Summary

By completing this project, Winnifred has learned the way public policy is made and how it influences health-care quality, safety, and practice. Of course, this influence varies somewhat according to the structure of the health-care delivery system. In the UK, for instance, the government (as the single payer in a single-payer system) has great influence on health-care practice. Conversely, the U.S. government (as part of a multipayer system) exerts influence on only a part of the health-care system. The influence often comes in the form of reimbursement ramifications or incentives, the reason that public policy is able to influence change that trickles down to the individual practice level. For example, a nurse who practices poor hand hygiene has the potential to increase the rate of surgical site infections in the institution; the individual practice of the nurse has become part of the institution's noncompliance with the policy or standard. This, in turn, has both cost and accreditation ramifications for the institution. Hopefully, this example never happens, and the nurse, aware of the evidence-based guidelines for hand hygiene, adheres to those guidelines and, through her individual practice, increases the potential for a safe patient outcome.

Finally, Winnifred recognizes that despite the differences, all health-care systems experience some of the same problems centered on issues of affordability, cost, quality, safety, and continuous improvement and monitoring (Box 15■11). There is growing global interest in evidence-based health- care as a way to address these concerns. This stems from the belief that use of the best available evidence will reduce errors, increase quality and safety, and result in better patient outcomes, while ultimately reducing both personal and fiscal costs.

BOX 15■10 Interdisciplinary Rounds

■ Pretend that you are responsible for putting a team together to plan and implement a hand hygiene program. How would you go about it? Who would you ask and why? What type of characteristics would you want the members of the team to have?

■ You are implementing a hand hygiene program and some of the physicians are not cooperating. What type of actions would you take to convince them of the value of the program?

■ What type of prompts would you design to remind everyone who enters the room to wash their hands?

BOX 15■11   **Tools for Learning and Practice**

- Go the CDC Web site and locate the available tools to implement a hand hygiene program.
- Using CINAHL and MEDLINE search for evidence on hand hygiene. See if you can find a systematic review.
- Go to the CDC Web site and sign up to be on their e-mail list.

CHAPTER QUESTIONS

1. Explain the process by which a policy is enacted into law.

2. Compare and contrast the U.S health-care system with one other health-care system.

3. Analyze the difference between single-payer systems and multipayer systems. Make an argument in favor of one over the other.

4. Explain the role of the Department of Health and Human Services (HHS) in regulating health-care quality.

5. What is the mission of the Agency for Healthcare Research and Quality (AHRQ), and how is it connected to evidence-based practice?

6. In your opinion, what should be the role of government in controlling quality and safety in health care?

7. Write a one-page paper explaining briefly the relationship of evidence-based practice to health-care quality and safety.

References

Agency for Healthcare Quality and Research. http://www.ahrq.gov/

Buse, K., Mays, N., & Watt, G. (2005). *Making health policy.* Maidenhead, UK: Open University Press.

Centers for Disease Control and Prevention. http://www.cdc.gov

Craig, J., & Smith, R. (2007). *The evidence based practice manual for nurses* (2nd ed.). London: Churchill Livingston Elsevier.

Davis, K., Schoen, C., Schoenbaum, S., et al. (2007). Mirror mirror on the wall: An international update on the comparative performance of American health care. The Commonwealth Fund.

Department of Health and Human Services. Medicare program; changes to the hospital inpatient prospective payment systems and fiscal year 2009 rates. Fed Regist: 2008;73:4843.

Dye, T. R. (1995). *Understanding public policy.* Englewood Cliffs, NJ: Prentice Hall.

Gray, M. (2009). *Evidence based health care and public health* (3rd ed.). London: Churchill Livingston Elsevier.

Inpatient Prospective Payment System (IPPS) 2009, Final Rule. Retrieved from (http://www.cms.gov/HospitalAcqCond/06_Hospital-Acquired_Conditions.asp#

Institute for Healthcare Improvement. http://www.IHI.org.

Institute of Medicine of the National Academy of Science. (2004). Insuring America's health: Principles and recommendations. Retrieved from www.iom.edu/.../Insuring-Americas-Health-Principles-and-Recommendations.aspx

Johnson, A. (2010). Recession swells number of uninsured to 50.7 million. *The Wall Street Journal,* p. A4. Retrieved from milliohttp://online.wsj.com/article/SB100014240527487043947045754960933 63948142.html

Kirpatrick. D., (2000). Definitions of Public Policy and the Law. Retrieved from www.musc.edu/vawprevention/policy/definition.shtml

Kaiser Commission on Medicaid and the Uninsured/Urban Institute Analysis of March, 2010. CPS. Retrieved from http://facts.kff.org/

Kaiser Commission on Medicaid and the Uninsured/Urban Institute Analysis. (2010). The uninsured and the difference health care insurance makes. Retrieved from http://facts.kff.org/

Martin, P. (2009). Health care profiteers: A billion dollar lobby. Retrieved from www.wsws.prg.

National Forum. http://www.nationalforum.org

Reid, T. R. (2010). *The healing of America: A global quest for better, cheaper and fairer health care.* New York: Penguin Press.

U.S. Census Report. (2009). Income, poverty and health insurance coverage in the U.S., 22–28.

U.S. Department of Health and Human Services. (n.d.). http://ASPE.hhs.gov/

Walt, G. (1994). *Health policy: An introduction to process and power.* London: Zed Books.

CHAPTER 16

Assess and Evaluate
Outcome Measurement and Revision of Plan

Michelle Block

LEARNING OBJECTIVES

- Describe process of using benchmarks in measuring outcomes.
- Identify organizations related to health-care quality that will assist in identifying benchmarks.
- Develop a plan for outcomes measurement within your institution.
- Examine the team needed to execute the outcomes.

KEY TERMS

Agency for Healthcare Research and Quality (AHRQ)
Benchmarking
Clinical nurse specialist (CNS)
Data
Institute for Healthcare Improvement (IHI)

Nurse-sensitive indicators
Nursing-sensitive patient outcomes (NSPOs)
Research knowledge
Review of the literature (ROL)
Standards of nursing practice

Clinical Story

Patricia is a new nurse manager on a medical-surgical unit. To address National Hospital Quality Measures proposed by the Joint Commission (JC), Patricia plans to assess and address the incidence of venous thromboembolism (VTE) on the unit. The presence of VTEs affects financial and human resources as well as the overall quality of patient care. Patricia starts by reviewing the incidence of VTEs on the unit over the past year. In addition, she begins reviewing current literature and national standards on VTE to implement a plan to improve these specific patient outcomes. ∎

Introduction

Evidence-based practice can effectively improve the quality of patient care and related outcomes. Because practice changes rapidly, it is always a challenge to solely incorporate research findings in a timely manner. On average, it takes 17 years for **research knowledge** to be integrated into practice (Balas and Boren, 2000). Therefore, additional sources of clinical knowledge are needed to inform bedside practice. For example, **benchmarking** and evaluating patient outcomes are necessary processes that affect practice and ultimately effect change.

Benchmarking

Benchmarking is a tool that has been used in the business world for many years. The Xerox Corporation used benchmarking in the 1970s to improve systemwide performance and implement the use of best practice in their industry (Tran, 2003). Benchmarking, also referred to as "standard setting," means the level of cost for a particular product (Rudy, Lucke, Whitman, et al., 2001). However, in health care, it is also related to quality care and best practices. The purpose of benchmarking is to establish a level of quality that can then be used to judge high-quality care. The focus on cost containment does not compromise care provided to the patient; rather, the idea is to save money while providing quality care to each patient.

Health-care officials can measure indicators of quality care in the following ways: actual cost, length of stay (LOS), complications, delays in recovery, and function status. To establish a benchmark in a given area, some type of comparison criteria must be identified. For example, in a clinical setting, **standards of nursing practice** are used to compare "what is" to "what ought to be." Benchmarking is a continuous and systematic process.

Establishing Benchmarks

There are many methods of establishing benchmarks, including cost, review of the literature, standards of care, imposed levels of care, hospital-specific, system-wide, problem-based, process-related, and performance-related. Often, multiple methods are used at the same time. Several of these methods are discussed below.

Because of increasing economic burden, cost containment has become even more important to long-term survival of health-care organizations. In addition to cost containment, there is an increasing need to prevent costs incurred from preventable complications. Avoidable complications increase hospital length of stay and related economic burden. Finally, attention must be given to third-party reimbursement. Benchmark data show how well an organization is meeting performance standards. The level of performance directly affects reimbursement from third-party payers (Brown and Golden, 2008). It literally pays to meet high performance standards.

A **review of the literature (ROL)** encompasses a strategic search for current knowledge on a given subject. You can search all literature on a specific topic to find out what has been published on the subject. Depending on the focus, your search may include multiple databases within multiple disciplines, and your search results may include informational articles, research findings, and theoretical papers. Published research is an example of previously generated knowledge—knowledge that is useful for setting benchmarks. For example, Rudy et al. (2001) outline how an ROL examining central line infections was used to establish a benchmark. The authors reviewed three published studies to draw a conclusion regarding central line infection occurrence. From this review, they established a benchmark. However, a benchmark is only as good as the accuracy and consistency in overall reporting. When using a review of the literature method, it is imperative that the authors carefully choose appropriate studies.

Benchmarking and the Nursing Process

Standards of nursing practice directly relate to nursing activities you carry out through the nursing process. This involves assessment, planning, implementation, and evaluation. As discussed in previous chapters, the nursing process is the basis for clinical decision making and drives all aspects of patient care. Standards of nursing practice are defined as "a set of guidelines for providing high-quality nursing care and criteria for evaluating care. Such guidelines help assure patients that they are receiving high-quality care" (Mosby's Medical Dictionary, 2009). Established standards are often recommended by professional organizations, working groups, state boards of nursing, and other overseeing governing bodies.

Imposed levels of care are those that strongly urge a standard for patient safety. If the suggested standard is not met, a payer may withhold reimbursement. In the United States, the Joint Commission proposed the idea of sentinel or never events, events that should never happen during a hospitalization (Agency for Healthcare Research and Quality, 2008). For example, a gross medication error such as giving the wrong medications to a patient that results in harm to that patient is considered a never event. If one of these events does happen, the facility will not be reimbursed for the costs incurred to treat the event as a penalty (Brown, Donaldson, Bolton, et al., 2010). In this case, physicians would treat the patient for the adverse effect of the medication, but the hospital would incur the cost of treating the complication. Obviously the idea of never events is to protect the patient, but the use of a pay-for-performance system acts as a greater motivator for facilities to meet safety standards and benchmarks of quality while adding financial impact.

Hospital-specific benchmarking occurs when a hospital assumes the risk of a given problem based on the numbers of exposure or line days. For example, Rudy et al. (2001) explain the process as it relates to central line infections. A hospital assumes the risk of a patient developing a central line infection based solely on the number of days the person has the central line. In addition, the hospital uses a mathematical formula to formulate intervals (benchmarks) once the incidence data are collected. The staff then plots the predicted intervals and the actual data to see if the actual data fall within the projected benchmarks.

These outline methods demonstrate the different methods that institutions use to set benchmarks. Benchmarking is part of the process to achieve outcomes (Box 16■1). No matter what outcome is chosen as the focus, the end result is meant to be the same: quality care provided to the patient.

Measuring Outcomes

Measuring outcomes in the clinical arena is important to understand the effects of an intervention or healthcare practices (Agency for Healthcare Research and Quality, 2008). Moreover, measuring outcomes can also reduce variability in practice (Deaton and Weintraub, 2002). For example, if a certain protocol is highly effective in preventing ventilator-associated pneumonia, it makes sense to use that protocol, thereby reducing variability in practice.

More recently, attention has turned to areas that measure how nurses function. These are called nursing process measures. In fact, the Institute of Medicine Committee on Quality Healthcare (2001) stated that intervention and outcome measures are integral to understanding the contribution nurses make to quality care. In turn, this understanding helps to establish **nursing-sensitive patient outcomes (NSPOs),** which confirm nurses' contributions to patient care in areas such as quality of life, symptom management, safety, functional status, and utilization of nursing resources (Given and Sherwood, 2005).

Outcomes can be examined from different perspectives (Box 16■2). For example, you can categorize outcomes as care-related, patient-related, and performance-related

---

BOX 16■1 **Why Is Outcome Measurement Important?**

- Cost containment
- Financial reimbursement from third-party payers
- Maintenance of managed care contracts
- Increased quality
- Enhanced patient safety
- Increased patient satisfaction
- Identification of staff training needs
- Validation that existing policies and procedures are on target

---

BOX 16▪2   **Common Foci for Clinical Outcomes**

- Urinary tract infections (UTIs)
- Patient falls
- Medication errors
- Venous thromboemboli (VTEs) and pulmonary emboli (PE)
- Pressure ulcers
- Central line infections (CLI)
- Hospital-acquired pneumonia
- Ventilator-associated pneumonia (VAP)
- Bloodstream infections/septicemia
- Nursing process measures: hand washing, wound dressings, adherence to care pathways/protocols, systematic skin inspections, and turning

---

(Kleinpell, 2001). The differences between these types using VTE and this chapter's clinical story are discussed below. Care-related outcomes focus on direct care provided to the patient. Therefore, the rate of VTE occurrence during a hospitalization is a care-related outcome. In contrast, patient knowledge regarding ambulation to prevent VTE is an example of a patient-related outcome. Finally, measuring a nurse's compliance to following best practice guidelines to prevent VTE is considered a performance-related outcome.

Ask/Assess

Patricia recognizes that every reported VTE could mean a longer LOS and potential complications, such as pulmonary embolism and death. In addition, there will be increased cost to the hospital, patient, and third-party payer(s). Patricia needs to create an effective and practical plan to improve patient outcomes on her unit.

Patricia begins to gather information to structure the overall project. She examines the **Agency for Healthcare Research and Quality (AHRQ)** Web site and finds information on VTE. She creates an information sheet on basic information related to VTE. On the sheet, she notes that VTE is considered one of the most preventable causes of death that occurs in the hospital (Heit, O'Fallon, Petterson, et al., 2002). In addition, Patricia identifies quality approaches to prevent VTE in hospitalized patients.

Next, Patricia communicates this cursory information and project idea to the chief nursing officer (CNO) and chief nursing executive (CNE) of the facility. Communication within an organization is important, and it is important to gain organizational support for the project (Tran, 2003). In addition, Patricia also informs the executives she intends to share the results with other units once the project is completed. Thus, any change on her unit will affect practice and outcomes on other units.

Once she has administrative approval, Patricia needs to educate the unit staff about the project. Patricia plans meetings so that staff on each of the shifts can learn about the undertaking. Because staff involvement is important to the overall success and integration of the project, conveying the reasons for improving this patient outcome is particularly helpful with staff acceptance of the project. Careful planning will help to ensure the success of the project.

Acquire/Diagnose

The first step in measuring outcomes is identifying a clinical problem; in this case: VTE. How does Patricia even know it is a problem? She is aware of the initiatives based on the National Quality Measures from the Joint Commission. In addition, a more extensive ROL reveals the breadth of problem. AHRQ (2008) reported that inpatient costs for persons with VTE are estimated to be as high as $10,000.00. In addition, approximately 1 in 10 of those who develop VTE will die from resulting pulmonary emboli. It makes sense to examine ways to reduce the incidence of VTE as it is a preventable problem.

Patricia also examines all available literature, including empirical studies, information articles, and national guidelines related to VTE. She quickly realizes there are inherent challenges in VTE prevention. Contributing variables are complex and can change during each hospitalization (White, 2003). In addition, successful prevention requires a multidisciplinary approach.

Patricia knows the data she must collect for this project will come from various sources. **Data** are facts that are collected for discussion or calculation, or for drawing conclusions (Encarta Dictionary, 2011). Patricia wonders how many VTEs occur on her unit. Data gathered on her unit are considered local data, whereas data available from databases and combined outside sources are national data. To collect unit data, she decides to conduct a chart audit for the past year. She determines this is the most efficient way to examine the occurrences of VTE under current patient care protocols. She enlists the help of the unit **clinical nurse specialist (CNS)** to review charts. Together they determine that 74 inpatients developed VTE during the past year. To put this number into perspective, Patricia needs to examine national data.

How often does VTE occur in other institutions? National data on VTE should give Patricia that information. However, Patricia is disappointed to find there is not an abundance of data to compare with. For example, White (2003) reported that VTE occurs on ~100 persons per 100,000 people each year in the United States. However, because several variables such as age, gender, race/ethnicity, risk factors, seasonal variation, acute and/or chronic illness, and comorbidities influence overall risk, it is difficult to determine the average number of VTEs for hospitalized patients. Therefore, Patricia opts to call some colleagues in nearby hospital systems to see if they are tracking VTE incidence. Using this information, she can ascertain what other units/institutions are doing to combat this potentially deadly issue. In talking with a colleague, she is told to check the Web site for **Institute for Healthcare Improvement (IHI).** This Web site does, in fact, have data to review from institutions of different sizes. However, the data are given in terms of problem reduction since a program was put in place to decrease VTE.

Patricia reviews unit policies and procedures, and she is surprised to find there is no established protocol for prevention of VTE. Aside from providing the usual and customary care to prevent pressure ulcers and post-operative complications, she finds nothing specific for VTE. Patricia is disheartened, but believes if she finds the right resources, she will be able to build an appropriate VTE prevention program.

Until now, Patricia was unaware of how much information is available to help her plan this project. There are a variety of Web sites related to health-care quality that are useful when planning to benchmark and measure outcomes in the clinical setting. Each one provides rich resources to improve patient outcomes (Table 16■1).

Appraise/Plan

Based on the literature, Patricia realizes that although putting a VTE prevention program in place will be challenging, existing guidelines and resources provide a usable framework to attain goals and create measurable outcomes. Patricia once again returns to searching for appropriate resources. She comes across several options.

Patricia returns to the IHI Web site and finds that many of the institutions listed are available to mentor others in areas of patient safety such as fall prevention, surgical complications, governance and improvement, and VTE, to name a few. Mentor names and contact information are available to Web-site visitors. This is a viable option to assist her to develop a nurse-driven prevention plan.

Another option is to adopt a ready-made package that addresses VTE prevention and treatment. For example, Zierler, Wittkowsky, Peterson, et al. (2008) used a multidisciplinary approach to develop a Venous Thromboembolism Safety Toolkit. The intent of the toolkit is to implement a systems-based method to intervene for those at risk for or those with VTE. The educational program includes both multidisciplinary health-care providers as well as patients. This comprehensive system is supported by AHRQ. There are 10 evidence-based components focused on preventing, diagnosing, treating, and educating patients and health-care providers about VTE. The toolkit is easily accessible and available free of charge. Patricia first notices that the materials are multidisciplinary. Because the toolkit has components

Table 16■1   **Organizations Related to Health-Care Quality**

Organization	Web Site
Agency for Healthcare and Research (AHRQ)	http://www.ahrq.gov
American Nurses Association (ANA)	http://www.nursingworld.org
American Society for Quality (ASQ)	http://www.asq.org
Institute for Healthcare Improvement (IHI)	http://www.ihi.org
Joint Commission	http://www.jointcommission.org
National Database for Nursing Quality Indicators (NDNQI)	http://www.nursingquality.org
National Quality Forum (NQF)	http://www.qualityforum.org

that are more appropriate for physicians or prescribing advanced practice RNs, Patricia needs to review all pieces to determine the appropriate nursing resources that will be most useful to implement in her project.

Finally, national organizations such as AHRQ, American Association of Critical Care Nurses (AACN), and Oncology Nurses Association (ONA) also provide background and literature that address VTE. Although some information is geared more toward a specialty area, other information is broad in scope and applicable to many areas of practice.

After considering her options, Patricia decides to combine them for this initial project. Her reasoning is that the first stage is going to be largely nurse-driven. Therefore, she focuses on implementing nursing interventions, or **nurse-sensitive indicators.** Another step Patricia must contemplate is whether to implement a screening checklist for nurses to use on each patient admission. Although it would be a good idea for all patients to be assessed for risk, it also means more paperwork for the nurses. Patricia reviews more literature on the use of checklists and finds that many institutions treat all patients admitted as high risk and does not spend the time or money to implement a checklist approach to VTE prevention. Patricia decides this approach would fit her unit and institution best. Instead of putting extra time into screening, she takes the approach to expend more effort into preventing VTE occurrence.

Based on these factors, Patricia realizes it is time to put the plan into action. She reviews the steps of her plan which include the following: (1) set up meetings with nursing and medical staff; (2) institute prevention program on all patients; (3) collect monthly data on VTE occurrence; (4) compare data collected using the prevention program to the previous year's occurrence numbers; and (5) reevaluate the prevention program.

Apply/Implement

Careful planning leads to successful implementation of any project. Reflecting on her checklist, Patricia sets the project in motion by setting up times to meet with nursing and medical staff. In each of the meetings, she provides information about the cost to treat VTE and the very real need to implement a plan to affect the number of VTEs occurring on the unit. Patricia emphasizes that all patients are to be addressed as at risk. Patricia also sets a 1-year time line for the project. This allows her to compare results for the previous year to determine if the new interventions have had a positive impact on the incidence of VTEs. However, she will also watch monthly trends; the previous year averaged out to approximately six VTEs per month.

During the meetings, Patricia outlines the role each person has in the project. Staff nurses will be implementing either sequential compression devices (SCDs) or anti-embolism hose on every patient. In addition, nurses will be responsible to document teaching regarding early ambulation and monitoring of patient ambulation.

The goal is to ambulate patients as early as possible with a minimum time of once per shift. In addition, the nurses will also check their patient charts to make sure a primary care provider has addressed VTE prevention from their perspective. These data will be tracked on a sheet each shift. The primary care providers will be asked to assess their patients for appropriate pharmacological intervention based on assessed risk. It will be their responsibility to communicate treatment through the use of orders. The charge nurses for each shift will be responsible to collect the shift data and put them in the manager's mailbox. Both the manager and the clinical nurse specialist will compile and track the data monthly on a spreadsheet.

After Patricia's plan goes into effect, data collected from the first month indicate six VTEs have occurred. However, in the second month, only four VTEs occurred. Although it appears that the vigilance with VTE prevention is making a difference, it may be too soon to tell. After 6 months, it is clear that the number of VTEs has decreased. Data reveal that in 6 months, only 26 VTEs have occurred. That means, on average, 4.3 VTEs occur per month, a decrease of almost 2 VTEs per month. Patricia relays this information to the staff.

Although only 6 months of data have been collected, it is important for Patricia to relay the results of the project at this time. In addition, it is helpful for her to get feedback from the nursing and medical staff to better understand the project from their roles. The nursing staff, overall, feels their responsibilities have been "folded in" to their routine at the bedside. As with anything else, it took time to get used to collecting the data.

However, one important piece of information emerges from Patricia's discussion with the staff: patients who transfer out of their unit to other intermediate care units (IMCUs) or intensive care units (ICUs) are no longer tracked. The nurses no longer follow their data and the patients do not always return to this unit. Patricia realizes this may be a source of lost data. Primary care providers report their routine has remained the same, although they are more vigilant regarding patients who may be at greater risk for VTE. Patricia decides to move forward using the same protocols. At this time, with positive results, there is no need to change what the staff is doing.

As the remaining 6 months tick by, the number of VTEs continues to remain lower than the previous year. The CNS compiles a monthly occurrence spreadsheet for the entire year. At the end of the year, the total number of VTEs is at 38, which is a 51% decrease in overall occurrence. Patricia plans to share the results with the CNO and the staff. It is very exciting to see that focused attention to prevention of VTE had such a large payoff. The outcome was successful and the results were positive.

Despite the success, it is still important to review the plan and make revisions if they are warranted (Box 16■3). For example, Patricia decides to track the number of patients who are transferred from the unit. In addition, she is working to obtain nursing input regarding ideas to streamline the process. Although there has been a decrease in VTE occurrence, it is necessary to continue to track this outcome. The overall plan for prevention may need to be changed based on patient differences, new clinical data, and/or new pharmacological measures. Vigilance is the key to maintaining positive trends in outcomes.

BOX 16■3 **Interdisciplinary Rounds**

- Plan a presentation in which you explain the concept of nursing-sensitive patient outcomes (NSPOs) to colleagues from other disciplines.
- Have a brainstorming session with several colleagues and discuss a benchmarking strategy to address an outcomes project.
- Compare and contrast the information for the following on multiple health-care quality Web sites: Hospital-acquired pneumonia and falls.
- Read B. K. Zierler, A. Wittkowsky, G. Peterson, et al., 2008, "Venous Thromboembolism Safety Toolkit: A Systems Approach to Patient Safety," found at http://www.ahrq.gov/qual/nurseshdbk/, and describe their multidisciplinary approach to the development of their tool kit.

■ Summary

Measuring and evaluating outcomes are integral to maintaining quality patient care. It is helpful to identify appropriate benchmarks to plan successful outcomes. Outcome results identify whether a process has made a positive influence in care. No matter the results, the processes will need to be reevaluated; measuring outcomes is a continual process (Box 16■4). This is necessary because health care is a constantly evolving entity influenced by new clinical knowledge, research knowledge, and patient variance.

BOX 16■4 **Tools for Learning and Practice**

- Read B. K. Zierler, A. Wittkowsky, G. Peterson, et al., 2008, "Venous Thromboembolism Safety Toolkit: A Systems Approach to Patient Safety," found at http://www.ahrq.gov/qual/nurseshdbk/. Describe their multidisciplinary approach to the development of their tool kit and discuss its usefulness for nursing practice.
- Identify a nursing practice problem; then search the Internet and see if you can find a standard of care that addresses the problem.

CHAPTER QUESTIONS

1. Explain the process of benchmarking.

2. Describe three ways that indicators of quality of care can be measured.

3. What is the purpose of standards of nursing practice?

4. Where might one find standards of nursing practice?

5. What do nursing-sensitive patient outcomes (NSPOs) confirm?

6. Give an example of a patient-related outcome.

References

Agency for Healthcare Research and Quality. (2008). *Patient safety and quality: An evidence-based handbook for nurses* (AHRQ Publication No. 08-0043). Retrieved from http://www.ahrq.gov/qual/nurseshdbk/

Balas, E. A., & Boren, S. A. (2000). Managing clinical knowledge for healthcare improvements. In V. Schattauer (Ed.), *Yearbook of medical informatics* (pp. 65–70). Stuttgart, Germany: Schattauer.

Brown, D., Donaldson, N., Bolton, L. B., et al. (2010). Nurse-sensitive benchmarks for hospitals to gauge high-reliability performance. *Journal for Healthcare Quality, 32*(6), 9–17.

Brown, P., & Golden, W. (2008). Benchmarking to high performers drives effective improvement. *Journal of the Arkansas Medical Society, 104*(8), 179–180.

Committee on Quality of Health Care in America and Institute of Medicine. Crossing the Quality Chasm: A New Health System for the 21st Century. National Academies Press, July 2001.

Deaton, M. & Weintraub, W. S. (2002). Outcome measurement: Evaluating evidence for managing patients with acute coronary syndromes. *Journal of Cardiovascular Nursing, 16*(4), 71–74.

Encarta. (2011). In *Encyclopædia Britannica*. Retrieved from http://www.britannica.com/EBchecked/topic/186436/Encarta

Farquhar, C. M., Stryer, D., & Slutsky, J. (2002). Translating research into practice: The future ahead. *International Journal for Quality in Health Care, 14*, 233–249.

Fineout-Overholt, E., & Johnston, L. (2006, 4th Quarter). Implementation of evidence: Moving from evidence to action. *Worldviews on Evidence-Based Nursing*, 194–206.

Given, B. A., & Sherwood, P. R. (2005). Nursing sensitive patient outcomes: A white paper. *Oncology Nursing Forum, 32*(4), 773–784.

Heit, J. A., O'Fallon, M., Petterson, T. M., et al. (2002). Relative impact of risk factors for deep vein thrombosis and pulmonary embolism: A population based study. *Archives of Internal Medicine, 162*, 1245–1248.

Joint Commission. (2007). *ORYX noncore measure information*. Retrieved January 12, 2011, from http://www.jointcommission.org/Perfromance Measurement/Performance Measurement. ORYZ+Non-Core+Measure+Information.htm

Kleinpell, R. (2001). Measuring outcomes in advanced practice nursing. In R. Kleinpell (Ed.), *Outcome assessment in advanced practice nursing* (pp. 1–50). New York: Springer.

Mosby's Medical Dictionary, 8th ed. (2009). St. Louis: Mosby.

Pearson, A. (2004). Getting research into practice. *International Journal of Nursing Practice, 10*, 197–198.

Rudy, E., Lucke, J., Whitman, G., & Davidson, L. (2010). Benchmarking patient outcomes. *Journal of Nursing Scholarship, 33*(2), 185–189.

Rycroft-Malone, J. (2008). Evidence-informed practice: From individual to context. *Journal of Nursing Management, 16*, 404–408.

Tran, M. J. (2003). Take benchmarking to the next level: Reach best practice status by heeding operational strengths and weaknesses. *Nursing Management, 34*(1), 19–23.

Wachter, R. M., Foster, N. E., & Dudley, R. A. (2008). Medicare's decision to withhold payment for hospital errors: The devil is in the details. *Joint Commission Journal on Quality and Patient Safety, 34*, 116–123.

White, R. H. (2003). The epidemiology of venous thromboembolism. *Circulation, 107*, I-1–I-5.

Zierler, B. K., Wittkowsky, A., Peterson, G., et al. (2008). Venous thromboembolism safety toolkit: A systems approach to patient safety. Retrieved from http://www.ahrq.gov/qual/nurseshdbk/

Putting It All Together

This unit provides practical examples of evidence-based decision making in specialty nursing areas. Each chapter is structured in a parallel fashion to illustrate how an evidence-based approach can address nurse-sensitive outcomes. Nurse-sensitive outcomes are those that confirm nurses' contributions to patient care in areas such as quality of life, symptom management, safety, functional status, and utilization of nursing resources. The chapters in this unit integrate the evidence based practice process from problem identification to outcome evaluation and quality improvement. The specialty topics that are covered in this unit are medical-surgical nursing, maternal health nursing, nursing of children, mental health nursing, nursing care of the older adult, and community health nursing. Each chapter provides a unique lesson in evidence-based decision making.

CHAPTER 17

Medical-Surgical Nursing

Lisa Hopp

LEARNING OBJECTIVES

- Given an ill-structured description of a common clinical case, apply all phases of the evidence-based practice process to guide decisions related to common medical-surgical nursing problems.

- Analyze the challenges to making evidence-based decisions in complex health-care environments.

- Generate next-step strategies to get better evidence into practice.

KEY TERMS

AGREE tool
Critical Appraisal Skills
    Program (CASP)
Hospital-acquired condition
    (HAC)
Incidence
National Guideline
    Clearinghouse (NGC)

Pay-for-performance
Pressure ulcer
Prevalence
Scale
Scope

Clinical Story

Sara has worked on an adult medical-surgical unit for 2 years. The patient population is a mixture of elderly, chronically ill patients with a variety of acute medical illnesses and general adult surgical patients. She is caring for LH, a 78-year-old female who is 5 days post-thoracotomy for lung cancer. LH was transferred from the intensive care unit to the Sara's unit 2 days ago. When helping LH to bathe, Sara noticed several areas of skin breakdown on her back and sacrum. The wounds on the skin covering her spine look as if a single layer of skin has been torn off, but the wound on her sacrum looks different. Sara observes that it is a shallow, full-thickness crater with a red to pink bed. Although LH walks about 15 feet twice per day and sits in a chair for 15 minutes after her walk, she spends the rest of the day in a standard hospital bed, requiring help to turn. She is still quite weak from her surgery and complicated early recovery, and requires oral pain medication every 4 hours. She is eating only clear liquids, tolerates them poorly, and has a distended abdomen. Sara wonders if there was something else that she and her fellow nurses could have done to prevent the breaks in LH's skin integrity. ■

Introduction

Skin care may seem like a very basic nursing task that does not merit a deep exploration of the evidence to support best practices. However, nurses should not reserve doing the right thing the right way only in complex interventions. Rather, nurses seek the best available evidence to support nursing care decisions and the best possible patient outcomes, regardless of how gripping the concern. In fact, often when you begin to think more about the reasons you do what you do, you find that there is more to understanding the simplest procedures than you had thought.

In this chapter, you will find a blueprint to apply the evidence-based practice process to one medical-surgical problem. To keep the focus sharp and the scenario as straightforward as possible, the chapter addresses only a small portion of the problem.

What Are the Key Issues?

According to international consensus, a **pressure ulcer** is a "localized injury to the skin and/or underlying tissue usually over a bony prominence, as a result of pressure, or pressure in combination with shear" (National Pressure Ulcer Advisory Panel, 2007). This definition provides hints about what a nurse needs to do to pay attention to and prevent pressure ulcers, but it will be the evidence that indicates the correct thing to do.

The evidence-based practice process begins by being curious and skeptical. You can use the nursing paradigm to organize how you think about the care you provide. You need to pay close attention to the patient, his or her state of health, the environment, and the usual nursing care. By assessing and examining each element of the nursing meta-paradigm, you can uncover the key issues related to your decisions. For example, think about how patient and health-related factors of aging enter into your decisions about skin care. Consider the person's ability to move or even shift his or her weight, skin condition, continence, sensory function, nutritional status, or other issues.

Part of thinking about the person is to understand the patient's preferences. For example, some bed surfaces may reduce pressure but the patient may find the surface uncomfortable. Patients have food preferences that can affect how to best meet their nutritional needs. It is important to find out and integrate patients' values, desires, and preferences in the decision-making process.

Next, question how the environment might influence your care. Is anything rubbing the skin to cause friction on the skin such as bed sheets, rails, or a device? What kind of surface is the patient sitting or lying on? Finally, consider how your nursing care can protect or pose a risk to the patient's skin integrity. For example, does the way you assist the patient to move in bed help or hurt? These are all key issues you must consider during the evidence-based practice process.

What Is the Scope and Scale?

When you have a curious attitude and are aware of how and why you make decisions, you can quickly become overwhelmed with the number of questions that underlie even basic nursing care. You can even run the risk of becoming paralyzed with inaction if you spend all of your time thinking rather than doing. That is not the intent of evidence-based nursing practice. Rather, you need thinking to be able to understand the **scope** (how big?) and **scale** (how much?) of the problem.

Scope

When you explore scope, you try to find the edges of the problem to determine its breadth. The "edges" may relate to age or risk groups, disease, functional ability, or even gender. In the case of skin integrity, the edges are very broad: all ages, all degrees of mobility, and risk. However, in this chapter's clinical story Sara can narrow her concern to frail, poorly mobile, elderly patients at high risk for impaired skin integrity because these factors all relate to LH's condition.

The scope of the question determines how you search and what type of evidence you find. For large questions, such as what is the best way to care for any patient at risk for skin breakdown, you are likely to find a clinical practice guideline that addresses many parts of the bigger problem. For smaller questions, such as what is the best bed surface to reduce pressure in at risk older patients, you are likely to find the answer in a systematic review of primary research or as part of a guideline.

Scale

To determine the scale of the problem, you need to determine if your observation is an isolated occurrence or if there is a trend that shows the nursing care simply isn't working. You may only focus on the care of particular patients for whom you are responsible, or you can expand your concern to a larger group of patients. To determine the scale of a problem in your unit, service line, or institution, you need to assess the **incidence** (the rate of new conditions) and/or **prevalence** (the rate of a condition at any point in time) of the condition, as well as the contexts in which it is occurring. For example, you might assess the problem on a smaller scale and ask: Are elderly patients recovering from significant surgery acquiring too many pressure ulcers on my unit? You may widen your view and ask: Are patients in certain areas such as the operating room or acute rehabilitation units acquiring too many pressure ulcers? These two questions illustrate how the scope and scale of your curiosity will drive you to ask questions and assess and search to uncover the evidence.

Ask/Assess

Both the nursing process and evidence-based practice process begin when nurses assess the problem and then ask questions that lead to the best available evidence to inform their decisions. Sara's skin assessment demonstrated that, at least in one patient, several skin tears and a stage II pressure ulcer occurred. Her next steps will determine both what she can do as an individual and how she might work with others to find out if the problem is bigger than a single patient.

First, find out if an evidence-based resource already exists. Sara checks her policies and finds out that although there is a skin-care policy, the policy lacks references or any mentions of the evidence that informs it.

Second, find out if someone else is already gathering data that can help you determine the scale of the problem. Often quality improvement nurses, unit managers, risk managers, or clinical nurse specialists gather data on outcomes such a pressure ulcer incidence and prevalence. Use these local data as clues to help you understand the problem. If the incidence is less than benchmarks or at the level required by regulators, you would not receive much support to change practice. However, if the local data indicate there is a problem, then you need to find how best to intervene.

In 2009, the Centers for Medicare & Medicaid Services (CMS), the U.S. governmental agency administering several health programs, implemented a rule that the federal government will not pay additional costs associated with certain **hospital-acquired conditions (HACs),** meaning complications that could otherwise be prevented. Stage III and IV pressure ulcers were among the first conditions that the CMS identified. This shift toward **pay-for-performance,** or reimbursement based on outcomes, makes pressure ulcer prevention a high priority for institutions and certainly for the patients themselves. In this case, any hospital-acquired pressure ulcer is unacceptable (Box 17■1).

> ### BOX 17■1 Significance of Pressure Ulcers
>
> ■ Overall prevalence of pressure ulcers = 11.9%
> ■ Overall facility acquired pressures ulcers = 5.0%
> ■ Facility acquired rates were highest in critical care units:
>   ■ 8.8% = general cardiac care units
>   ■ 10.4% = surgical ICUs
>   ■ 6% in medical and surgical step-down units
> ■ In 2007, pressure ulcers were estimated to cost $2.41 billion (Healthgrades, 2009)
> ■ Pressure ulcers cause pain and can lead to infection and sepsis

From VanGilder, C., Amlung, S., Harrison, P., et al. (2009). Results of the 2008–2009 International Pressure Ulcer Prevalence™ survey and a 3-year, acute care, unit-specific analysis. *Ostomy Wound Management, 55,* 39–45. Retrieved from http://www.o-wm.com/content/results-2008-%E2%80%93-2009-international-pressure-ulcer-prevalence%E2%84%A2-survey-and-a-3-year-acute-care

In the clinical story, the phrase "at-risk frail, elderly patients who are hospitalized in acute care areas" describes the scope of the problem. Using this scope, Sara talks with the quality officer, who provides her with the following data for the acute medical-surgical units in the facility:

■ Monthly prevalence of all-stage hospital acquired pressure ulcer rates on the medical-surgical units ranged from 5% to 12% over the past 6 months, compared with 1.3% to 4% hospital-wide rates and a national benchmark of 5.0% for all types of U.S. hospitals in 2009 (VanGilder, Amlung, Harrison, et al., 2009).
■ When stage I pressure ulcers were excluded from the data, the units had hospital-acquired prevalence ranging from 3.2% to 7% compared with the national rate of 3.1% (VanGilder et al., 2009).
■ Most pressure ulcers in this hospital were on the sacrum or heels.

Given these data, Sara has good reason to pursue evidence to determine if her nursing practice needs to change. To find the evidence, she needs to ask a well-formed question that points her to the target evidence. She decides that although all of the care related to preventing pressure ulcers is important, she will begin with a limited focus.

The patient, LH, told Sara that she was on a different type of bed in the ICU. Sara suspects that transferring to a standard mattress in the medical-surgical unit may have contributed to the problem. Because the patient is weak and still experiencing pain, she does not move easily in bed; Sara often finds her crumpled at the bottom of the bed, needing a boost up toward the head of the bed. She assesses the patient's risk factors according to the hospital's policy and she finds this patient is at high risk for pressure ulcers due to limited activity, mobility, and nutrition and increased friction and shear (National Pressure Ulcer Advisory Panel and European Pressure Ulcer Advisory Panel, 2009).

As Sara did, you will start with very broad questions that usually begin with "What is the best way to...?" As you define the focus, ask increasingly narrow questions until you can state the questions in a typical population, intervention, comparison and outcome (PICO) format (Table 17■1).

Acquire/Diagnose

Sara suspects that her patient has impaired skin integrity related to inadequate pressure reduction and friction injury. Her diagnosis is based on her assessment of the patient's key risk factors: very limited mobility, increased friction caused by frequent repositioning, and very poor nutrition. Although Sara is not prepared to address the problems of the patient's nutrition, she recognizes the patient's poor intake contributes to her risk for skin breakdown. Sara's next step is to acquire the best available evidence based on her diagnosis and questions she suspects relate to caring for the patient's specific risk factors. She may search herself or call upon a librarian or more experienced searcher to help her.

Based on your PICO questions generate a list of key words and ideal sources of evidence. Take your PICO question apart, finding the main words that will help you reach your target, and think about synonyms and alternate spellings for each (Table 17■2).

Now you are ready to search for your ideal source. Sara's questions relate to the effectiveness of interventions, so her ideal source would be an excellent clinical practice guideline based on systematic reviews of randomized controlled trials that tested the interventions. If no guidelines exist that meet her requirements, she

Table 17■1 **Narrowing the Focus and Generating Questions**

Question Type	Example	
Broad	What are the best practices for preventing pressure ulcers?	
Narrow	What are the best bed surfaces for at-risk elderly patients?	
Narrow	What is the best way to help patients move up in bed to reduce friction?	
Searchable PICO	What is the effectiveness of pressure-reducing specialty beds versus standard hospital mattresses in elderly, at-risk patients on the incidence of pressure ulcers?	P = elderly, at-risk patients I = pressure-reducing specialty beds C = standard hospital beds O = incidence of pressure ulcers
Searchable PICO	What is the effectiveness of slip sheets versus helping elderly, at-risk patients move up in bed on the incidence of pressure ulcers?	P = elderly, at-risk patients I = slip sheets C = helping patients move up in bed O = incidence of pressure ulcers

Table 17■2   **Keywords and Search Strategy for the Cochrane Library or a Bibliographic Database**

PICO	Synonyms	Search Strategy
What is the effectiveness of pressure-reducing specialty beds versus standard hospital mattresses in elderly, at-risk patients on the incidence of pressure ulcers?		
I = pressure-reducing specialty beds	beds support surface specialty bed overlay sport bed gel bed low pressure static air pressure alleviat* pressure support pressure reliev* pressure reduc* waffle mattress alternat* pressure water suspension	Link with OR
C = standard hospital beds	bed foam standard	Link with OR
O = incidence of pressure ulcers	pressure ulcer decubitus pressure sore skin tear	Link with OR
I + C + O		Link with AND
I = slip sheets	reposition mobility aid slip sheet	Link with OR
O = incidence of pressure ulcers	pressure ulcer decubitus pressure sore skin tear	Link with OR
I + O		Link with AND

would need to search for systematic reviews or individual studies using bibliographic databases such as the Cumulative Index to Nursing and Allied Health Literature (CINAHL) or MEDLINE.

If you are consulting with a librarian, take your question and list of keywords and synonyms with you. If you are searching yourself, start by searching the "best bet" sources. One place to begin searching for a clinical practice guideline is the online **National Guideline Clearinghouse** (NGC) (http://www.guidelines.gov). This collection is made up of full-text and abstracted versions of guidelines that societies, governmental groups, and agencies voluntarily submit. You can conduct basic or more detailed searches in the NGC, but the database does not use controlled language words (MeSHs). It does allow you to use a Boolean search and/or filters to limit the search. Not all topics and interventions are covered in the collection and some topics have many related guidelines you must sort through.

If Sara starts her basic search of the NGC with "pressure ulcer prevention," she finds 78 guidelines. This means she needs to use a more specific approach. Using the "detailed search" tool, you can select options that filter and narrow the guidelines that you find. You need to use some trial and error to be sure you are not missing important results by using too many filters. For her detailed search, Sara uses the keyword "pressure ulcer"; selects "bed" as her intervention; and then filters by "prevention" and "nurses" as intended user, and picks age groups to capture anyone 65 years of age and older. She nets three practice guidelines: the Registered Nurses' Association of Ontario (RNAO) 2005 update, the American Medical Directors Association—Professional Association 2008 update, and the Australian National Stroke Foundation 2007 guideline that includes pressure ulcer prevention. At this point, you need to scan the links to see if the guidelines address the correct context, patient group, and, ultimately, if the guidelines fit your question. When Sara scans the guidelines, she discards two of the three because they do not address the correct context or population and did not make recommendations about bed surfaces or how to move patients in bed. Sara retains the RNAO best practice guideline because it fits her population, setting, and intervention. However, the guideline was last updated in 2005 (Registered Nurses' Association of Ontario [RNAO], 2005).

Sara broadens her search of the literature to include guidelines published after 2005 or outside the NGC. When Sara searches the Internet for international professional societies that address pressure ulcer prevention, she finds two organizations that look as though they are authorities. The two organizations, the National Pressure Ulcer Advisory Panel (NPUAP) and the European Pressure Ulcer Advisory Panel (EPUAP), collaborated to produce one practice guideline in 2009 (National Pressure Ulcer Advisory Panel and European Pressure Ulcer Advisory Panel [NPUAP-EPUAP], 2009). After scanning the guideline for relevance, she retains this guideline to appraise.

Finally, Sara searches the Cochrane Library to see if any more recent systematic reviews have been published. If Sara uses the basic search using just "pressure ulcer" as the search term, she gets over 6000 results. She needs to narrow the search using the advanced search tools. If she uses the advanced search and some logic, she can narrow the results quickly. She uses the following Boolean strategy to first capture common terms for the outcome and intervention and then to link them together in the same review: ("pressure ulcer" OR decubitus) AND (bed OR "support surface" OR mattress OR lift OR reposition) AND prevention. She also selects "search all text" in case these words were not mentioned in the title or abstract. Finally, she is looking only for systematic reviews so she filters the search to the Cochrane Database of Systematic Reviews *(Cochrane Reviews)* and the Database of Reviews of Effects (reviews other than Cochrane). She nets 12 reviews, but only seven are completed reviews. Of these, only two are clearly relevant and published after the practice guidelines.

Busy clinicians usually do not have time to conduct exhaustive searches using all of the potential synonyms and spellings. Your librarians can help you search the bibliographic databases if you can articulate what evidence you are looking for. It is helpful to talk with them to help them discover the words that might be used in various evidence sources. To obtain the right results, the search experts will link synonyms and alternate spellings for each key element together with the Boolean operator "or" to expand the search and they will glue the PICO elements together with "and" to narrow the search towards your target (see Table 17■2).

Appraise/Plan

Sara has selected two clinical practice guidelines and two systematic reviews to evaluate to determine if the recommendations represent the best available evidence. The comprehensiveness of the search determines the *available evidence.* Now Sara will need to appraise the evidence to find out if it is the *best evidence.* Because she has searched at the top of the effectiveness hierarchy (guidelines as meta-sources and systematic reviews), she has already obtained a more powerful type of evidence. But she still needs to appraise the evidence before she can use it to inform her nursing practice.

To appraise evidence, you will use a standardized tool that matches the type of evidence you have selected. In Sara's case, she will evaluate these basic questions of the practice guideline and the systematic review (Public Health Research Unit [PHRU], 2007):

- How clear is the focus?
- How transparent and rigorous were the methods?
- Can I apply the recommendations to these patients?

When Sara appraises the two practice guidelines and the systematic review, she uses two tools that others have developed and validated. The **AGREE tool** (a standardized appraisal tool for practice guidelines, rigorously developed by an international group of experts) and the tools from the **Critical Appraisal Skills Program (CASP)** (standardized appraisal instruments for systematic reviews and primary research developed by the Public Health Research Unit in the United Kingdom) tools make it easier because they have hints about what to look for as she reads the guidelines and review (AGREE Collaboration, 2003; PHRU, 2007). When Sara appraises both practice guidelines using the AGREE tool, she finds that both were strong in all of the following criteria:

- Scope and questions are clear and focused.
- Diverse stakeholders were an integral part of the process.

- Both used rigorous and transparent methods including systematic methods to search and appraise the evidence.
- A panel of experts reviewed the appraised and extracted evidence and considered the benefits and risks to reach a consensus on recommendations.
- Both identified the levels of evidence or recommendations and used external reviewers.
- Both have an update plan, but the RNAO guideline is now past the renewal date.
- Both are clear and have synopses that are freely available online, but the full NPUAP-EPUAP guideline requires purchase, whereas the entire RNAO guideline and implementation toolbox are free online.

Next, Sara uses the CASP tool for systematic reviews (PHRU, 2007) to appraise the meta-analysis of support surfaces, published after the most recent practice guideline. She finds the following strengths of the review by McInnes, Cullum, Bell-Syer et al. (2009), in which the authors evaluated the effectiveness of various support surfaces for preventing pressure ulcers:

- Objectives were clear and the authors selected appropriate study designs to include in the review (randomized controlled trials).
- Comprehensive search of four databases and hand searching were used.
- Study appraisal and data extraction were fairly strong, although a second author was used to check decisions rather than a blinded, dual reviewer method; the authors transparently identified and used rigorous criteria to decide what to include in the study.
- The authors used appropriate statistical methods to determine the effectiveness of different surfaces with good precision (using confidence intervals).
- Because of study designs, the authors were unable to find significant benefit among the various mattresses and overlays, but they did find that some kind of pressure support device is superior to standard foam mattresses.
- The studies did not consistently address patient comfort or caregiver preferences; therefore, the authors could not address these outcomes.

Once you have appraised your sources, you need to look for consistencies, summarize the bottom-line recommendations, and identify the strengths of each recommendation. For her question, Sara combines recommendations from the two practice guidelines and the systematic review to answer the questions about support surfaces and how to decrease friction during repositioning. Her bottom-line determination for patients at risk for pressure ulcers is the following:

- Do not use a standard foam hospital mattress (level A) (McInnes et al., 2009; NPUAP-EPUAP, 2009; RNAO, 2005).
- Use a mattress or overlay that reduces interface pressures, such as high-density foam. In patients at higher risk, consider an active support surface (e.g., alternating pressure, air fluidized or low-air-loss beds). There is no good evidence to recommend one of these higher technology surfaces over the others (level A) (McInnes et al., 2009; NPUAP-EPUAP, 2009; RNAO, 2005)
- Use lifting devices or slip sheets; avoid dragging the skin over another surface to reduce friction and shear (level C) (NPUAP-EPUAP, 2009; RNAO, 2005).

You will note that each recommendation has a rating of the level of recommendation. As you learned in Chapter 11, many systems exist to represent levels of evidence and strength of recommendations. Levels of evidence usually indicate the degree of confidence you can have in the underlying approach to answer the question. Degrees may vary from strong—a systematic review—to weak—an expert opinion. Grades of recommendations should relate to the level of evidence and usually make a qualified statement about how urgently you should adopt the practice or avoid the practice altogether. International efforts exist to standardize the rating of evidence and recommendations but they are not yet universally accepted (GRADE Working Group, 2004).

Sara's institution uses an A through D hierarchy in which recommendations are based on the body of the evidence:

- Grade A = strong support that merits application; evidence from a systematic review or precise randomized controlled trial
- Grade B = moderate support that merits consideration; evidence from single, well-designed studies
- Grade C = Moderate support that merits consideration: evidence from case series or expert consensus
- Grade D = Evidence cannot support the adoption of the practice

Apply/Implement

Armed with evidence about support surfaces and how to move patients in bed, Sara can now make decisions when she intervenes with at-risk patients. Sara recognizes that these are just two of a larger set of interventions to prevent pressure ulcers, but she can still individualize her care by assessing each person's risk and preferences. Because the best available evidence does not indicate that one surface is superior to another, she can offer alternatives based on the availability of different products at her facility. When patients are at risk, she offers one of the support surfaces available and includes their preferences in her selection decision. When patients need to move in the bed, she makes sure she uses a slip sheet to avoid any friction or shear, enlists help, or uses a lift device to avoid dragging the patient over the bed surface.

Implementation within a system is complex. If Sara is the only nurse making decisions based on the evidence, her impact will be limited. She will need to work with a team to change the practices of others (Box 17■2). You will need to seek out a clinical nurse specialist or skin care advanced practice nurse to aid the practice change throughout the hospital. If advanced practice nurses use the Promoting Action on Research Implementation in Health Service (PARIHS) Framework, they will assess the strength of the context and evidence to determine how to facilitate the practice change (Kitson, Rycroft-Malone, Harvey, et al., 2008). Nurses who deliver bedside care are key stakeholders and need to be involved in the process of changing practices system wide.

In Sara's situation, the evidence has already been appraised as strong. The advanced practice nurses may use tools that are just being developed to assess the context based on characteristics that will either help or hinder implementation of the evidence. These characteristics relate to a system's leadership, evaluation systems,

BOX 17◼2 **Interdisciplinary Rounds**

Pressure ulcer prevention is a team effort. Involve the following members in your plans:

- Registered nurses providing professional nursing care at the bedside
- Nursing assistants who contribute to patient hygiene and mobility
- Physiotherapists who intervene to progress mobility
- Wound and ostomy specialists with expert knowledge
- Clinical nurse specialists with expert knowledge and change and project management skills
- Hospitalists or other physicians with vested interest
- Safety and quality officers
- Clinical educators
- Risk managers

Ensure that the key stakeholders have a voice and engage their clinical expertise appropriately.

and organizational culture. If the context is strong, advance practice nurses can best facilitate practice change by enabling and empowering others to use the evidence. If the context is weaker, they may need to facilitate practice change by providing more directions and technical, practical, and task-driven help (Kitson et al., 2008).

Advanced practice nurses could also develop evidence-based strategies to help the organization adopt the guidelines in nursing practice. For Sara's question about pressure ulcer prevention or any other guideline implementation, the following are some examples of research-based strategies to move evidence into practice. You may use them alone but they may be more effective in combination:

- Interactive education sessions about when and how to use support surfaces and lift devices (Forsetlund, Bjørndal, Rashidian, et al., 2009; O'Brien, Rogers, Jamtvedt, et al., 2007)
- Educational outreach via one-on-one education and support at the bedside from the clinical nurse specialist or skin-care specialist (Forsetlund et al., 2009; O'Brien et al., 2007)
- Prompts or reminders as simple as a magnet on the door signifying the patient within is at high risk for pressure ulcers or as high-tech as a pop-up electronic reminder when a patient reaches high risk as well as some type of visual prompt in the care plan (O'Brien et al., 2007)
- Audit and high-intensity feedback about how frequently the unit uses the proper surface and lift devices in at-risk patients (Jamtvedt, Young, Kristoffersen, et al., 2006)
- The Apply phase of the evidence-based practice process includes both application of the evidence supporting the nursing intervention and the evidence supporting strategies to change practice

Assess/Evaluate

Both the nursing and evidence-based practice processes require assessment to evaluate the effectiveness of interventions used with patients. Sara assesses all of LH's skin but carefully focuses on the pressure points like her sacrum, heels, scapula, hips, elbows, ears, and occipital region. She also follows the stage II pressure ulcers to make sure that they begin to heal. If the depth, color, or size of the ulcers worsen, she will need to intensify her efforts and consult further with wound specialists.

Patient outcomes are the highest priority, but the process of care is important to assess as well. The manager or advanced practice nurse will help audit the key interventions to determine if the right patients receive the right care at the right time.

■ Summary

Every day, nurses make both basic and complex clinical decisions. In this chapter's clinical story, Sara systematically assessed the patient and determined if the problem was an isolated event or part of a trend. She asked the questions to find the best available evidence. She searched and acquired the evidence to fit her diagnosis. She appraised the relevant evidence and was able to select synthesized sources to help her plan. Finding similar answers among those sources that met her criteria of excellence, she implemented the evidence and considered patient preferences when making decisions with other at-risk patients. Beyond her individual application of the evidence, she consulted with advanced practice nurses and wound and skin specialists for their clinical expertise and their influence over change on a larger scale within the institution. Finally, Sara evaluated the effectiveness of implementing the evidence in her individual patients by following the important clinical outcomes, and she helped monitor how other nurses used the evidence-based guidelines (Box 17■3). Thus, the evidence-based nursing practice and the nursing process aligned to produce optimal patient outcomes.

BOX 17■3 **Tools for Learning and Practice**

- Generate additional PICO questions related to pressure ulcer prevention.
- Search for additional evidence based on the key words in your PICO question using the strategy supplied in this chapter as a template.
- Go to international guideline repositories such as the National Institute for Clinical Excellence (http://www.nice.org.uk/) and compare the guideline recommendations with those from the National Pressure Ulcer Prevention Advisory Panel (http://www.npuap.org) and the Registered Nurses' Association of Ontario's Nursing Best Practice Guidelines (http://www.rnao.org). Use the AGREE collaboration tool to appraise the guidelines (http://www. agreecollaboration.org/ instrument/).
- Compare and contrast levels of evidence and levels of recommendations from organizations such as the RNAO, the Joanna Briggs Institute, and the Centers for Disease Control and Prevention.

BOX 17▪3 **Tools for Learning and Practice** (continued)

- Help gather data by participating in the national pressure ulcer prevalence study.
- Develop a simple audit tool that allows you to observe for adherence to key evidence-based strategies or use criteria that may already have been developed.
- Conduct an audit, summarize the data, and present feedback to colleagues.
- When mentoring other nurses, discuss the evidence related to pressure ulcer prevention with mentees; role-model best practices such as selecting appropriate pressure-reducing surfaces and using friction-reducing techniques to reduce sheer.

CHAPTER QUESTIONS

1. In this chapter's clinical story of pressure ulcer prevention, what were the steps of nursing process that Sara took? What were the steps of the evidence-based process?

2. What were the strengths of the evidence that Sara found?

3. What were the differences in how Sara approached the problem of pressure ulcer prevention as an individual nurse and when she consulted with advance practice nurses to solve the problem on a broader scale?

4. Understanding that there is more to pressure ulcer prevention than support surfaces and how to move a patient in bed, what are other PICO questions that you could ask?

5. Using these PICO questions, search for a practice guideline and a systematic review. Using the criteria for critical appraisal, make a decision to use or discard the evidence you found. Support your reasoning and identify the strength of the evidence using a hierarchy.

6. If you found more than one guideline or systematic review, compare them and identify if they found similar recommendations or differed.

7. Given the implementation strategies that were listed, what are some creative ways that you could put these strategies into practice?

8. Consider a scenario in which the evidence indicates that a certain bed surface is effective in preventing pressure ulcers but the patient refuses to use it because it is uncomfortable. What would you do next?

(continues on page 248)

CHAPTER QUESTIONS (continued)

9. Given the evidence that Sara found, construct a simple audit tool to observe adherence to these interventions. Make sure that your criteria can be observed or identified in documentation and that they can be answered with a simple yes or no. Determine what the next steps would be to improve performance on those items where adherence was low. For high-performing criteria, plan a creative celebration to acknowledge good work among your peers.

References

AGREE Collaboration. (2003). Development and validation of an international appraisal instrument for assessing the quality of clinical practice guidelines: The AGREE project. *Quality and Safety in Health Care, 12,* 18–23.

Centers for Medicare & Medicaid Services. (2008). Hospital acquired conditions: Statute regulations program instructions. Retrieved from http://www.cms.hhs.gov/HospitalAcqCond/02_Statute_Regulations_Program_Instructions.asp

Forsetlund, L., Bjørndal, A., Rashidian, A., et al. (2009). Continuing education meetings and workshops: Effects on professional practice and health care outcomes. *Cochrane Database of Systematic Reviews, 2.* Art. No.: CD003030. doi:10.1002/14651858.CD003030.pub2

GRADE Working Group. (2004). Grading quality of evidence and strength of recommendations. *British Medical Journal, 328,* 1490–1497. doi:10.1136/bmj.328.7454.1490

HealthGrades. (2009). The sixth annual HealthGrades patient safety in American hospitals study. Retrieved from http://www.healthgrades.com/media/dms/pdf/PatientSafetyInAmerican HospitalsStudy

Jamtvedt, G., Young, J. M., Kristoffersen, D. T., et al. (2006). Audit and feedback: Effects on professional practice and health care outcomes. *Cochrane Database of Systematic Reviews, 2.* Art. No.: CD000259. doi:10.1002/14651858.CD000259.pub2

Joanna Briggs Institute. (2009). JBI approach to evidence based practice. Retrieved from http://www. jbiconnect.org/connect/info/about/jbi_ebhc_approach.php#LEGR.FAME

Kitson, A., Rycroft-Malone, J., Harvey, G., et al. (2008). Evaluating the successful implementation of evidence into practice using the PARIHS framework: Theoretical and practical challenges. *Implementation Science, 3.* doi:10.1186/1748-5908-3-1

McInnes, E., Cullum, N.A., Bell-Syer, S. E.M., et al. (2008). Support surfaces for pressure ulcer prevention. Cochrane Database of Systematic Reviews, Issue 4. Art. No.: CD001735. doi: 10.1002/14651858.CD001735.pub3

National Pressure Ulcer Advisory Panel. (2007). Pressure ulcer stages revised by NPUAP. Retrieved from http://www.npuap.org/pr2.htm

National Pressure Ulcer Advisory Panel and European Pressure Ulcer Advisory Panel. (2009). Pressure ulcer prevention guide: Quick reference. Retrieved from http://www.npuap.org/Final_Quick_Prevention_for_web_2010.pdf

O'Brien, M.A., Rogers, S., Jamtvedt, G., et al. (2007). Educational outreach visits: Effects on professional practice and health care outcomes. *Cochrane Database of Systematic Reviews, 4.* doi:10.1002/14651858.CD000409.pub2

Public Health Research Unit. (2007). Critical appraisal skills program. Retrieved from http://www. phru.nhs.uk/pages/phd/resources.htm

Registered Nurses' Association of Ontario. (2005). Risk assessment and prevention of pressure ulcers [Nursing best practice guidelines]. Retrieved from http://www.rnao.org/Page.asp?PageID=924& ContentID=816

VanGilder, C., Amlung, S., Harrison, P., et al. (2009). Results of the 2008–2009 International Pressure Ulcer Prevalence™ survey and a 3-year, acute care, unit-specific analysis. *Ostomy Wound Management, 55,* 39–45. Retrieved from http://www.o-wm.com/content/results-2008-%E2%80% 93-2009-international-pressure-ulcer-prevalence%E2%84%A2-survey-and-a-3-year-acute-care-

CHAPTER 18

Evidence Implementation to Provide Safe Nursing Care to Laboring Women

Cheryl Moredich, Beth Vottero

- Examine the role of evidence-based practice in the promotion of patient safety in the context of caring for a laboring mother.

- Analyze the effect of ethical principles on evidence-based decision making.

- Establish a prototype for change toward evidence-based practice.

- Facilitate collaborative communication as a means toward implementing evidence in the workplace.

Advocate
Autonomy
Beneficence
High-alert medications

Moral decision making
Nonmaleficence
Professional standards

Clinical Story

Freda is caring for a 26-year-old nulliparous woman who is at 38 weeks' gestation. The patient has not experienced complications during this pregnancy and is excited about her labor being induced today. Both her mother and husband are accompanying her. Her mother asks you if you think it is a good idea for her daughter to be induced. Her mother states, "Back in my time, you just waited until the baby was ready." Freda has worked in labor and delivery for over 3 years, witnessing both positive and negative responses to induction of labor. According to the patient's gestational age, Freda questions the order for induction in this apparently healthy pregnant woman. When Freda asks the patient why her labor is being induced today, she states, "My husband has a business trip next week and will be out of the country. We wanted him to be here for the birth." Freda already has one patient in early labor, making this her second labor patient.

Introduction

The goal of any elective induction of labor is to facilitate a vaginal birth without causing harm to the mother or fetus. Medical indications for inducing labor exist; however, when induction of labor is implemented solely for provider or patient convenience, it is termed *elective*. Although a variety of methods are available for induction of labor, we focus here on the use of oxytocin. Oxytocin is used to induce labor in over 30% of U.S. pregnant women; it has been on the high-alert medication list since 2007; and it has no universal, formal policy for its safe use (Hayes and Weinstein, 2008). **High-alert medications** are those medications that can cause significant harm if administered incorrectly. Because oxytocin is a high-alert medication, prescribing it in error can be particularly dangerous. Medication errors make up the most common form of inpatient error, injuring 1.5 million hospitalized patients each year (National Academies of Science, 2006).

Professional organizations have developed recommendations to promote the safe use of oxytocin in induction of labor (Agency for Healthcare Research and Quality [AHRQ], 2009b; American Congress of Obstetricians and Gynecologists [ACOG], 2009; Association of Women's Health, Obstetric, and Neonatal Nurses [AWHONN], 2009). However, administration decisions for oxytocin have traditionally been at the discretion of the individual obstetrician. Breaking away from tradition and moving toward evidence-based practice will facilitate safety in elective induction of labor.

This chapter's clinical story demonstrates the immediate and subsequent actions that the nurse can take to safely deliver care to the laboring patient. Immediate actions occur as the clinical story unfolds, steps that can be taken immediately to correct a safety concern. Subsequent actions are those taken after the identification of a clinical problem, but will take time to develop and implement. This chapter provides a depiction of how the identification and selection of resources lays the foundation for providing the best patient care. Freda uses the processes of ask, acquire, appraise, apply, and assess as she builds a plan for safe patient care.

Ask/Assess

Freda is trying to reconcile what she believes to be safe patient care with the current clinical situation. Freda questions whether the patient truly understands the risks of elective induction of labor, especially before 39 gestational weeks. Freda questions if she is adequately prepared to **advocate** for the patient's wishes. To advocate is to champion or support the patient to meet her needs and wishes. Was this choice the best for the baby? Could she advocate on behalf of the unborn child? What about the unit policies regarding induction? Was it ethical to follow her unit's policies that might be out of date? All of these thoughts raced through Freda's mind as she assessed the situation.

Freda wants to provide safe, evidence-based, quality patient care. She knows the desired outcome, yet has many questions concerning the care of this patient. The significance of the problem is discussed in Box 18■1.

BOX 18■1 **Significance of the Problem**

- Thirty percent of pregnant women in the United States receive oxytocin to induce labor; it is the most common method to induce labor worldwide.
- Oxytocin is used most commonly in developed nations once the membranes have ruptured.
- Oxytocin is used to induce labor, either alone, or in combination with amniotomy or other pharmacologic agents.
- When comparing intravenous oxytocin to expectant management (waiting to see if labor starts naturally), fewer women failed to deliver within 24 hours; however, there is an increase in the number of women requiring epidural analgesia cesarean births with oxytocin use.
- While a systematic review of trials comparing oxytocin with expectant management found no differences in tachysystole, uterine rupture and other complications, nurses who help mothers labor while on oxytocin must be highly vigilant for these potentially catastrophic complications
- Adequate nursing staffing is highly important to insure safe use of oxytocin to induce labor.

From Alfirevic Z., Kelly A., & Dowswell, T. (2009). Intravenous oxytocin alone for cervical ripening and induction of labour. *Cochrane Database of Systematic Reviews, 4.* Art. No.: CD003246. doi:10. 1002/14651858.CD003246.pub2

The first question is the rationale for this patient's ordered induction of labor. Freda recalled reading a recent peer-reviewed article that suggested that elective induction of labor before 39 completed gestational weeks is not advisable. Freda is also aware that because oxytocin is a high-alert medication, she needs to be particularly cautious and informed about how to use the drug safely. She wonders if the unit's oxytocin protocol matches those written in national guidelines. Staffing patterns also concern Freda. If this patient becomes her second labor patient, Freda worries that she will not be able to be adequately vigilant, which could jeopardize the patient's safety. She wants to be proactive in creating an environment that promotes the safe use of oxytocin in laboring patients, but how does this journey begin?

To begin, Freda takes immediate action by informing her charge nurse, nurse manager, or nurse supervisor about her concerns regarding safe patient care. Following her chain of command, Freda knows that the first line of help comes from those in a direct supervisory position closest to the point of care. When critical incidents escalate, a formalized channel of communication helps stakeholders interact cooperatively. Frequently, immediate actions are taken to minimize patient risk and maximize safe patient care. Changing Freda's assignment to reflect the acuity of care required by the patient is one immediate action that could affect patient safety. Freda could also call the physician to question the rationale for inducing this patient. Another post-critical incident channel is to take the case to the ethics committee for discussion and ruling. Some organizations have specific committees designed to come together when a critical incident arises. Such committees allow a real-time decision on a patient care issue. The benefits include working through a critical issue as it occurs rather than afterward.

Freda questions whether the oxytocin protocol on her unit mirrors the national guidelines. Because the scope and scale of her concerns are broad, Freda's question is quite comprehensive. Her question is, "What is the best available evidence for safe delivery in healthy, non–full-term mothers when requesting elective induction of labor?" Potential roadblocks to safe administrations of oxytocin include outdated protocols that do not reflect the evidence, less than adequate staffing, and inappropriate patient selection. On review, Freda realizes that her unit protocol is missing gestational age limits and staffing guidelines, and has not been updated in 5 years. Freda hears other nurses voice a concern that this oxytocin protocol is sometimes forfeited in favor of physician preference.

Based on the evidence she has gathered, Freda has good reason to question the clinical practice on her unit. She decides to ask her supervisor if she can form a team of nurses to investigate the evidence. This would be considered a subsequent action.

Acquire/Diagnose

As described in Chapter 17, Freda's next step is to acquire the best available evidence relating to her question and diagnosis. She can conduct a search herself or consult with a more experienced person such, as a librarian. Freda is fortunate that she has access to professional recommendations that address her clinical problem. She finds an AWHONN recommendation stating that elective induction of labor should be reserved for patients who are at 39 completed weeks' gestation unless medically indicated (AWHONN, 2009). Another recommendation from AWHONN addresses appropriate staffing patterns for laboring patients (AWHONN, 2010). Freda continues her search of the literature. She finds an *Elective Induction of Labor* bundle that matches AWHONN's recommendation from the Institute for Healthcare Improvement (IHI) Web site (IHI, 2009). She found a systematic review in the Cochrane Library that compares expectant management of labor with oxytocin use (Alfirevic, Kelly, and Dowswell, 2009).

In every patient situation, nurses are obliged to follow the principles of the ANA Code of Ethics (ANA, 2001). The ethical concepts of **beneficence** and **nonmaleficence** must govern when nurses participate in elective induction of labor. Simply put, beneficence is a moral obligation to help another, and nonmaleficence is a moral obligation not to harm (Beauchamp and Childress, 2009). If induction of labor may cause undue risk to the mother or baby, then, ethically, the nurse must act. Informed consent requires that we fully disclose to the patient, who is competent to make a consent decision. In the case of a pregnant woman, the patient is making a decision for both herself and her unborn baby. Therefore, we must be sure that a health professional provided her full disclosure about the risks and benefits of elective induction.

Autonomy in health care is respected and honored as a basic ethical right of the patient. In 2009, the Agency for Healthcare Research and Quality (AHRQ) published a comprehensive guide for pregnant women who are considering having their labor induced with an accompanying evidence-based guide for professionals (AHRQ, 2009a; AHRQ, 2009c). Recognizing that patient autonomy requires informed consent, nurses must be proactive in developing a consent form that the patient understands. It needs to match the literacy level of the patient and address the risks to both the mother and baby. Once fully informed, the patient and her preference should be respected, as long as the recommendations for elective induction of labor are met. In the clinical story, Freda recognizes the presence of a moral dilemma. She can use an ethical guide to help her sort out the best solution (Table 18■1).

Appraise/Plan

Freda thinks about her role as a professional nurse and the strength of her **professional standards.** Professional organizations develop appropriate standards of care based on the *Nursing Scope and Standards of Practice* (ANA, 2010). This document provides a framework for each state's professional practice act, which defines the legal obligation for nursing. Each state prescribes an appropriate scope of practice for a registered nurse. When confronted with a complex nursing situation, these documents help determine the best course of action.

According to the ANA Code of Ethics (2001), nurses have a duty to participate in advancement of the profession through contributions to practice and collaboration

Table 18■1   **Guide for Moral Decision Making**

Step	Guideline	Relevance to Clinical Situation
Recognizing the moral issue	Understanding that there is a moral/ethical issue	Current practice is not based on the best evidence and could cause harm
Identifying the participants/ stakeholders	Identify those who have a stake in the issue. Consider those with obligations or special considerations to the issue.	Mother, baby, father, patient's mother, physician (OB-GYN and Peds), nurse, unit director, charge nurse, nursing assistants, pastoral care, patient advocate (if present), ethics committee representative
Distinguish the values involved	Think through the values associated with the issue (autonomy, justice, advocacy, beneficence, nonmaleficence, confidentiality)	Autonomy, advocacy, beneficence, nonmaleficence
Weigh the benefits and burdens	Benefits include outcomes from choices that are positive. Burdens involve results from actions that cause physical, emotional, or other pain/suffering.	Positives: Patient satisfaction, convenience for mother/father and physician Negatives: Increased risk to the baby both immediate and later developmentally
Look for analogous situations	Identify similar cases; examine the decisions made and outcomes. Was it a good decision? Look at the similarities and differences between the cases.	Freda can consult with the ethics committee, unit director, and charge nurse as well as her professional organization to identify similar situations.
Discuss with appropriate people	Time permitting, discussing the case with as many participants as possible to understand their opinions of the case. Rules of confidentiality must be adhered to.	Freda needs to discuss with the physician, ethics committee, charge nurse, unit director, and unit practice council.
Ascertain organizational rules and legal codes	Consider the legality of the case and options, ethics of the professional organization, and institutional policies.	Freda should consult the policies, her professional organization (AWHONN), and, if possible, the legal and ethical departments.
Examine own comfort with the decision	Questions to be asked in this regard might include the following: 1. If I carry out this decision, would I be comfortable telling my family about it? My pastor? My mentors? 2. Would I want children to take my behavior as an example? 3. Is this decision one that a wise, informed, virtuous person would make? 4. Can I live with this decision?	While making a decision about the ethical issue, Freda should consider her responses to the questions.

Adapted from http://www.ethicsweb.ca/guide/

with other health professionals (provisions 7 and 8). Just as Freda began by examining current practice and comparing it to national recommendations, an interdisciplinary committee on policies and procedures for the obstetric unit should do the same. In the clinical story, members could include Freda, the nursing assistant, charge nurse, nurse manager, respiratory therapist, obstetrician, neonatologist, pharmacist, social worker, pastoral care, and other stakeholders.

A multidisciplinary team can support collaboration among stakeholders by enhancing communication. Neonatologists and obstetrician/gynecologists provide knowledge and clinical expertise from a medical perspective. The inclusion of physicians into clinical care committees minimizes physician resistance to change, opens channels of communication with physician committees, and creates opportunities for a physician "champion" to support the initiative throughout the organization (Mandel, Pirko, Grant, et al., 2009). Inclusion of physician stakeholders from conception through completion of the project enhances collaboration between physicians and nurses.

Collaborating with other disciplines brings a multidimensional aspect to the provision of care. Each perspective provides valuable insights on facets of the clinical concern. To support the use of interdisciplinary collaboration, the Institute of Medicine's (2010) consensus report, *The Future of Nursing: Leading Change, Advancing Health,* advocates for nurses to work with others to support quality patient care. Nurses are positioned at the forefront of direct patient care; it is at this level that practice issues become apparent (Box 18■2).

BOX 18■2 Interdisciplinary Rounds

Safe delivery of mother and baby during oxytocin-induced labor should involve these members of the team:

- A fully informed mother
- The nursing team that includes the registered professional nurse and possibly a nurse midwife or clinical nurse specialist
- The physician team of obstetrician, pediatrician, and neonatologist in complex cases joins the nursing team, the patient, and the patient's family to make the best decision regarding inducing labor
- If you are faced with an ethical decision, many hospitals have an ethics team to consult, which will help resolve dilemmas

Teams that function well:

- Use excellent communication that is well timed, accurate, mutually respectful, and efficient and includes the key stakeholders
- Engage the patient in real-time discussion to include preferences in the decision making
- Use the best available evidence gleaned from multiple practice guidelines

Armed with the clinical recommendations and the best available evidence, the committee can appraise the literature. Freda appraises the practice recommendations using the AGREE tool; she determines that the recommendations were strong in all of the following criteria:

- Scope and questions are clear and focused with a definitive population.
- Appropriate multidisciplinary stakeholders were part of the process and included a variety of professional organization recommendations.
- A risk/benefit analysis for recommendations is included.
- The developers identified both the levels of evidence and recommendations and they used external reviewers.
- The recommendation includes a post-test, tables, and a sample policy. The full recommendations require purchase.

After appraising the recommendations using the AGREE tool, the team can construct a new protocol on elective induction of labor, one that reflects the best available evidence.

Apply/Implement

Once they write a new protocol, the team can begin the process of implementing it. Dissemination of the new protocol will need to be well thought out and involve the entire perinatal team. All members need to be educated about the new oxytocin guideline. Producing a clinical checklist that reflects the new protocol can serve as a reminder to staff (Fig. 18■1). In fact, although imperfect, evidence supports that using clinical prompts such as checklists helps nurses and physicians use evidence-based guidelines (Grimshaw, Thomas, MacLennon, et al., 2004).

A challenge exists for nurses and physicians to clearly communicate as the new oxytocin protocol is implemented. A common goal, understood by all parties (nurses, physicians, midwives, parents, etc.), is the foundation for communication. For example, in the clinical story, Freda and the other stakeholders clearly understand the common goal of safely delivering the mother without harming either the mother or baby. AHRQ identified process problems with communication and suggested ways to address such issues. According to AHRQ (2002), communication should be timely, complete, and accurate and come to closure. Multiple structured channels are fundamental to effective communication. A primary tool for nurse–physician communication is situation-background-assessment-recommendation (SBAR). The use of this tool structures communication to enhance its effectiveness. Figure 18■2 contains a full description of what the SBAR tool entails. Box 18■3 provides an example of Freda's use of the SBAR tool to communicate information from the clinical story to her supervisor.

Another tool that enhances clear communication is multidisciplinary rounding. Rounding brings the various stakeholders together within the context of care needs for the individual patient. The patient is a part of the care team and she should

Elective Induction of Labor Safety Checklist

Patient selection appropriate

    ☐ Gestational age 39 completed weeks as evidenced by _____

    ☐ No contraindications to induction of labor

Consent guidelines followed

    ☐ AHRQ pamphlet given to patient to read

    ☐ Risks and benefits of elective induction of labor discussed by primary care provider (PCP)

    ☐ Signed consent on the chart

AWHONN staffing guidelines of registered nurses followed

    ☐ 1:1 patient ratio for woman receiving oxytocin for labor induction

Standardized oxytocin protocol followed

    ☐ _____ units of oxytocin mixed in _____ mL of _____

    ☐ Initial dose started at _____ milliunits per minute

    ☐ Increase by _____ milliunits per minute every _____ minutes

    ☐ Maximum dose not exceeded _____ milliunits per minute

Perinatal care team approach to adverse changes in patient status

    ☐ Nursing intervention with tachysystole
       Tachysytole defined as _____

    ☐ If tachysystole is recognized, the nurse will:

    ☐ Nursing intervention with NICHD Category II fetal heart rate patterns
       NICHD Category II fetal heart rate patterns include:

    ☐ If Category II fetal heart rate patterns are recognized, the nurse will:

    ☐ Nursing intervention with NICHD Category III fetal heart rate patterns
       NICHD Category III fetal heart rate patterns include:

    ☐ If Category III fetal heart rate patterns are recognized, the nurse will:

Respectful perinatal care team communication

    ☐ PCP notified about adverse changes in patient status and action taken

        ☐ PCP will be available at cell number: _____

    ☐ Neonatal care unit notified of patient status

    ☐ Chain of command will be followed in the event of disagreements

FIGURE 18■1 Sample elective induction of labor safety checklist.

Situaton

I am calling about <patient name and location>.

The patient's code status is <code status>

The problem I am calling about is _____.

> I am afraid the patient is going to arrest.

I have just assessed the patient personally:

Vital signs are: Blood pressure _____/_____, Pulse _____, Respiration_____ and temperature _____

I am concerned about the:

> Blood pressure because it is over 200 or less than 100 or 30 mmHg below usual
>
> Pulse because it is over 140 or less than 50
>
> Respiration because it is less than 5 or over 40.
>
> Temperature because it is less than 96 or over 104.

Background

The patient's mental status is:

> Alert and oriented to person place and time.
>
> Confused and cooperative or non-cooperative
>
> Agitated or combative
>
> Lethargic but conversant and able to swallow
>
> Stuporous and not talking clearly and possibly not able to swallow
>
> Comatose. Eyes closed. Not responding to stimulation.

The skin is:

> Warm and dry
>
> Pale
>
> Mottled
>
> Diaphoretic
>
> Extremities are cold
>
> Extremities are warm

The patient is not or is on oxygen.

> The patient has been on _____ (l/min) or (%) oxygen for _____ minutes (hours)
>
> The oximeter is reading _____%
>
> The oximeter does not detect a good pulse and is giving erratic readings.

Assesment

> **This is what I think the problem is:** <say what you think is the problem>
>
> **The problem seems to be cardiac infection neurologic respiratory** _____
>
> **I am not sure what the problem is but the patient is deteriorating.**
>
> **The patient seems to be unstable and may get worse, we need to do something.**

Recommendation

I suggest or request that you <say what you would like to see done>.

> Transfer the patient to critical care
>
> Come to see the patient at this time.
>
> Talk to the patient or family about code status.
>
> Ask the on-call family practice resident to see the patient now.
>
> Ask for a consultant to see the patient now.

Are any tests needed:

> Do you need any tests like CXR, ABG, EKG, CBC, or BMP?
>
> Others?

If a change in treatment is ordered then ask:

> How often do you want vital signs?
>
> How long to you expect this problem will last?
>
> If the patient does not get better when would you want us to call again?

FIGURE 18■2 SBAR tool. (Courtesy of Kaiser Permanente.)

> ## BOX 18■3 SBAR Use in the Clinical Story
>
> "Hi Ann (nursing supervisor), I am calling about a situation that is occurring on the OB unit. I need some guidance on how to proceed."
>
> ### Situation
>
> "I received a patient for an elective induction, and I just don't feel right about it. The problem is she is at 38 weeks' gestation, and Dr. Z is planning on inducing her with oxytocin today. This is my second patient. I am concerned that the patient is not an appropriate candidate for elective induction and I do not feel she has been properly informed of her options."
>
> ### Background
>
> "The patient is here with her husband and mother. She is excited about the birth of the baby and seems oblivious that she is being induced early. She cares only that her husband will be present for the birth."
>
> ### Assessment
>
> "Her informed consent is signed, physical assessment is normal, and the baby is presenting appropriately."
>
> ### Recommendations
>
> "I request that there is documentation of my concern about inducing this patient and concern for both the mother and baby's safety."

be included when the health-care professionals discuss her care. When real-time discussion occurs among the disciplines and includes the patient, care becomes individualized and patient centered. Multidisciplinary rounding encompasses the elements of evidence-based practice—best available evidence, clinical expertise of all professionals, and the patient's preferences.

Assess/Evaluate

The effect of the new practice guideline implementation requires assessment to evaluate outcomes in elective induction processes. In this chapter's clinical story, a key element is the auditing of interventions to determine that the right patient receives the right care at the right time. The clinical nurse specialist, manager or even staff nurses may audit key interventions that include safe oxytocin administration to the appropriate patient, and staffing ratios that reflect the care required when patients receive oxytocin. Chart audit reviews provide evidence of safe oxytocin administration to the appropriate patient. Cross-referencing daily staffing and team assignment with oxytocin patients provides evidence of safe staffing levels that adhere to the guidelines. Finally, safe delivery of a healthy baby and mother are the most important clinical outcomes.

■ Summary

In the clinical story, ethical considerations confounded the complexity of everyday nursing decisions. Knowing and doing what is right for the patient conforms to our guiding principles for ethical nursing practice (Box 18■4). Freda identified a clinical problem and employed the systematic process of ask, acquire, appraise, apply, and assess to change practice. Throughout the process, Freda maintained a focus on her ethical obligations to provide optimal care, ensured that the patient understood the ramifications of choices, promoted the voice of the unborn child, and collaborated with others to establish guidelines based on the best available evidence.

BOX 18■4   **Tools for Learning and Practice**

- To find comprehensive evidence related to a problem such as maternal labor, search AWHONN guidelines; compare them with guidelines from the National Institute of Clinical Excellence (NICE), American Congress of Obstetricians & Gynecology, and other organizations.
- Appraise the guidelines using the AGREE tool.
- Checklists, reminders, and alerts help health-care providers implement evidence-based guidelines.
- Communication tools such as SBAR help to provide structure and develop routines.
- Use guides such as Table 18■1 to help structure ethical thinking and decision making.
- Audit criteria based on the evidence and feedback directly to those engaged in the care to improve implementation.
- Know your unit's performance related to patient outcomes such as safe delivery rates, complications, and vaginal delivery rates.

CHAPTER QUESTIONS

1. Apply the ethical principles from the ANA *Code of Ethics* to Freda's clinical situation.

2. Discuss how knowledge of the ANA's ethical principles and evidence-based nursing practice can facilitate working through the following clinical situations:
   a. The patient signs for a tubal ligation because she knows this can be easily reversed.
   b. The physician orders 50 mg of a pain medication that is usually given at a dose of 25 mg.
   c. Dr. X prescribes oxytocin that contradicts the newly established protocol without medical indication.

3. You know that a policy guiding the care of the postpartum patient is outdated. Develop a plan to address the issue.

4. Select one of your patients from a recent clinical experience. Using the SBAR format, create a report to a physician.

5. Interdisciplinary rounding is described as a functional method to enhance communication. How would you participate in the clinical rounds? Create a plan for communicating your perspective to the interdisciplinary group.

References

Agency for Healthcare Research and Quality. (2002). *A toolkit for redesign in health care. Final report* (prepared by Denver Health under Contract No. 290-00-0014; AHRQ Publication No. 05-0108-EF). Rockville, MD: Author. Retrieved from http://www.ahrq.gov/qual/toolkit/

Agency for Healthcare Research and Quality. (2009a). *Elective induction of labor: Safety and harms* (Publication No. 10-EHC004-3). Retrieved from http://www.ncbi.nlm.nih.gov/books/NBK45288/

Agency for Healthcare Research and Quality. (2009b). *Standardized protocols and processes enhance compliance with recommended care, improve staff perceptions of patient safety at a birthing center.* Retrieved from http://www.innovations.ahrq.gov/content.aspx?id=2362

Agency for Healthcare Research and Quality. (2009c). *Thinking about having your labor induced? A guide for pregnant women* (Publication No. 10EHCO004-A). Retrieved from http://effective-healthcare.ahrq.gov/index.cfm/search-for-guides-reviews-and-reports/?pageaction=displayproduct&productID=353

Alfirevic, Z., Kelly, A., & Dowswell, T. (2009). Intravenous oxytocin alone for cervical ripening and induction of labour. *Cochrane Database of Systematic Reviews, 4.* Art. No.: CD003246. doi:10.1002/14651858.CD003246.pub2

American Congress of Obstetricians and Gynecologists. (2009). *Induction of labor* (Practice Bulletin No. 107). Washington DC: Author.

American Nurses Association. (2001). *Code of ethics for nurses with interpretive statements.* Silver Springs, MD: Author. Retrieved from www.nursingworld.org/mods/mod580/code.pdf

American Nurses Association. (2010). *Nursing scope and standards of practice* (2nd ed.). Silver Spring, MD: Nursebooks.org.

Association of Women's Health, Obstetric, and Neonatal Nurses. (2009). *Cervical ripening and induction and augmentation of labor* (3rd ed.). Washington, DC: Author.

Association of Women's Health, Obstetric, and Neonatal Nurses. (2010). *Guidelines for professional registered nurse staffing for perinatal units.* Washington, DC: Author.

Beauchamp, T., & Childress, J. (2009). *Principles of biomedical ethics* (6th ed.). New York: Oxford University Press.

Frederico, F. (2007). Preventing harm from high-alert medications. *The Joint Commission Journal on Quality and Patient Safety, 3*(9), 537–542.

Friesen, M. A., Farquhar, M. B., & Hughes, R. (2008). The nurse's role in promoting a culture of patient safety. American Nurses Association. Retrieved from http://www.nursingworld.org/mods/mod780/cerolefull.htm-pdf

Grimshaw, J. M., Thomas, R. E., MacLennon, G., et al. (2004). Effectiveness and efficiency of guideline dissemination and implementation strategies. *Health Technology Assessment, 8*(6), vii–352.

Hayes, E., & Weinstein, L. (2008). Improving patient safety and uniformity of care by a standardized regimen for the use of oxytocin. *American Journal of Obstetrics & Gynecology,* 622e1–622e7. doi:10.1016/j.ajog.2008.01.039

Institute for Healthcare Improvement. (2009). *Elective induction and augmentation bundles.* Retrieved from http://www.ihi.org/IHI/Topics/PerinatalCare/PerinatalCareGeneral/EmergingContent/ElectiveInductionandAugmentationBundles.htm

Institute of Medicine. (2010). *The future of nursing: Leading change, advancing health.* Retrieved from http://www.iom.edu/Reports/2010/The-Future-of-Nursing-Leading Change-Advancing-Health.aspx

Institute of Safe Medication Practice. (2008). *ISMP's list of high-alert medications.* Retrieved from http://www.ismp.org/Tools/highalertmedications.pdf

Joint Commission on Accreditation of Healthcare Organizations. (2008). *Behaviors that undermine a culture of safety.* (Sentinel Event Alert No. 40). Oakbrook Terrace, IL: Author.

Mandel, D., Pirko, C., Grant, K., et al. (2009). A collaborative protocol on oxytocin administration: Bringing nurse, midwives, and physicians together. *Nursing for Women's Health, 13,* 482–485. doi:10.1111/j.1751-486X.2009.01482.x

National Academies of Sciences. (2006, July 20). *Office of News and Public Information.* Retrieved from http://www8.nationalacademies.org/onpinews/newsitem.aspx?RecordID=11623

CHAPTER 19

Nursing Care of Children

Marsha Ellett

LEARNING OBJECTIVES

- Given a clinical case, apply all phases of the evidence-based practice process to guide decisions related to common pediatric nursing problems.

- Analyze the challenges to making evidence-based decisions in complex health-care environments.

- Generate next-step strategies to get better evidence into practice.

KEY TERMS

**Nasogastric/orogastric
(NG/OG) tube**
Regression equation

Clinical Story

Anthony has worked on a pediatric unit of a major academic-affiliated medical center for almost a year. The unit's patient population includes a mixture of mostly acute care patients; a few are chronic care infants having medical or surgical problems. He recently admitted EB, a 6-week-old African-American full term male infant with respiratory distress, possibly the result of respiratory syncytial virus (RSV). Exhausted from the admission assessment, EB is sleeping peacefully with 1 L of oxygen by nasal cannula (30% oxygen) showing only minimal tachypnea at 68 breaths per minute; his mother and grandmother are at his side. His pulse oximetry reading is 92%. EB has an order for a nasogastric/orogastric (NG/OG) tube to be placed to facilitate feeding.

Anthony remembers the last time he placed a feeding tube in an infant: the radiologist called the unit to tell him the tube needed to be pushed in 2 cm to position it appropriately in the stomach. Previously, he had followed the hospital policy of measuring from the nose to the earlobe to the xiphoid (cartilage at the lower border of the sternum) to predict the insertion length. Insertion length is to the number of centimeters the tube needs to be pushed in to place the tip and all the openings on the tube from which the liquid feeding flows in the stomach. Anthony knows it is important not to stress EB any more than necessary while placing the tube, so he decides to search for evidence regarding the insertion length of a gastric tube so the tube is likely be placed in the stomach on the first attempt. ■

Introduction

Respiratory syncytial virus (RSV) is a common virus that leads to mild, cold like symptoms in adults and older healthy children. It can be more serious in young infants leading to respiratory distress and decreased oral intake (Centers for Disease Control and Prevention, 2010). Sometimes an infant with RSV can either breathe or suck, but not both, leading to decreased oral intake. At other times, the infant is too ill to breathe adequately, as occurred with EB. In this chapter, you will find a blueprint to apply the evidence-based practice process to one pediatric problem—inserting a nasogastric/orogastric tube and testing placement at the bedside during its use.

What Are the Key Issues?

A **nasogastric/orogastric (NG/OG) tube** is a soft, flexible tube inserted through the nose or mouth into the stomach for feeding, decompression, medication instillation, or lavage (irrigation of the stomach). It is usually used on a short-term basis for 6 weeks or less. In this chapter's clinical story, EB is likely to need feeding assistance for only a few days because, according to his mother's report, he was healthy and feeding well before this respiratory illness. With the understanding that the viral respiratory illnesses will usually resolve in a few days to about a week, placing an NG/OG tube is appropriate (Box 19■1).

Considering the nursing meta-paradigm, there are some nursing care issues to consider: how to safely insert the tube and how to maintain the tube. The first decision to make is whether to insert the tube through the nose or through the mouth. Practical issues influence your decisions as well as the evidence. For example, you need to be able to secure the tube and the infant's nostrils need to be big enough to accommodate both the NG tube and an oxygen nasal cannula if the baby is receiving oxygen. Anthony knows that most gastric tubes on his unit are inserted through the nose because it is easier to tape the tube in place. Saliva in the mouth can cause the tape securing the tube to become wet, thus allowing the tube to slip through the tape unnoticed and become partially dislodged. If the tube does not stay in the proper position, the infant could be at risk to aspirate formula. EB's nostrils appear large enough to accommodate both a tube of small diameter (probably 8 Fr.) and the nasal cannula.

During the insertion procedure, you must decide how far to insert the tube so that it reaches the stomach. Then you need to verify that it is in the right place. It is possible that you could insert the tube into the lungs instead of the esophagus and stomach. The key nursing care issues relate to the following broad question: In an infant who requires supplemental feeding through an NG or orogastric tube, what is the best way to insert and maintain the tube safely?

Ask/Assess

You will most likely consult the hospital policy when you are unsure about how to proceed. In the clinical story, Anthony looks up his hospital's NG/OG tube policy, but he finds there is no evidence to support about how he should determine how far to insert the tube. He is aware of method called the nose-earlobe-xiphoid (NEX) method of predicting the length to insert an NG/OG tube. To determine how far to

---

BOX 19■1 **Significance of Nasogastric/Orogastric Tube Placement in Infants**

- Infants with respiratory conditions may not be able to both breathe and suck to take in nutrition and fluids.
- NG/OG tubes are a very common method to feed infants unable to take in adequate oral nutrition and fluids because of a variety of conditions.
- Two key issues related to nursing care are determining proper insertion length and verifying placement of the tube in the gastrointestinal tract.
- Tube placement poses two safety threats to the infant:
  - Improper insertion length: too short, leading to potential aspiration, or too deep, impairing normal digestion (too long)
  - Insertion in the respiratory tract, leading to catastrophic aspiration and pneumonia if infant is fed through an improperly placed tube

insert the tube using this method, you first measure the length from the infant's nose to the earlobe and ends at the xiphoid process.

When you determine the scope and scale of the problem, you consider how frequently the nursing care issue arises in everyday practice and what aspects of care you need to address for an infant with a feeding tube. Anthony knows that nurses on his unit are likely to place or change an NG tube in an infant at least once per day. Given how frequently nurses are caring for these tubes and the opportunity for a poor outcome, the problem certainly merits a thorough examination of the best available evidence. There are several aspects of care to consider; for instance, what types of tubes are best, what the indications for using a feeding tube are, what the best way to check placement is, and how the tube should be secured. In the clinical story, Anthony is most concerned with issues of safety, namely, how to estimate the insertion length and how to check the placement of an NG tube.

The first step in evidence-based practice is to write down the clinical questions that will lead to the evidence you need. For this particular issue, you might write a general question: "What is the best method to predict the insertion length to place an NG tube in hospitalized infants?" If you have an idea about an intervention that might work, you can narrow the question when you create a PICO question. However, if you do not know alternative interventions, you may not be able to state both a comparison and an intervention. In this case, the population of interest (P) is hospitalized infants, the intervention (I) is a better method to predict the insertion length to place an NG/OG tube, the comparison (C) method is NEX, and the outcome (O) is safe placement of the tube tip and all openings in the stomach. Putting the parts together, Anthony's PICO question is, "In hospitalized infants, is there a better method to predict the insertion length to successfully place an NG/OG tube in the stomach than NEX?"

Acquire/Diagnose

After you have formed your question based on your assessment of the nursing-relevant problems, the next step is to find the evidence. You may be like Anthony and have only a short time to search for evidence when you are at the point of care. When pressed for time, you will likely use a broad search using the key terms that come to mind. For example, you might use a search strategy that links synonyms for "nasogastric tube" and "orogastric tube" with the idea of placement. Anthony found 81 articles when he used a quick strategy of combining these key words: "nasogastric tube" OR "NG tube" OR "orogastric tube" OR "OG tube" with place*. This search strategy will find both articles with the full name or common abbreviation for naso-gastric tube or orogastric tube. By combining "place*" with the key words represent-ing the tube, you will find articles that address both the tube and placement. In the MEDLINE database, the * symbol truncates words and allows you to find articles with any form of the word "place," such as "placement," "placing," "placed," and so on.

Table 19■1 provides the currently available evidence for predicting the length of gastric tubes for insertion in children. Anthony is able to find only part of this evidence, here listed in order of publication, on his first search of the literature because he only has time to search the MEDLINE database—Ziemer and Carroll (1978); Weibly, Adamson, Clinkscales, et al. (1987); Gallaher, Cashwell, Hall, et al. (1993); Tedeschi, Atimer, and Warner (2004); and Beckstrand, Ellett, and McDaniel (2007). As you can see, three of the studies were published more than 10 years prior to the more recent studies.

Anthony works at a major medical center that is affiliated with a school of nursing. Researchers from the school typically carry out their clinical research in the university hospital. In fact, Anthony remembers that one of the faculty members had recently completed a study about NG tube placement. He searches again for articles with the author's name but did not find anything published yet. He asks the advanced practice nurse (APN) who had helped with the study how to find the information. The APN says that the data were analyzed and the articles are nearly ready to be

(text continues on page 270)

Table 19■1 **Research Evidence for Predicting the Length to Insert a Nasogastric/ Orogastric Tube in Children**

Authors (Year)	Sample/ Design	Results	Conclusions	Strengths/ Weaknesses	*LOE
Royce et al (1951)	30 premature infants <1800 g/ retrospective descriptive	NG tube was inserted until it was "estimated by rough measurement to have entered the stomach" (p. 79).	28/30 premature infants survived	Early documentation of how an NG tube was inserted/ method of predicting the length for placing the NG tube was not the focus of the study.	Background
Ziemer and Carroll (1978)	Unreported number of infants at autopsy/ prospective descriptive	NG tube inserted using the NEX method reached just past the cardiac sphincter. If the tube was inserted using the NEMU method, the tube was properly positioned.	The NEMU method should be used to predict the insertion length to place NG tubes in infants.	First study comparing NEX and NEMU prediction methods in infants/ number of infants studied not reported. A red rubber tube was used.	3

(continues on page 268)

Table 19■1   **Research Evidence for Predicting the Length to Insert a Nasogastric/ Orogastric Tube in Children** (continued)

Authors (Year)	Sample/ Design	Results	Conclusions	Strengths/ Weaknesses	*LOE
Weibly et al (1987)	30 premature infants (28–36 weeks' gestational age)/ Prospective within subject comparison	NEX length was too short in 55.6% of the infants, and the NEMU length was too short in 39.3% of infants.	NEMU was superior to NEX, but neither was optimal.	Study was stronger using infants as their own comparison, as all infants received both the NEX and NEMU method/ no random-ization	3
Gallaher et al (1993)	171 x-rays in of 31 very low-birth-weight infants were reviewed retrospec-tively. Then, after insti-tuting the new guide-lines, 117 x-rays from 27 infants were reviewed/ retrospec-tive and prospective review of x-rays	Recommended the following minimal inser-tion lengths: 13 cm for infants (<750 g), 15 cm (750–999 g), 16 cm (1000–1249 g), and 17 cm (1250–1499 g)	Using these insertion lengths, they were able to de-crease the error rate in their neona-tal intensive care unit from 38% to 14%.	Study focused on very low-birth-weight infants. First study to in-vestigate weight as a method of predicting OG tube insertion length.	3
Tedeschi et al (2004)	43 tubes in-serted in 38 premature infants (25–35 weeks' gestational age)/prosp ective de-scriptive	NEMU method resulted in only two tubes (5%) being located in the distal esophagus and 41 (95%) accurately located in the stomach.	Recom-mended use of NEMU to predict the length to insert an NG tube.	Found NEMU to be a bet-ter predictor than Weibly et al had/no comparison.	3

Authors (Year)	Sample/ Design	Results	Conclusions	Strengths/ Weaknesses	*LOE
Beck-strand et al (2007)	Studied 20 external measures including NEX, NEMU, age, height, and weight as possible insertion length predictors in 494 children 2 weeks to 19 years (231 months) undergoing upper gastroin-testinal en-doscopy or esophageal manometric studies/ descriptive.	Regression equa-tions using height in age groups (ARHB) were found to be the best predic-tors of optimal placement of the endoscope or manometric probe in the stomach. Ages: 1–28 months, –100 months, 100121 months, and >121 months.	Age-specific regression equations using the child's height/ length accurately predicted the dis-tances to the stomach in 98.8% of children ages 0.5– 100 months and in 96.5% of children older than 100 months. The next best choice was the NEMU length.	Large sample size with sophisti-cated data analyses/ researchers did not use recom-mended method to insert NG/OG tubes. They also did not present the regression equations in a form eas-ily usable in practice.	3
[1]Ellett, Smith, Cohen, Perkins, Lane et al. (2010)	165 hospital-ized neonates ≤1 month of age requir-ing place-ment of a NG/OG tube/RCT	Both NEMU and ARHB methods were the supe-rior insertion length predictors. NEX was too short in 39% of cases. Using both NEMU and ARHB methods, there were sta-tistically signifi-cant differences from NEX, but there was no statistically sig-nificant differ-ence between the two.	Use either NEMU or ARHB method (in infants over 47 cm in length) to predict the insertion length to place NG/OG tubes in neonates.	First RCT. A new equa-tion based on length was devel-oped specif-ically for neonates. New ARHB method pro-vided as nomogram for easy use by health-care pro-viders. Origi-nal ARHB equation could not be used for pre-mature in-fants less than 44.5 cm in length.	2

(continues on page 270)

Table 19■1   **Research Evidence for Predicting the Length to Insert a Nasogastric/ Orogastric Tube in Children** (continued)

Authors (Year)	Sample/ Design	Results	Conclusions	Strengths/ Weaknesses	*LOE
[1]Ellett, Smith, Cohen, Perkins, et al. (2010)	95 children 1 month to 18 years of age/RCT	Both ARHB and NEMU methods were superior to NEX as insertion-length predictors. NEX was too short in 41% of cases. Using both ARHB and NEMU methods, there were statistically significant differences from NEX, but there was no statistically significant difference between the two.	Use either NEMU or ARHB method to predict the insertion length to place NG/OG tubes.	Part of the same RCT as above. ARHB method provided as a nomogram making it easier for healthcare providers to use.	2

ARHB = age-related, height-based; NEMU = nose-earlobe-midumbilicus; NEX = nose-earlobe-xiphoid; NG/OG = nasogastric/orogastric tube; RCT = randomized controlled trial

[1]Acknowledgement: This study was supported in part by the National Institute of Nursing Research R01 NR00811. (From Ellett, M. L. C., Smith, C.E., Cohen, M.D., et al. (2010). Gastric tube placement in neonates. Manuscript in preparation; Ellett, M. L. C., Smith, C. E., Cohen, M. D., Perkins, S. M., Lane, K., Austin, J. K., et al. (2010). Gastric tube placement in children 1 month to 18 years of age. Manuscript in preparation.

*LOE = Levels of evidence (Joanna Briggs Institute, 2010), where 1 = meta-analysis with homogeneity of RCTs with concealed randomization OR one or more large RCT with narrow confidence limits; 2 = one or more smaller RCTs with wider confidence intervals OR quasi-experimental study without randomization; 3 = cohort study with a control group or case-controlled or observational studies without a control group; 4 = expert opinion or physiology bench research or expert opinion.

sent to journals for peer review. The APN asks the faculty member to present her studies of neonates and children older than 1 month to the unit. The researcher gladly shares her data and the findings from the studies (Ellett, Smith, Cohen, Perkins, et al., 2010; Ellett, Smith, Cohen, Perkins, Lane, et al., 2010). Based on his conversation with the APN and the investigator, Anthony is satisfied that he has found all of the available evidence, so it is time to appraise its quality and plan the intervention.

Appraise/Plan

When you do not have access to a high-quality, summarized, and pre-appraised evidence source, you need to critique the primary studies. Anthony asked the APN to help him organize the information from the studies and to rate their quality. Most are descriptive (lower level of evidence) but the more recent, prepublication articles look as though they represent stronger research methods. For example, the methods include one comparative study and one randomized controlled trial (higher levels of evidence).

When Anthony looks over the evidence table (see Table 19■1) and scans the abstracts of these articles, he is pleased to see that many of the researchers studied infants, most of whom were premature. He notices that none of the researchers recommended using NEX as the insertion-length predictor. Measuring from the nose to the earlobe to a point midway between the xiphoid process (the tip of the sternum) and the umbilicus was suggested in the oldest article (Ziemer and Carroll, 1978) and was tested in five subsequent articles. Weibly et al. (1987) found the nose-earlobe-midumblicus (NEMU) insertion-length predictor was too short but the other four found it to be either the best or second best choice (Beckstrand et al., 2007; Ellett, Croffie, and Beckstand, 2005; Gallaher et al., 1993; Tedeschi et al., 2004). Beckstrand et al. proposed a new insertion-length predictor using a regression equation based on the child's length/height in age groups (age-related, height-based [ARHB] method). **Regression equations** come from a statistical analysis that allows you to predict the dependent variable based on two or more independent variables. In this example, insertion length (the dependent variable) can be predicted based on an equation that factors in the baby's length and age. Ellett, Smith, Cohen, Perkins, Lane et al. (2010) tested NEX, NEMU, and ARHB in a large sample of 276 children and found NEMU to be superior to NEX in neonates (infants less than 1 month old corrected age, including premature infants) and both ARHB and NEMU to be superior in children 1 month of age or older (Ellett, Smith, Cohen, Perkins, et al., 2010). Anthony notices that the most recent studies were also conducted with the strongest designs.

The APN wanted to make sure that they found all of the literature and expanded the quick search to include more databases (Cochrane Database of Systematic Reviews, Cochrane Database of Randomized Clinical Trials, MEDLINE, CINAHL, and National Guidelines Clearing House). She found other evidence and added them to the evidence table (see Table 19■1).

The APN also uncovered the probable origin of the NEX insertion-length predictor when she found the Ziemer and Carroll (1978) article. These authors cited the Royce, Tepper, Watson, et al. (1951) article that seemed to form the basis for the use of the NEX method for predicting the insertion length to a place an NG/OG tube. Anthony was taught the NEX method in nursing school and it formed his hospital's policy. But the earlier publications did not mention the NEX method by name nor was it the focus of the study being conducted. Subsequently, authors/editors of nursing textbooks probably either cited this article as a reference for using the NEX method to predict the length to insert an NG/OG tube or cited previous editions of theirs or others' nursing textbooks (Ellett, Smith, Cohen, Perkins, Lane, et al., 2010).

Apply/Implement

Based on his initial appraisal of the evidence, Anthony would like to use the NEMU insertion-length predictor to insert EB's NG tube; however, the policy of his hospital states that the NEX insertion-length predictor should be used. He knows he could get into trouble if he does not follow hospital policy. Anthony remembers that EB is scheduled to receive a chest x-ray in about 20 minutes. Because of EB's mild tachypnea that worsens when disturbed, he is justified in requesting a portable chest x-ray be done at the bedside. This will allow Anthony to ask the x-ray technician to take the film in such a manner that the tip of the NG tube should be visible because he wants to be sure it is placed correctly in the stomach. Anthony quickly assembles the equipment he will need to place the NG tube, explains the procedure including the need for the tube to EB's mother and grandmother, and gives them permission to either leave or stay while he inserts the tube. The mother has been up with EB for 24 hours, so she decides to make a trip to the hospital cafeteria for something to eat, while the grandmother decides to stay to make sure nothing happens to her grandson. Anthony wraps EB securely in the blanket on which he is lying. He does this so that there will be minimal disturbance to the sleeping EB. Anthony will not have to deal with flying arms and legs while inserting the tube. He prepares his supplies for easy access, puts on clean gloves, and estimates the insertion length using the NEMU method—he measures the length from the baby's nose to the earlobe and to the midpoint between the xiphoid and umbilicus. He holds the tube at the spot he measured so he knows how far to insert, wrapping the tube around his hand so he can control the tube. He places one hand on EB's head to keep his neck slightly flexed toward his stomach (to keep the airway closed), lubricates the distal part of the tube with sterile water, and gently but continuously inserts the tube into one nostril. This awakens EB, who cries as the tube is inserted the desired distance. Anthony encourages EB's grandmother to talk to her grandson. She begins to sing a special song that she sings to EB most evenings before he goes to sleep; this immediately focuses EB's attention on her and calms him.

Anthony tapes the tube in place and tests placement by injecting a small amount of air (0.5 to 1 mL) into the tube while listening over the epigastrium (region over the stomach) for a "whish." He hears the sound loud and clear. He makes sure the tube is taped securely to the skin protector he places on EB's cheek and directs the rest of the tube down the infant's back into the blanket. Then Anthony leaves the room briefly to order the film.

Anthony waits for about 15 minutes after the x-ray has been taken and then calls the radiology department to see if it has been read. The clerk answering the telephone reports that the pediatric radiologist is reading it now and transfers his call to the radiologist. Anthony asks about the position of the NG tube. The radiologist reports the tip of the tube is at the lower border of the diaphragm, indicating that it is likely at the gastroesophageal junction (the point where the esophagus and stomach join). Although any openings on the tube are not visible, they would likely be in the esophagus. He suggests Anthony advance the tube 2 to 3 cm deeper. Anthony knows he should be relieved for a break soon, so he asks if the radiologist will show him the film if he comes by on his break. The radiologist agrees.

Anthony returns to the bedside to explain to EB's mother and grandmother that the tube is headed in the right direction but needs to be pushed in about an inch. As EB is again sleeping, Anthony carefully loosens the tape on the tube so as not to disturb EB because the tape is adhered to the skin-protective barrier rather than his cheek. Anthony pushes in the tube 2.5 cm, causing EB to stir briefly, and then he quickly retapes the tube. Both EB's mother and grandmother relax as EB drifts off to sleep again.

About an hour later, Anthony is relieved for break. He heads to the radiology department and asks for the radiologist. The radiologist shows him EB's film and briefly explains the anatomical landmarks he uses to determine placement (lower border of the diaphragm, gas bubble in the stomach, lungs, and vertebral column). He shows Anthony where the tube was and where it is likely to be now after he pushed it in 2.5 cm. Anthony realizes that safe and effective NG tube placement and care require more than the nursing team (Box 19■2).

Assess/Evaluate

The next step in the evidence-based practice and nursing process is to evaluate the implementation of the evidence and care plan. In the clinical story, Anthony needs to assess the effectiveness of how he estimated how far to insert the NG tube. The proper evaluation of the plan also requires knowing what the best evidence is to assess your care.

BOX 19■2   **Interdisciplinary Rounds**

- Nurses are accountable and responsible for inserting tube properly and maintaining proper placement of the tube.
- Work with parents to help them understand the reason that the tube is necessary.
- If the mother is breastfeeding, it's possible to provide her milk through the NG/OG tube.
- The gold standard for verifying placement of NG/OG tubes remains a chest x-ray, which requires a physician's order and interpretation and working with the radiology technician to capture the tube placement.
- Partner with clinical nurse specialists to help you manage the evidence.
- Other stakeholders in the insertion and maintenance of NG/OG tubes in infants include the following:
  - Nutritionists—determine optimal feeding protocols
  - Skin specialists—advise on maintaining skin integrity when securing the tube
  - Respiratory therapists—coordinate and manage oxygen delivery whether it be through a nasal cannula, mask, or ventilator
  - Occupational therapists—help restore effective sucking
- Engage with nurse researchers and or any discipline that shares interest in nursing problems to gain access to cutting-edge research.

Anthony is now curious about the best way to check the placement of the tube. Why did the bedside method he used to test placement fail to tell him the tube was not yet in the stomach and needed to be pushed in further? Thus, his second clinical question is, "Is injecting air through the tube while auscultating over the epigastrium the best bedside method available for monitoring tube location?" Anthony decides to search for information to answer this second clinical question, so he places it in PICO format. His population of interest (P) remains hospitalized infants, the intervention (I) is to see if there is a better bedside method to determine the internal location of an NG/OG tube, the comparison (C) method is auscultation over the epigastrium, and the outcome (O) remains successful placement of the tube tip and all openings in the stomach. Putting the parts together, his PICO question is "In hospitalized infants, is there a better method to determine the internal location of an NG/OG tube in the stomach than auscultation over the epigastrium?" He repeats his search using the same databases as before and finds the resources summarized in Table 19=2. He prints the articles so that he can read them carefully.

Anthony is surprised to find no support for injecting a small amount of air through the tube with a syringe while listening for sound over the epigastrium, as this was the method recommended in his hospital's policy and the method he was taught in nursing school for checking NG/OG tube placement (Bankhead et al., 2009; Ellett and Beckstrand, 1999). He also notices that no studies specific to children were found before 1999. It appears that unsuspected respiratory placements in children occur rarely, as none were documented in any of the published studies. Multiple researchers have studied the effectiveness of measuring the pH (the degree of acidity) of tube aspirate (fluid removed the tube) using a cutoff of pH greater than 5 in fasting children and greater than 6 in fed children. But they found little success of this technique in predicting when an NG/OG tube is not inserted in the stomach (Ellett, Croffie, Cohen, et al., 2005; Ellet, Smith, Cohen, Perkins, Lane, et al, 2010; Ellett, Smith, Cohen, Perkins, Lane, Poindexter, et al., 2010). Likewise, measuring bilirubin (a secretion typical of the small intestine) of tube aspirate using the cutoff of 5 mg/dL or greater has had limited success in predicting when an NG/OG tube is located in the small intestine. Also, the visual bilirubin scale tested in the research studies is not commercially available. Measuring pepsin and trypsin (enzyme secretions found in the stomach and small intestine, respectively) shows promise as an indicator of enteral tube placement (Westhus, 2004); however, no bedside tests are currently available for either of these enzymes. Thus, radiographic verification of proper placement, done at the time of initial NG/OG tube insertion or change in position is necessary to ensure that the tube has not been misplaced. Assessing that the tube insertion length has not changed and assessing the color (gastric fluid is usually white, tan, colorless, or green) and consistency (gastric fluid is usually cloudy) of tube aspirate along with pH testing appear to be the best bedside methods currently available for interim monitoring of NG/OG tube location (Ellet, Smith, Cohen, Perkins, Lane, et al., 2010; Ellett, Smith, Cohen, Perkins, Lane, Poindexter, et al., 2010; Westhus, 2004).

During his next shift, Anthony asks his fellow nurses whether any of them has received a call from the radiology department telling them to push in the NG tube on any of their patients. Most of them admitted that they had but thought it was

(text continues on page 283)

Table 19■2   **Research Evidence for Bedside Methods Used to Verify the Internal Location of Nasogastric/Orogastric Tubes in Children**

Authors (Year)	Sample/ Design	Results	Conclusions	Strengths/ Weaknesses	*LOE
Ellett and Beckstrand (1999)	39 hospitalized children (6 days to 13 years of age, mean = 20.1 months) having 46 enteral tubes (35 NG, 3 OG, 8 nasointestinal)/ prospective descriptive	Studied three bedside placement screening methods: (a) submerging the open end of the enteral tube in water and observing for bubbles during expiration; (b) auscultating the epigastrium and all four abdominal quadrants for the loudest sound; and (c) aspirating tube contents and testing pH. Enteral tube placement errors were observed on 22/101 (20.9%) x-rays. For NG tubes, pH of tube aspirate >4 had the PPV) for predicting tube placement error on x-ray, as 9/21 (42.8%) of tubes having a pH value >4 were found not to be located in the stomach. This compares with PPVs of 6/17 (35.3%) for hearing sound on auscultation over the epigastrium and 1/5 (20.0%) hearing sound on auscultation over the left upper quadrant on x-ray.	None of the bedside placement-screening methods were adequate in detecting enteral tube placement errors.	First study to prospectively document tube placement error rate in children/ Because the x-rays compared with beside placement screening assessments of tube locations were done for medical reasons within 12 hours, tube location potentially could have changed from the time of assessment.	3

(continues on page 276)

Table 19■2   **Research Evidence for Bedside Methods Used to Verify the Internal Location of Nasogastric/Orogastric Tubes in Children** (continued)

Authors (Year)	Sample/ Design	Results	Conclusions	Strengths/ Weaknesses	*LOE
Metheny, Eikov, Roundtree, et al (1999)	39 critically ill neonates (4 to 182 days of age, mean = 59 days)/ Prospective descriptive	Mean pH of aspirates from 88 gastric aspirates was 4.32 and mean pH of 2 intestinal aspirates was 7.80. 47/88 (53.4%) of neonates were fasting ≥4 hours and 41/88 (46.6%) were being continuously fed at the time tube aspirates were obtained. 75% of neonates were receiving acid-inhibiting medications. The neonates' mean fasting gastric pepsin concentration (76.1 mcg/mL) was much lower than that of adults.	pH and concentrations of trypsin and bilirubin in feeding tube aspirates from neonates were similar to those of adults. Gastric pepsin values were much lower than adults. Further research is needed to determine cutoff values of pH, pepsin, trypsin, and bilirubin concentrations in feeding tube aspirates in children of all ages.	Study was done by an experienced research team that has completed many similar studies in adults/ Too few intestinal aspirates were available for recommendations to be made. Bedside tests for bilirubin, pepsin, and trypsin are not currently available.	3
Gharpure et al (2000)	53 critically ill children (8 days to 19 years of age, mean = 2.5 years) providing 96 gastrointestinal aspirates/ Prospective descriptive	68% of children were fasting when aspirates were obtained, and all were receiving acid-inhibiting medications. pH of tube aspirate ≥6 had a low PPV and high NPV for pospyloric tube placement. Bilirubin ≥5 mg/dL had	Simple bedside assessment of gastrointestinal aspirate color, pH, and bilirubin concentration is useful for predicting feeding tube position. Use of	First study to specifically look at postpyloric tube placement. There are currently no bedside tests for bilirubin, pepsin, or trypsin.	3

Authors (Year)	Sample/ Design	Results	Conclusions	Strengths/ Weaknesses	*LOE
		a high PPV and a low NPV for post-pyloric tube placement. Overall efficiency for predicting postpyloric placement of the tube was best for the combination of a clear yellow aspirate, pepsin concentration ≤20 mcg/mL, and trypsin concentration ≥50 mcg/mL.	these tests may reduce the number of x-ray studies needed to confirm postpyloric positioning.		
Westhus (2004)	56 critically ill children (birth to 14 years of age, mean = 3.1 years)/ prospective descriptive (validation) study	49 (87.5%) feeding tubes were placed in the stomach and 7 (12.5%) were placed in the duodenum. 38/49 gastric aspirates (77.6%) had pH meter readings ≤6 in spite of 23/49 children (49%) receiving acid-inhibiting medications. The mean trypsin concentration was 70.4 mcg/mL. Gastric aspirates were most frequently colorless, green, tan/offwhite, or brown in color and cloudy in consistency; small bowel aspirates were usually yellow to bile colored and clear in consistency.	A pH <6, trypsin <50 mcg/ mL; pepsin ≥20 mcg/ mL; and clear, tan, or green color of aspirate predict placement of the enteral tube in the stomach >90%. However, a negative result is not a good indicator that the tube is in the intestine (NPV <63%). Negative results require the x-ray determination of tube location.	Validates that current bedside methods available to the healthcare providers (pH and color of tube aspirate [NPV 36.8%]) are clinically inadequate in predicting tube placement errors.	3

(continues on page 278)

Table 19■2   **Research Evidence for Bedside Methods Used to Verify the Internal Location of Nasogastric/Orogastric Tubes in Children** (continued)

Authors (Year)	Sample/ Design	Results	Conclusions	Strengths/ Weaknesses	*LOE
		NPVs, indicating the ability to predict when the enteral tube was not located in the stomach, were 35.2% for pH <6, 50% for trypsin <50 mcg/ mL, and 25% for pepsin >20 mcg/ mL; 62.5% for color (yellow or bile-stained).			
Ellett et al (2005)	72 hospitalized children (3 days– 7 years 4.4 months, M = 11.4 months) having 68 NG tubes [94.4%] and 4 OG tubes [5.6%])/ Prospective, descriptive	NG/OG placement errors occurred in 15/72 tubes (20.8%). In 13/15 (86.7%), the tube tip and/or orifices were in the esophagus, and in 2/15 (13.3%), the tip and at least one of the tube's orifices were beyond the pyloric sphincter into the duodenum. Mean pH values ranged from 4.3 in bolus-fed children to 4.7 in intermittent and continuously fed children. Using the suggested adult pH cutoff of 5, pH monitoring correctly predicted only 7/28 (25.0%) of tubes shown to be incorrectly placed outside the	Used the following algorithm: (a) if the pH of tube aspirate was ≤5, assume correct placement in the stomach (34 children correctly identified), and (b) if either pH was >5 (28 children) or no aspirate was obtained (4 children), obtaining an abdominal x-ray to determine tube position, would have resulted in 66/72 (92%) eventually	Recommended an algorithm for practice that had the potential of being 92% accurate in predicting tube placement errors. There were no respiratory misplacements to adequately test the ability of CO_2 monitoring to detect unsuspected respiratory misplacement. Measuring of pH of tube aspirate alone was clinically inadequate in	3

Authors (Year)	Sample/ Design	Results	Conclusions	Strengths/ Weaknesses	*LOE
		stomach (PPV). There was an adequate amount of aspirate obtained for bilirubin determination in 62/72 (86.1%). Using the suggested adult bilirubin cutoff of ≥5 mg/dL, bilirubin monitoring failed to predict either of the two incorrectly placed tubes. In addition, two tubes having a bilirubin level >5 mg/dL (7.3 and 11.6 mg/dL) were found to be correctly placed in the stomach on x-ray. No tubes were placed in the respiratory tract on radiograph. CO_2 readings were obtained in all 72 children. The values were 0 mm Hg in 71 (98.6%) and 2.0 mm Hg in the 1 (1.4%) remaining child. These values were well below the suggested adult cutoff of ≤15 mm Hg.	having correct placement in the stomach. Alternatively, obtaining an abdominal x-ray on all NG/OG tubes on insertion would result in nearly 100% accuracy.	predicting tube placement errors.	

(continues on page 280)

Table 19■2　**Research Evidence for Bedside Methods Used to Verify the Internal Location of Nasogastric/Orogastric Tubes in Children** (continued)

Authors (Year)	Sample/ Design	Results	Conclusions	Strengths/ Weaknesses	*LOE
Bankhead et al (2009)		Confirmation of correct position of a newly inserted enteral tube is mandatory before feedings or medications are administered. The gold standard for confirming correct placement of a blindly inserted enteral tube is a properly interpreted x-ray that visualizes the entire length of the tube. Multiple case reports clearly indicate that clinicians cannot differentiate between respiratory and gastric placement by the auscultatory method. Fasting gastric fluid typically is clear and colorless or grassy green with a pH of ≤5 with or without the use of gastric acid suppression. When the pH is ≥6, the pH method is of no benefit in predicting tube location in either the gastrointestinal or respiratory tract.	In pediatrics and neonates, all methods but x-ray verification of enteral tube placement have been shown to be inaccurate. X-ray use in children should be as judicious as possible given the radiation exposure. Among bedside methods that may be useful for interim monitoring of tube location between x-rays are (a) determining if the external length of the tubing has changed since the time of a confirmatory x-ray and (b) measuring the pH of the tube aspirate.	Recent practice recommendations from the professional group specializing in enteral nutrition.	4

Authors (Year)	Sample/ Design	Results	Conclusions	Strengths/ Weaknesses	*LOE
Ellett, Smith, Cohen, Perkins, Lane, Poindexter, et al, 2010; Ellet, Smith, Cohen, Perkins, Lane, Austin, et al, 2010	276 hospital-ized children (28.7 weeks' gestation corrected to 17 years 8 months)/ (RCT)	Tested using CO_2 monitoring to detect unsus-pected respira-tory placement of NG/OG tubes and measuring pH and bilirubin of tube aspirate to determine the internal location of the tube. In 275/276 children, CO_2 readings were 0. One infant had a reading of 32 mm Hg. Within 24 hours of the tube being placed in the fundus of the stomach on radi-ograph, that infant was being watched for necrotizing ente-rocolitis. There were no respira-tory placements on x-ray. Of the 41 tube place-ment errors in neonates, using the adult fasting pH cutoff of ≤ 5 suggested by Metheny et al (1999), only two tubes placed in the esophagus were detected. The pH readings of both tube as-pirates were 6. Likewise, of the 22 tube place-ment errors in children >1 month of age,	Inability to aspirate fluid from the NG/OG tube to be an indicator of mis-placement into the esophagus. Both pH and biliru-bin alone and in com-bination performed poorly in children as indicators of NG/OG tube mis-placement. Radio-graphic verification at the time of initial NG/OG tube inser-tion or change is necessary to ensure that the tube has not been misplaced. Using a combina-tion of as-sessing that the tube inser-tion length has not changed and as-sessing the color (gas-tric fluid is	First RCT in-volving a large sample of children. Recom-mendations for practice provided. No unsus-pected res-piratory placements occurred so the CO_2 monitoring could not be ade-quately tested.	2

(continues on page 282)

Table 19■2   **Research Evidence for Bedside Methods Used to Verify the Internal Location of Nasogastric/Orogastric Tubes in Children** (continued)

Authors (Year)	Sample/ Design	Results	Conclusions	Strengths/ Weaknesses	*LOE
		using the fasting adult pH cutoff of ≤5, three tubes placed in the esophagus were detected. The pH readings of the three tube aspirates were 7, 8, and 9. No aspirate was obtained from 16/41 (39.0%) misplaced tubes in neonates. All of the tubes were placed in the esophagus. Likewise, no aspirate was obtained from 8/22 (36.4%) misplaced tubes in older children. Again, all eight tubes were misplaced into the esophagus. None of the tubes misplaced into the duodenum in either age group (10/41 [24.4%] tubes in neonates and 4/22 [18.2%] in older children) were detected by either a pH >5 or a bilirubin >5 mg/dL.	usually white, tan, colorless, or green) and consistency (gastric fluid is usually cloudy) of tube aspirate along with pH testing are the best bedside methods currently available for interim monitoring of NG/OG tube location.		

ARHB = age-related, height-based; NEMU = nose-earlobe-midumbilicus; NEX = nose-earlobe-xiphoid; NG/OG = nasogastric/orogastric tube; NPV = negative predictive value; PPV = positive predictive value; RCT = randomized controlled trial

[1]Acknowledgement: This study was supported in part by the National Institute of Nursing Research R01 NR00811. (From Ellett, M. L. C., Smith, C. E., Cohen, M. D., Perkins, S. M., Lane, K., Poindexter, B., et al. (2010). Gastric tube placement in neonates. Manuscript in preparation.; Ellett, M. L. C., Smith, C. E., Cohen, M. D., Perkins, S. M., Lane, K., Austin, J. K., et al. (2010). Gastric tube placement in children 1 month to 18 years of age. Manuscript in preparation.

because they had done something wrong, although they had heard sound when they injected air and listened over the epigastrium or left upper quadrant of the abdomen. Anthony knew he was scheduled for his first annual review with his unit director the following week, so he plans to take this information from fellow nurses and his articles to this meeting. He thinks his hospital has an evidence-based practice committee and he plans to discuss joining this committee with his unit director. Possibly this problem is already on the committee's "radar screen"; if not, he can bring it to their attention and entreat them to put discussion of it on their agenda. In the meantime, he can help with other evidence-based practice projects that the committee has under way. Anthony feels good about the possibility of moving from being a novice nurse providing good care to his assigned patients to being a nurse working to influence the quality of care patients receive throughout his hospital.

■ Summary

Predicting the insertion length of an NG/OG tube is only one example of the way nurses have practiced based on tradition rather than on the best available evidence. When the usual way does not work adequately, nurses might think they personally have done something wrong. Therefore, they do not talk about it with their colleagues. Often, it is not their fault but the fault of the method they are using. Becoming involved in evidence-based practice committees at your place of employment that are actively involved in searching for answers to clinical problems important to your practice can be interesting and give you the satisfaction that you are truly supporting quality care for your patients (Box 19■3).

BOX 19■3 Tools for Learning and Practice

- Craft other questions related to the care of NG/OG tubes in infants.
- Analyze NG/OG insertion and care recommended in textbooks and compare the information with the current best available evidence.
- Compare policies related to NG/OG care on your clinical unit with current best available evidence.
- Work with an advanced practice nurse and/or a nurse researcher to develop an algorithm to help nurses make decisions for estimating insertion length and checking placement if they suspect the tube has moved, including how to assess the color of the aspirate.
- NG/OG tube placement should be verified by an x-ray and a mark should be placed externally on the tube so that nurses know when the tube may have moved.

CHAPTER QUESTIONS

1. What kinds of decisions did Anthony face when taking care of the baby EB's NG tube? How did these decisions relate to the nursing process and the evidence-based practice process? How would you have approached these same decisions?

2. What dilemma did Anthony face when he was preparing to pass EB's NG tube? Do you think he would have made the same decision if EB had not been scheduled for an x-ray soon? Why or why not?

3. What other ways could Anthony have brought the problem and the evidence he found to the attention of the nurses on his unit?

4. What do you find when you search the literature for risk factors for NG/OG tube misplacement (a tube placement error occurring on insertion) in children?

5. What do you find when you search the literature for risk factors for NG/OG tube displacement (migration of the tube from its original correct position) in children?

6. How did Anthony's access to the nurse researcher make a difference in how he approached the evidence? How might his decision have been different if he were not aware of the cutting-edge research?

References

Bankhead, R., Boullata, J., Brantley, S., et al. (2009). Enteral nutrition practice recommendations. *JPEN: Journal of Parenteral and Enteral Nutrition, 33,* 122–167.

Beckstrand, J., Ellett, M. L. C., & McDaniel, A. (2007). Predicting internal distance to the stomach for positioning nasogastric and orogastric feeding tubes in children. *Journal of Advanced Nursing, 59,* 274–289.

Centers for Disease Control and Prevention. (2010). Respiratory syncytial virus infection (RSV). Retrieved from http://www.cdc.gov/rsv/index.html

Ellett, M. L. C., & Beckstrand, J. (1999). Examination of gavage tube placement in children. *Journal of the Society of Pediatric Nursing, 4,* 51–60.

Ellett, M. L. C., Croffie, J. M. B., Cohen, M. D., et al. (2005). Gastric tube placement in young children. *Clinical Nursing Research, 14,* 239–252.

Ellett, M. L. C., Smith, C. E., Cohen, M. D., Perkins, S. M., et al. (2010). Gastric tube placement in children 1 month to 18 years of age. Manuscript in preparation.

Ellett, M. L. C., Smith, C. E., Cohen, M. D., Perkins, S. M., Lane, K., et al. (2010). Gastric tube placement in neonates. Manuscript in preparation.

Ellett, M. L. C., Smith, C. E., Cohen, M. D., Perkins, S. M., Lane, K., Rust, J. E., et al. (2010). The ability of bedside methods to determine the internal location of nasogastric/orogastric tubes in children. Manuscript in preparation.

Gallaher, K. J., Cashwell, S., Hall, V., et al. (1993). Orogastric tube insertion length in very low weight infants. *Journal of Perinatology, 13,* 128–131.

Gharpure, V., Meert, K. L., Sarnaik, A. P., et al. (2000). Indicators of postpyloric feeding tube placement in children. *Critical Care Medicine, 28,* 2962–2966.

Joanna Briggs Institute. (2010). JBI levels of evidence. Retrieved from http://www.joannabriggs.edu.au/pubs/approach.php

Metheny, N. A., Eikov, R., Rountree, V., et al. (1999). Indicators of feeding-tube placement in neonates. *Nutrition in Clinical Practice, 14,* 307–314.

Royce, S., Tepper, C., Watson, W., et al. (1951). Indwelling polyethylene nasogastric tube for feeding premature infants. *Pediatrics, 8,* 79–81.

Tedeschi, L., Atimer, L., & Warner, B. (2004). Improving the accuracy of indwelling gastric feeding tube placement in the neonatal population. *Neonatal Intensive Care: The Journal of Perinatology-Neonatology, 17,* 16–18.

Weibley, T. T., Adamson, M., Clinkscales, N., et al. (1987). Gavage tube insertion in the premature infant. *MCN: The American Journal of Maternal/Child Nursing, 12*(1), 24–27.

Westhus, N. (2004). Methods of testing feeding tube placement in children. *MCN: The Journal of Maternal Child Nursing, 29,* 282–287.

Ziemer, M., & Carroll, J. S. (1978). Infant gavage reconsidered. *American Journal of Nursing, 78,* 1543–1544.

CHAPTER 20

Psychiatric—Mental Health Nursing

Leslie Rittenmeyer

LEARNING OBJECTIVES

- Given an ill-structured description of a serious clinical problem, apply all phases of the evidence-based practice process to guide decisions related to the psychiatric—mental health domain.

- Analyze the challenge of making evidence-based decisions in complex health-care environments.

- Generate next-step strategies to get better evidence into practice.

KEY TERMS

Acute care setting
Joint Commission Performance
   Standard EP 4
Joint Commission Performance
   Standard EP 5
Local data

Occupational hazard
Occupational Safety and Health
   Act (OSHA) of 1970
PARIHS framework
Workplace violence

Clinical Story

Adam is a psychiatric liaison nurse at a large, acute care hospital. He provides services to the medical-surgical acute care units, including nursing staff consultation and education. During a weekly meeting with the nurse managers, Adam expresses concern about three different incidents of aggressive behavior in the past 6 weeks for which security staff presence was required. Two incidents were patient-related, and one was family-related. In the first case, the patient was transferred to the psychiatric unit; in the second case, the patient was given anti-anxiolytic medication; and in the third case, the offending family member was banned from visiting. In one incident a staff nurse sustained an injury when she was shoved against a wall. The nurse managers share Adam's concern but they fear the staff is ill equipped to provide intervention that prevents or manages aggressive behaviors. They feel this is an increasing problem and admit they lack a cohesive plan for addressing the issue. They ask Adam to assist them in addressing this vexing problem. ■

Introduction

Internationally, workplace violence is an increasing problem in the health-care environment (Beech and Leather, 2005). According to McPaul and Lipscomb (2004), it is a complex one as well, presenting an **occupational hazard** (danger of sustaining harm because of one's occupation) for nurses and other health-care workers. McPaul and Lipscomb believe that the complexity is due, in part, to a health-care culture that resists the idea that health-care workers are truly at risk and that treats workplace violence as part of the job. Lack of formal training in violence prevention and intervention adds to the problem and leaves the nursing staff with few resources to combat this growing issue.

As Adam starts developing a plan to address the increasing violence in the medical-surgical units at his facility, he realizes he needs to search for the best available evidence before he can make any recommendations about the right thing to do and the right way to do it. He also realizes that this is a complex problem because it affects both the well-being and safety of patients and the staff. Adam wants to ensure he uses the best available evidence when crafting his recommendations because he understands that any recommendations he makes will likely lead to changes in facility policy and new program development.

In this chapter, you will find guidelines for applying the evidence-based practice process to a growing mental health problem: workplace violence. To manage the complexity of this problem, the focus here is on the effectiveness of prevention and management interventions for aggressive behaviors in patients in the **acute care setting.** An acute care setting, such as a medical or surgical unit, provides services to patients with acute needs as opposed to chronic, rehabilitative, or palliative needs.

What Are the Key Issues?

Searching for information that will help solve clinical problems begins by asking basic questions. When considering the problem of workplace violence in the health-care setting, a list of initial questions might include the following:

1. What is workplace violence?
2. What is the scale and scope of the problem in the health-care setting?
3. Are there prevention guidelines already in place?
4. If there are guidelines in place, what type of evidence informed those guidelines?
5. Are there systematic reviews available to inform this topic?
6. What does the primary research literature say about this topic?
7. What do the experts say about this topic?

To start gathering information to answer these questions, you might first search the Internet for societies and groups that consider workplace violence in the health-care setting a problem. In doing so, you would find entities such as the World Health Organization (WHO), the United States Department of Labor Occupational Safety and Health Administration (OSHA), the Canadian Centre for Occupational Health and Safety (OSH), National Institute for Occupational Safety and Health (NIOSH), the American Nurses Association (ANA), the American Association of Occupational Health Nurses (AAOHN), and the U.S. Department of Justice (DOJ). All of these organizations consider workplace violence a serious problem in the health-care setting and recognize the need for prevention and education.

Although the wording might vary slightly, the definition of **workplace violence** is consistent across the organizations. The term is defined as any act in which a person is abused, threatened, intimidated, and/or assaulted as a result of his or her employment. The acts that constitute workplace violence include being threatened, either verbally or in writing; harassment; verbal abuse; or physical attack. Workplace violence is not just limited to the traditional workplace and can occur off site; for example, employees receiving threatening phone calls at home. Workplace violence can result in injury, psychological distress, and, in some cases, even death.

The next step is to identify the scale and scope of the problem. *Scope* is identifying the breath of the problem, and *scale* is determining if the problem is an isolated experience. In the case of workplace violence, the DOJ and the Bureau of Labor Statistics (BLS) gather relevant national statistical data related to the problem. Available data from the DOJ and BLS reveal that health-care workers are at increased risk to become victims of workplace violence. BLS reports that there were 69 homicides in health services from 1996 to 2000, and in 2000, 48% of all nonfatal injuries from occupational assault occurred in health care and social services (U.S. Department of Labor and Occupational Safety and Health Administration [OSHA], 2004). These data suggest that workplace violence in the health-care setting is not unique to Adam's institution in this chapter's clinical story. Adam begins to see that the problem is large in both scope and scale. Having gathered some baseline data and having a better idea of the scale and scope of the problem, Adam begins to develop a question that will guide him in his search for the best available evidence.

Ask/Assess

Both the nursing process and the evidence-based practice process begin with assessment, which should result in questions that lead to the best available evidence. To begin his assessment, Adam attempts to find out how many aggressive incidents occurred at his facility over the past 2 years. In most facilities, the risk management department should have a reliable system in place for recording and storing this type of data. These data would constitute **local data** and can provide a better understanding of the problem at Adam's particular institution. Unfortunately (and to his disappointment), Adam finds the record-keeping in his facility has been somewhat lax. The most he can ascertain is that security was called to the medical-surgical units 26 times in the past 2 years for reasons ranging from theft to threats of aggression. Adam makes a mental note to recommend more accurate and verifiable reporting mechanisms for aggressive incidents at his workplace. He knows that good local data lead to better planning and policies.

The next step is to find out if there is an existing policy on workplace violence prevention at the institution. Once existing policies are located, they can be evaluated to determine what type of evidence, if any, informed the policy. In some cases, policies are produced without being informed by any evidence, usually leading to ineffective programs or infrastructure. On searching the procedure manuals of his facility, Adam finds policies that generally address issues of patient and employee safety, as well as policies that outline procedures for dealing with aggressive incidents after they occur. However, none of the policies specifically addresses workplace violence prevention and intervention before or as it occurs.

While searching for more information, Adam finds that OSHA (2004) published *Guidelines for Preventing Workplace Violence for Healthcare and Social Service Workers.* He is surprised to learn OSHA does not have a mandatory compliance standard for the prevention of workplace violence because the guidelines are only advisory in nature. The compliance standard is the **Occupational Safety and Health Act (OSHA) of 1970.** This act mandates that, in addition to compliance with hazard-specific standards, all employers have a general duty to provide their employees with a hazard-free workplace. Adam also discovers that, although there is no federal standard that specifically requires workplace violence protections, the Joint Commission instituted a new leadership standard (LD 03.01.01) (effective January 1, 2009) that addresses disruptive and inappropriate behavior in two of its elements of performance. **Joint Commission Performance Standard EP 4** states the hospital/organization must have a code of conduct that defines acceptable and disruptive and inappropriate behavior, and **Joint Commission Performance Standard EP 5** states that leaders need to create and implement a process for managing disruptive and inappropriate behavior.

After reviewing this information, Adam believes he has ample reason to pursue the development of a policy and program aimed at the prevention of workplace violence. He is ready to ask a well-formed question that will help him find the best available evidence to accomplish his task. After some thought, he forms the following two PICO questions (Table 20■1):

1. What is the effectiveness of interventions in the prevention of aggressive behaviors in patients admitted to an acute care hospital setting?
2. What is the effectiveness of interventions in the management of aggressive behaviors in patients admitted to an acute care hospital setting?

Acquire/Diagnose

Once you have used the assessment data to identify a problem and you have clarified your question, you begin to pursue the next step of the process: how to acquire the best available evidence. Based on your PICO questions, you generate a list of keywords to start a search. If your questions are based on the effectiveness of interventions, the ideal source of evidence is a clinical practice guideline based on systematic reviews of randomized controlled trials (RCTs) that tested the interventions. If no such guidelines exist, search for systematic reviews or individual studies using bibliographic databases such as CINAHL and MEDLINE. It is usually wise to ask the hospital librarian to assist you in searching. This is what Adam did, and Table 20■2 provides an outline of Adam's search strategy and keywords.

Table 20■1 **Narrowing the Focus and Generating Questions**

Broad	What are the best practices for preventing workplace violence?	
Narrow	What are the best practices to prevent and manage workforce violence in the health-care sector?	
Narrow	What is the best way to prevent and manage aggressive behaviors in the acute care setting?	
Searchable PICO	What is the effectiveness of interventions in the prevention of aggressive behaviors in patients admitted to an acute care hospital setting?	P = admitted patients I = interventions to reduce aggressive behavior C = no comparison O = reduction of aggressive behavior
Searchable PICO	What is the effectiveness of interventions in the management of aggressive behaviors in patients admitted to an acute care hospital setting?	P = admitted patients I = interventions to manage aggressive behaviors C = no comparison O = management of aggressive behavior

Table 20■2   **An Example of Keywords and Search Strategy for Searching the CIHAHL Bibliographic Database for a PICO Question**

What is the effectiveness of interventions in the prevention and management of aggressive behaviors in patients admitted to an acute care hospital setting?

1.	(MH "Nurses") or MH "Nurse Patient Relations")
2.	Nurs*
3.	S1 or S2
4.	(MH "Violence") or (MH "Workplace Violence")
5.	Aggress* or abus* or violen* or danger* or assault*
6.	S4 or S5
7.	(MH "Patients")
8.	Patient*
9.	S7 or S8
10.	(MH " Hospitals") or (MH "Hospital Units")
11.	(acute, or medical surgical) (ward* or hospital or setting*)
12.	S10 or S11
13.	(MH "Psychotherapy") or (MH "Chemical restraint") (MH "Psychopharmacological treatment") ("Physical restraint") (MH "Music therapy") (MH "Staff education")
14.	Intervention or prevention or restrain*
15.	S13 or S14
16.	S3 and S6 and S9 and S12 and S15
17.	S3 and S6 and S9 and S12 and S15

Adam has already identified that OSHA (2004) published the *Guidelines for Preventing Workplace Violence for Healthcare and Social Service Workers*. He is now interested in determining how these guidelines were developed. A good guideline will demonstrate validity, reliability, reproducibility, and transparency. In examining the OSHA (2004) guidelines, Adam observes that they might not have been developed by the use of synthesized evidence, despite the fact that they were informed by individual research studies and the opinion of experts. Synthesized evidence is the effect of pooling the results of research findings to make a judgment about what interventions, activities, or phenomena the evidence supports. He notes it is difficult to see the transparency in the guideline development process, and the research processes to identify best available evidence should be transparent.

"Synthesized evidence" is the effect of pooling the results of research findings in order to make a judgment about what interventions, activities or phenomena the evidence supports. Adam decides to broaden his search and look for available synthesized evidence to help with his task. The hospital librarian assists him in broadening his search and the results reveal what he previously observed: there is more evidence that addresses violence prevention in the mental health setting than in the acute care setting. Finally, after conducting an extensive search, Adam finds a systematic review on the prevention and management of workplace violence in the acute care setting. The objective of the review was to establish best practice in the prevention and management of aggressive behaviors in patients admitted to acute care settings, and Adam hopes the systematic review will report reliable synthesized evidence.

As a last step, Adam asks the librarian to search the Cochrane Library and Joanna Briggs Institute Library of Systematic Reviews for any other systematic reviews that will assist him. Finding none, he selects the OSHA guideline and the systematic review to critically appraise. He chose the OSHA guideline because it was the only practice guideline he found related to his question and the systematic review because it provided the most complete form of synthesized evidence. Adam is confident that his comprehensive search has led him to available evidence, but now he needs to appraise the evidence to find out if it is the best.

Appraise/Plan

There are numerous tools available for the critical appraisal of clinical guidelines. Standardized appraisal tools assist with evaluating practice guidelines and systematic reviews to answer the following basic questions (Public Health Research Unit [PHRU], 2007):

- How clear is the focus?
- How transparent and rigorous were the methods?
- Can the recommendations be applied to this situation?

Adam appraises the OSHA (2004) guideline first. Although there are numerous tools available for the critical appraisal of clinical guidelines, he chooses the Appraisal of Guidelines Research and Evaluation tool (AGREE) (AGREE Collaboration, 2003). This tool was developed by an international collaboration of researchers and policy makers whose goal was improve the quality and effectiveness of clinical practice guidelines (Box 20■1).

Adam appraises the OSHA guideline against the AGREE criteria and found the following:

- The scope and questions seemed clear and focused.
- Diverse stakeholders such as doctors, nursing, academics, researchers, psychologists, and consumers were an integral part of the process.

BOX 20■1 AGREE Appraisal Instrument

Scope and Purpose

■ The potential health impact of a guideline on society and populations of patients has been identified.
■ A detailed description of the clinical questions is provided.
■ A clear description of the target population to be covered by the guideline is included.

Stakeholder Involvement

■ The guideline development group includes individuals from all the relevant professional groups.
■ Information about patients' experiences and expectations of health care should inform the development.
■ The target users of the guideline are clearly defined.
■ The guideline has been piloted among target users.

Rigor of Development

■ Systematic methods were used to search for evidence.
■ The criteria for selecting the evidence are clearly described.
■ The health benefits, side effects, and risks have been considered in formulating the recommendations.
■ There is an explicit link between the recommendations and the supporting evidence.
■ The guideline has been externally reviewed by experts prior to its publication.
■ A procedure for updating the guideline is provided.

Clarity and Presentation

■ The recommendations are specific and unambiguous.
■ The different options for management of the condition are clearly presented.
■ Key recommendations are easily identifiable.
■ The guideline is supported with tools and applications.

Applicability

■ The potential organizational barriers in applying the recommendations have been discussed.
■ The potential cost implications of applying the recommendations have been considered.
■ The guideline presents key criteria for monitoring and/or audit purposed.

Editorial Independence

■ The guideline is editorially independent from the funding body.
■ Guideline development members' conflicts of interest have been recorded.

- The use of rigorous and transparent methods, including systematic methods to search and appraise the evidence, was not readily evident. Research was used to develop the guideline but it was not synthesized research.
- Although stakeholders and experts were involved in the development of the guideline, there did not appear to be a formal process in which a panel of experts appraised and extracted the evidence, considered the benefits and risks, and reached consensus on the recommendations.
- The level of evidence was not identified in the guideline.
- The U.S. Inspector General's office performed an evaluation of OSHA's handling of workplace violence issues and made recommendations. There seems to be no formal update plan.
- The guideline is understandable and readily available online.

Adam chooses the Critical Appraisal Skills Program (CASP) tool for systematic reviews (PHRU, 2007) to appraise the systematic review (Box 20■2).

He identifies the following strengths of the review:

- The review asked two clearly focused PICO questions and selected appropriate study designs to include in the review (RCTs, controlled prospective, prospective cohort)
- There was a comprehensive search of eight databases and the gray literature as well as hand searching.
- The study appraisal and data extraction were strong. The authors used a blinded duel review method and transparently used rigorous criteria to include in the study.
- The researchers used appropriate data analysis techniques. Because of the type of studies conducted, a meta-analysis was not undertaken, but as there was considerable variation in the measured outcomes in the trials identified, data were therefore presented in a narrative summary.

BOX 20■2   Critical Appraisal Skills Program (CASP)

Critical Appraisal of Systematic Review Criteria:

- Did the review ask clearly focused questions?
- Did the review include the right type of study?
- Is the appraisal worth continuing?
- Did the reviewers try to identify all relevant studies?
- Did the reviewers assess the quality of the included studies?
- If the results of the studies have been combined, was it reasonable to do so?
- How are the results presented and what is the main result?
- How precise are the results?
- How can the results be applied to the local population?
- Were all important outcomes considered?
- Should policy or practice change as a result of the evidence contained in this review?

- The results of the study were reported according to the study intervention participants (e.g., staff training program, music, chemical restraint).
- There is limited evidence to support the use of staff training, chemical and/or physical restraint, and music therapy.
- The results of this study could be applied to a local population.

After reviewing the evidence he has gathered, Adam is disappointed that there is not more synthesized evidence but is confident that this is the best evidence available to him at this time. He agrees with the conclusions in the systematic review that state that "further quality research is needed to assist staff with identifying appropriate interventions to prevent and manage aggressive behavior in acute hospitalized patients" (Kynoch, Wu, and Chang, 2009, p. 196).

Because the systematic review represents stronger evidence than the OSHA (2004) guideline, Adam compares the two to look for consistencies in recommendations. From both the OSHA guideline and the systematic review, Adam identified the following bottom-line recommendations:

- A training program for staff about managing patient aggression improves self-efficacy and assists staff in managing aggressive and/or violent patients (Kynoch et al., 2009 p. 195).
- Effective violence preventions programs have the following components (OSHA, 2004):

  1. Management commitment and employee involvement
  2. Worksite analysis
  3. Hazard prevention and control
  4. Safety and health training
  5. Record-keeping and program evaluation

- Administration of medication reduces the incidents of aggressive and/or violent behavior in patients in the acute care setting (Kynoch et al., 2009, p. 195).
- Physical restraints are effective in reducing harm to patients and staff and have minimal complications when used for short periods of time (Kynoch et al., 2009 p. 195).
- Individual interventions such as music therapy have been shown to decrease aggressive/and or agitated behaviors (Kynoch et al., 2009, p. 195).

Apply/Implement

The next step in the process is planning to implement changes in policy or programs. Remember that the whole point of evidence-based practice is to move evidence to the point of care. Because the evidence illustrates the benefits of staff training programs, Adam thinks he will focus his efforts on staff training. He begins thinking about how he can best facilitate this process, He decides to use the **PARIHS framework** (Promoting Action on Research Implementation in Health Services) (Kitson, Harvey, and McCormack, 1998; Kitson, Rycroft-Malone, Harvey, et al., 200'.

The PARIHS framework provides a way to implement research into practice. The framework posits that the successful implementation of evidence into practice has as much to do with context or setting where the new evidence is being introduced and how the evidence is introduced (facilitated into practice) as it has to do with the quality of evidence (Kitson et al., 1998). The PARIHS framework then looks at the type of evidence, the context in which the evidence is to be implemented, and the way in which the process is facilitated. Adam realizes that because of the size of his facility, the success of any program he wishes to implement will likely be compromised if he is the sole planner (Box 20■3). He knows, as the OSHA (2004) guideline suggests, that he needs to elicit management commitment and employee involvement. Adam proceeds to create a steering committee with broad representation of upper management, risk control staff, unit managers, professional nurses, and other staff. He knows that initially, as Kitson et al. (2008) suggest, he will need to facilitate change by providing direction along with technical, practical, and task-driven help. Eventually, he hopes his role will be to support and empower others to facilitate and evaluate the workforce prevention-training program.

With the emphasis on the development of a training program, Adam wants to discuss with others what he is envisioning. He knows he must provide strong leadership to create a culture sympathetic to the creation and implementation of the program.

As the systematic review did not make specific recommendations about the content of a training program, Adam focuses on the recommendations in the OSHA (2004) guideline. Although he would prefer to have a guideline developed with stronger synthesized evidence, he knows that this guideline is the best evidence that is available to him at this time. Adam also understands that time is of the essence with this problem, and he cannot afford to wait for better evidence to emerge. He reviews the OSHA (2004) recommendations related to essential training program content, as listed below:

- Presence of a workplace violence prevention policy
- Risk factors that cause or contribute to assaults
- Early recognition of escalating behavior or recognition of warning signs or situations that may lead to assault

---

BOX 20■3   **Interdisciplinary Rounds**

In the acute care setting it is essential to involve a diverse group of stakeholders. Participation by the following is vital. Can you think of any others?

- Vice-president of nursing service
- Nurse managers of the acute care units
- Registered nurses providing professional nursing care at the bedside
- Licensed practical nurses providing technical nursing care at the bedside
- Nursing assistants
- Risk managers

- Ways to prevent or diffuse volatile situations or aggressive behavior, manage anger, and appropriately use medications as chemical restraints
- A standard response action plan for violent situations, including the availability of assistance, response to alarm systems, and communication procedures
- Ways to deal with hostile people other than patients and clients, such as relatives and visitors
- Progressive behavior control methods and safe methods to apply restraints
- The location and operation of safety; devises such as alarm systems, along with required maintenance schedules and procedures
- Ways to protect oneself and coworkers, including the use of a buddy system
- Policies and procedures for reporting and recording
- Information on multicultural diversity to increase staff sensitivity to racial and ethnic issues and differences
- Policies and procedures for obtaining medical care, counseling, workers' compensation, or legal assistance after a violent episode or injury

Adam uses his own clinical knowledge and expertise to judge the OSHA recommendations, and he finds them theoretically consistent with what he believes should be part of an effective training program. In addition, although he does not want to recommend more than the steering committee can handle at one time, Adam feels that designing a better record-keeping system to gather better local data is also a priority. He also knows that they must design a good program evaluation system so that they can measure the effectiveness of their program. He is confident that he can successfully navigate the complexities of implementing evidence into practice and improve staff and patient safety at his facility (Box 20■4).

BOX 20■4 **Tools for Learning and Practice**

- Generate PICO questions that narrow the focus of prevention/management of workplace violence in acute care settings.
- Generate your own list of keywords and search for evidence in CINHAIL and Medline pertaining to prevention/management of workplace violence in acute care settings.
- Search the Internet for the AGREE Collaboration tool.
- Search the Internet for the CASP tool.
- Find OSHA's (2004), *Guidelines for Preventing Workplace Violence for Healthcare and Social Service Workers* (no. OSHA 3148-01R) and appraise them using the AGREE Collaboration tool.
- Conduct a search for workplace violence prevention and management programs and assess what evidence the program is based on.
- Search the Centers for Disease Control and Prevention (CDC) Web site and see if it has any data about workplace violence in the heath-care setting.

■ Summary

As Adam searched for the best available evidence, he discovered there is often a need for more primary research that can be pooled on a particular subject. Research generation is part of the evidence-based practice model and is certainly vital to Adam's quest for evidence about the prevention and management of aggressive patients in acute care settings. One of the benefits of an evidence-based practice model is that it identifies when there is a need for more evidence generation. Another common problem Adam encountered was learning there are instances when guidelines are based more on expert opinion than they are on more highly graded, synthesized research. Although research is generally considered the more highly regarded evidence and often possesses a higher level of quality and validity than expert opinion, in its absence expert opinion may be the best available evidence. Some (Pearson, Fields, and Jordan, 2004) feel that in the absence of rigorously derived research, it is not defensible to discount expert opinion as nonevidence.

CHAPTER QUESTIONS

1. How do the steps of the nursing process and the evidence-based process align in this chapter's clinical story?

2. How did Adam judge the strength and quality of the evidence? Do you agree with his assessment?

3. Justify the position of using a guideline that was developed from the evidence of expert opinion.

4. Considering that you might want to narrow the focus of your search, what other PICO questions could you ask about prevention and/or management of workplace violence in health care?

5. Adam chose to focus on developing an education program as his first priority. Considering the best available evidence, do you agree with that decision?

6. Given Adam's recommendations from the evidence, how would you prioritize an implementation plan?

7. Develop a written implementation plan using the PARIHS framework.

8. Develop a plan to gain acceptance of your implementation plan from a diverse group of stakeholders.

References

AGREE Collaboration. (2003). Development and validation of an international appraisal instrument for assessing the quality of clinical practice guidelines: The AGREE project. *Quality and Safety in Health Care, 12,* 18–23.

Beech, B., & Leather, L. (2006). Workplace violence in the health care sector: A review of staff training and integration of training evaluation model. *Aggression and Violent Behavior, 11,* 27–43.

Grade Working Group. (2004). Grading quality of evidence and strength of recommendations. *British Medical Journal, 328,* 1490–1497. doi:10.1136/bmj.3328.7454.1490

Joint Commission. (2009). National patient safety goals. Retrieved from http://www.jointcommission.org/

Kitson, A., Harvey, G., & McCormack, B. (1998). Enabling the implementation of evidence based practice: A conceptual framework. *Quality Health Care, 7,* 149–158. doi:10.1136/qhsc.7.3.14.9

Kitson, A., Rycroft-Malone, J., Harvey, G., et al. (2008). Evaluating the successful implementation of evidence into practice using the PARIHS Framework: Theoretical and practical challenges. *Implementation Science, 3.* doi:10.1186/1748-5908-3-1

Kynoch, K., Wu, J., & Chang, A. M. (2009). The effectiveness of interventions in the prevention and management of aggressive behaviors in patients admitted to an acute hospital setting. A systematic review. *JBI Library of Systematic Reviews, 7*(6), 175–223.

McPaul, K., & Lipscomb, J. (2004). Workplace violence in healthcare: Recognized but not regulated. *Online Journal of Issues in Nursing, 3*(9), Manuscript 6.

Pearson, A., Fields, J., & Jordan, Z. (2007). *Evidence-based clinical practice in nursing and health care: Assimilating research, experience and expertise.* Oxford: Blackwell.

Public Health Research Unit. (2007). Critical appraisal skills program. Retrieved from http://www.phru.nhs.uk/pages/phd/resources.htm

U.S. Department of Labor, Bureau of Labor Statistics. (2001). *Survey of occupational injuries and illnesses, 2000.* Retrieved from http://www.bls.gov/

U.S. Department of Labor and Occupational Safety and Health Administration. (2004). *Guidelines for preventing workplace violence for healthcare and social service workers* (No. OSHA 3148-01R). Washington, DC: Author. Retrieved from http://www.OSHA.gov/

CHAPTER 21

Nursing Care of the Older Adult

Jane Walker, Peggy Gerard

LEARNING OBJECTIVES

- Apply the evidence-based practice process to identify suitable printed medication information materials to use with elderly patients.

- Analyze the role of an evidence-based practice committee in using the evidence-based practice process to address an identified clinical problem.

- Develop strategies to improve the readability of written patient information material using recommended evidence.

KEY TERMS

Critical Appraisal Skills
  Program (CASP)
Easy-to-read
Health literacy
Patient education
Printed medication information
  sheets

Promoting Action on Research
  Implementation in Health
  Services (PARIHS)
  framework
Readability

C l i n i c a l S t o r y

David, a nurse manager on a cardiac step-down unit, is making telephone calls to recently discharged patients to check on how they are doing and to answer questions they might have about discharge instructions. He finds that many of the elderly patients are asking questions about how to take their medications. Although patients tell him they received a written medication instruction sheet at discharge, they are having trouble reading and understanding the information.

After compiling the feedback from several calls, David presents his findings to the nurses during a unit meeting. Ainsley, one of the more experienced nurses, voices a concern about the way the information on the medication instruction sheets is formatted and written. The standard hospital medication information sheets are formatted using single spacing and small fonts. In addition, the instruction sheets use generic terms for the medications and include complicated medical terminology. Sentences are long, and many of the terms are multisyllabic. The staff questions whether elderly patients are able to read and understand the information. Because taking the correct dose of medications on the right schedule is important, the manager asks Kristin, the unit's representative to the hospital's evidence-based practice committee, to take this problem to the next committee meeting. By doing so, the committee members can review the scope and scale of the problem and explore current evidence related to the readability of instruction material written for elderly patients. ■

Introduction

Nurses working in acute care settings are usually responsible for teaching patients about medications and providing printed information sheets describing their medications before the patients go home. This information typically includes the purpose of each medication, major side effects, schedule for taking the medications, and dosage instructions. The goal of giving **printed medication information sheets** to patients is to help them safely take their medications independently when they are home. However, if patients are not able to read and understand the written material, they might not take their medications correctly, which may place them at risk for serious adverse effects. Elderly patients who frequently take multiple medications can be at an even greater risk for problems if they have difficulty reading and understanding printed medication instructions.

This chapter helps you apply the evidence-based practice process to identifying suitable printed materials for medications for elderly patients. This process includes exploring the scope and scale of the problem, generating a PICO question, searching for and evaluating the evidence, and translating the evidence into practice. You will also learn more about health literacy and the elderly.

What Are the Key Issues?

Patients' ability to read and understand the printed materials you give them is influenced by their **health literacy** level as well as the readability of the information. The most widely used definition of health literacy is the one developed by Ratzan and Parker (2000) for the National Library of Medicine. According to this definition, health literacy is "the degree to which individuals have the capacity to obtain, process and understand basic health information and services needed to make appropriate health decisions" (Introduction section, para. 7). Health literacy affects patients' ability to perform a number of health-related tasks, including how to monitor their health conditions, schedule appointments with their doctors and other health-care providers, and understand why each medication is being used as well as when and how to take the medications (Box 21■1).

The most recent National Assessment of Adult Literacy study (NAAL), published in 2003, assessed the literacy levels of adults in the United States and included an assessment of health literacy. Findings demonstrated that 35% of the population has health literacy abilities that are in the *below basic* and *basic* ranges. Among those age 65 years and older, 59% read at *below basic* and *basic* levels (Kutner, Greenberg, Jin, et al., 2003). At *below basic* and *basic* levels of ability, individuals are able to read and understand simple health information only. For example, individuals who read *below basic* level can understand how often they should have a medical exam from reading clearly written material. They can also circle dates for medical

---

BOX 21■1　Significance of Health Literacy

- Thirty-six percent of the population has health literacy abilities that are in the *Below Basic* and *Basic* ranges (Kutner, Greenberg, Jin, et al., 2003).
- Adults over age 65 have literacy abilities lower than do younger adults (Kutner et al., 2003).
- Adults living below the poverty level have lower health literacy than do those living above the poverty level (Kutner et al., 2003).
- In 2007, the cost of low health literacy to the U.S. economy was estimated to range between $106 to $238 billion annually (Vernon, Trujillo, Rosenbaum, et al., 2007)
- Adults with limited health literacy reported poorer health status and lower use of preventive health services (Institute of Medicine [IOM] of the National Academies, 2004).
- Within a Medicare managed care setting, low health literacy was associated with higher mortality rates (Baker, Wolf, Feinglass, et al., 2007).
- Adults with low health literacy are less likely to follow prescribed treatment and self-care regimens, more likely to make more medication errors, and lack the skills needed to effectively use the health-care system (Weiss, 1998)

follow-up on an appointment slip (Kutner et al., 2003). At the *basic* level, when individuals read a clearly written pamphlet, they can identify at least two reasons for obtaining screening related to a specific disease. However, individuals who read at *basic* and *below basic* levels cannot read and follow instructions on a prescription drug label that relate to timing medication doses in relation to eating. They also cannot identify drug interactions based on over-the-counter drug labels (Kutner et al., 2003). This means many patients in these two health literacy categories may have difficulty understanding and acting on printed medication information.

Readability is the other piece of the equation related to a person's ability to comprehend information they are attempting to read. *Readability* commonly refers to how easy it is to read and understand written material (Harris and Hodges, 1995). Sometimes the phrase **easy-to-read** is used in place of *readability*. One way to help your patients understand printed medication information may be to use easy-to-read printed educational materials using evidence-based guidelines.

Ask/Assess

At the hospital evidence-based practice committee meeting in this chapter's clinical story, Kristin describes the problem her unit is experiencing with elderly patients who do not understand their medications or how to take them after going home. She also shares the nurses' suspicion that the cause of the problem could be the format and reading level of the medication instruction sheets. She distributes samples of the unit's medication instruction sheets to the committee members. After reviewing the sample instruction sheets, the members of the evidence-based practice committee question whether there is a mismatch between the format of the hospital's current medication information sheets and the health literacy ability of many elderly patients. The committee decides the next step is to determine the scope and scale of this potential problem. The members establish a task force to work with Kristin to continue the investigation into this issue.

To describe the scope of the potential problem (the inability to understand printed health information), the task force searches the Internet to locate information from national institutes and organizations that addresses issues related to health literacy and readability of written health materials. They discover the Institute of Medicine (IOM) of the National Academies (2004) reported that more than 90 million people in the United States have difficulty reading and understanding health information. The NAAL data also include statistics addressing the relationship between age and health literacy abilities, which show that adults older than age 65 years have lower average health literacy abilities than do younger adults (Kutner et al., 2003). In addition to national statistics, the committee members are also able to locate state information pertaining to general literacy levels for their locale. They find approximately 60% of their local population reads at a level below that of the eighth grade.

The task force also identifies several Web sites that provide background information related to the problem of health literacy and readability. These include the

National Institutes of Health's Clear Communication Web site; the Office of Disease Prevention and Health Promotion's Web site related to health communication, literacy and older adults; and the U.S. Department of Health and Human Services Centers for Medicare & Medicaid Services' (CMS) tool kit for writing clear written materials. You can find a listing of these helpful Web sites and others in Box 21■2.

To determine the scale of the problem, Kristin conducts an audit on her unit to assess how well the recently discharged elderly patients understood their medication regimen. The nurses indicate that the majority of the discharged patients were older than 65 years, and 80% of them were not able to answer simple questions about their medications after leaving the hospital, despite the answers to these questions being readily available in the printed medication information material the patients

---

BOX 21■2   Selected Web Sites Containing Health Literacy and Readability Information

- Office of Disease Prevention and Health Promotion: "Health Communication Activities"
  http://www.health.gov/communication/literacy/
- Office of Disease Prevention and Health Promotion: "Quick Guide to Health Literacy and Older Adults"
  http://www.health.gov/communication/literacy/olderadults/default.htm
- National Network of Libraries and Medicine
  http://nnlm.gov/outreach/consumer/hlthlit.html
- The National Cancer Institute: "Clear and Simple: Developing Effective Print Materials for Low-Literate Readers" (includes a specific guide)
  http://www.cancer.gov/cancerinformation/clearandsimple
- National Institutes of Health: "Clear Communication: An NIH Health Literacy Initiative"
  http://www.nih.gov/clearcommunication/
- Harvard School of Public Health
  http://www.hsph.harvard.edu/healthliteracy/resources/glossaries/index.html
- Plain Language.gov
  http://www.plainlanguage.gov/populartopics/health_literacy/index.cfm
- California Health Literacy Initiative
  http://cahealthliteracy.org/rc/4.html
- Partnership for Clear Health Communication
  http://www.npsf.org/askme3/PCHC/
- Canadian Public Health Association: "Good Medicine for Seniors: Guidelines for Plain Language and Good Design in Prescription Medication"
  http://www.cpha.ca/uploads/portals/h-l/goodmed_e.pdf
- Centers for Medicare & Medicaid Services: "Toolkit for Making Written Material Clear and Effective"
  http://www.cms.gov/WrittenMaterialsToolkit/01_Overview.asp#TopOfPage

were given. Meanwhile, the task force finds that the majority of patients admitted to the hospital are also over the age of 65 years and that this problem of lack of understanding of printed medication information could be widespread. According to the Joint Commission (2007), hospitals must provide written health information that is age appropriate, clear, and understandable. In addition, the IOM (2004) recommends that health-care institutions develop strategies to address problems with health literacy. Based on all of this information, the task force recognizes the need for further action related to printed medication information.

To more fully assess the scale of the problem, the task force members test the readability of the most frequently used medication instruction sheets. Testing readability involves assessing the reading level as well as the overall suitability of the printed materials. To assess the reading level of the instruction forms, the task force uses the Fry formula (1977), which is a widely accepted and easy-to-use method. The Fry method involves testing sample text from three sections of a document. Sentences and syllables are counted in these samples and averaged. Users then plot the results on a graph to identify a readability level, which reflects a grade level from first grade to a post-college grade of 17 (Doak, Doak, and Root, 1996). To assess suitability of the medication sheets, they chose the frequently used Suitability Assessment of Materials (SAM) tool, which is also considered reliable and valid (Doak et al., 1996; Wallace, Rogers, Turner, et al., 2006). Suitability factors addressed by the SAM tool include content, literacy demand (e.g., grade level, writing style, learning aids), graphics, layout, learning stimulation through the use of interaction and self-efficacy, and cultural appropriateness (Doak et al., 1996). Reviewers use criteria related to each factor to assign points related to an assessment of written material, and the final suitability assessment results are reported as percentages. Superior ratings range from 70% to 100%, adequate ratings range from 40% to 69%, and materials that receive scores lower than 40% are considered not suitable (Doak et al., 1996). Based on members' evaluation of the printed medication sheets, the task force finds the average reading level of the medication sheets was grade 13 and the average suitability score was 34%, indicating the materials are not suitable for patients as written.

As a result of this assessment, the task force determines the scale of the problem is quite large, and the members need to find a way to provide elderly patients with printed medication information that is easy to read. The task force's broad background question initially focuses on identifying the best types of printed medication information materials to use with elderly patients. After further discussion, they identify a narrower question to better focus their search for best evidence. This narrower question addresses the best way to format written medication information material so elderly patients can understand it more easily. This question is then further refined into a PICO format to guide the search for evidence (Table 21■1).

Acquire/Diagnose

At the next evidence-based practice committee meeting, the task force presents its recommendations. First, members discuss the information they have collected

Table 21 ■1   **Narrowing the Focus and Generating the PICO Question**

Broad	What are the best types of printed medication information materials to use with elderly patients?	
Narrow	What is the best way to format written medication information material that can best be understood by elderly patients?	
Searchable PICO	What is the effectiveness of using easy-to-read written medication information material compared with standard written medication information material on knowledge and understanding among elderly hospitalized patients?	P = elderly hospitalized patients I = easy-to-read written medication information material C = standard written medication information material O = knowledge, understandability

regarding the scope and scale of the problem. Based on this information, they suspect the lack of understanding of the medication regimen by elderly patients is likely the result of a mismatch between the readability and suitability of the medication information sheets and the health literacy abilities of their elderly patient population. Second, the task force presents the recommendation to conduct a search of the literature to identify the most appropriate strategies for writing and formatting written medication information materials for elderly patients. The task force also present its PICO question to the committee. The evidence-based practice committee agrees with the task force's assessment of scope and scale, their PICO question, and the plan to search the literature for best evidence.

After receiving support from the evidence-based practice committee to proceed, the task force meets with the hospital's medical librarian to develop a plan to search for the evidence. Their goal is to identify the best evidence-based methods for selecting written medication information that can be easily read and understood by elderly hospitalized patients. The librarian helps the group use its PICO question to create a list of search terms (Table 21 ■2) and to decide on a strategy to locate the best sources of evidence.

Using the hierarchy of evidence (see Chapter 11), the task force begins searching for evidence that is already pre-appraised and synthesized. Therefore, its first search is the National Guideline Clearinghouse (NGC). If the search for a practice guideline is unsuccessful, to the task force will search for systematic reviews in the Joanna Briggs Institute (JBI) Library of Systematic Reviews and the Cochrane Library of Systematic Reviews as well as in CINAHL and MEDLINE. If systematic reviews are not available, controlled trials in CINAHL and MEDLINE will be sought. If adequate controlled trials are not present, the task force plans to seek expert opinion by searching the Web sites of government agencies and health literacy organizations, associations, and foundations.

To locate guidelines, the task force searches the NGC using the key words "easy to read." With this strategy, the task force obtains 94 guidelines. Of these, one guideline focuses on adherence to medications (National Collaborating Center for Primary

Table 21 ■2 **Key Search Terms and Search Strategies for Medical/Nursing Databases**

PICO*	Synonyms	Search Strategy
What is the effectiveness of using easy-to-read written medication information material compared with standard written medication information material on knowledge and understanding among elderly hospitalized patients?		
P = elderly hospitalized patients	1. elder* 2. aged 3. hospitali*	Link 1 through 3 with OR
I = easy to read written medication information material	4. easy-to-read 5. plain language 6. teaching material* 7. print material* 8. written information 9. written medication information 10. pamphlet 11. brochure	Link 4 through 11 with OR
O = knowledge, understandability	12. knowledge 13. medication knowledge 14. suitab* 15. comprehen* 16. understand*	Link 12 through 16 with OR
P + I + O		Link with AND

* Note that there was no need to include the comparison (C) in the search because the process of searching on standard materials would not yield additional information.

Care, 2009). The authors of this evidence-based guideline recommend providing easily understood information to patients and to avoid using medical jargon. In addition, the authors advise health-care providers not to assume their patients can understand patient information leaflets that are given out with the medications (National Collaborating Center for Primary Care, 2009). Unfortunately, no information is included in this guideline that specifically addresses easy-to-read guidelines in relation to understandability. The task force is not able to locate any other guidelines in the NGC specifically focused on their topic, and moves on to searching for systematic reviews on this topic.

In order to search for additional sources of synthesized evidence, the task force then searches the JBI Library of Systematic Reviews and the Cochrane Library of Systematic Reviews using the key words "written information," "easy-to-read," and "health literacy." Using this strategy, the task force is not able to locate a systematic review in the JBI Library. However, the Cochrane Library has a systematic review completed by Nicolson, Knapp, Raynor, et al. (2009) that addresses the impact of written information about medications. But the focus of this review does not fully address the task force's question. The task force is not able to locate any additional systematic reviews in Cochrane that is focused on their question.

The task force meets again with the librarian to ask for help with the Medline and CINAHL search. Seeking help from your librarian is a strategy you may also find useful due to the expertise and time required to perform a thorough search. The librarian performs a search using the search terms in Table 21■2. The MEDLINE search yielded 564 articles when limiting the search to English language and to the years 1995 to 2010. The librarian tries to limit the MEDLINE search using the filter of "controlled clinical trial," but that search yields too few relevant articles.

The number 564 is higher than desirable. However, the librarian feels it is somewhat difficult to identify optimal search terms for this topic, and she decides to review all of the titles and abstracts as necessary. As a result of this manual review of titles and abstracts, she finds 31 potentially relevant articles in Medline. Within the CINAHL database, she finds 253 potential titles, which she narrows to 37. In addition to these potential articles, she locates a systematic review pertaining to the role and effectiveness of written medication information. At this point, the librarian gives the list of titles and accompanying abstracts to the evidence-based practice committee task force.

After reviewing the abstracts, the task force asks the librarian to retrieve full text versions of several articles. The task force is comfortable with the results of the search that yielded one systematic review, one narrative literature review, and 16 articles of primary research. Of the 16 articles of primary research, only one has been published after the systematic review's publication date. After further review, the committee finds the remaining 15 articles are not closely related to their PICO question. Therefore, they decide to evaluate the systematic review, the narrative review, and the one primary research article published after the publication date of the systematic review.

Appraise/Plan

Although members of the task force are not able to locate guidelines or systematic reviews that specifically match their PICO question, they are able to locate one systematic review that is closely related to their question. This review also contains a synthesis of texts that provides recommendations for designing print materials. Based on what you have learned, you know that the task force will need to examine the quality of the systemic review before they can confidently rely on information it contains.

The systematic review that the task force has located focuses on the effectiveness of written medication information to convey knowledge and understanding (Raynor, Blenkinsopp, Knapp, et al., 2007). The task force decides to also review the quality of the individual studies that have been published after the systematic review publication date.

When you evaluate the quality of a systematic review, an appropriate tool to use is the **Critical Appraisal Skills Program (CASP)** evaluation checklist for systematic reviews (PHRU, 2007). This tool is reliable, concise, and easy to use. Because of these factors, the task force uses the CASP tool to evaluate the quality of the systematic review conducted by Raynor et al. (2007). The purpose of the review by Raynor et al. (2007)

was to determine to what extent patients, caregivers, and health professionals rated the role and value of written information pertaining to medications. Findings most closely related to the evidence-based practice task force's area of interest include patient concerns about the use of complex language and the poor appearance of written materials. The authors conclude that a gap exists between provided print information and the type of information patients would like to have (Raynor et al., 2007).

When the task force evaluates this systematic review using the CASP criteria, members conclude that the quality of this systematic review is high. The review's questions were clearly written, appropriate types of studies were included, the search was exhaustive, and there was a clear method for evaluating the quality of each included study. Because of the nature of the evidence included in this systematic review, the authors appropriately performed a narrative analysis of the evidence. They carefully considered all important outcomes, and the results can be applied in the local setting.

In addition to the high quality of this systematic review, the task force finds that the review by Raynor et al. (2007) contains a synthesis of texts devoted to information design. These texts were nominated by a panel of six experts from the information design field who agreed on a final selection of six texts. The panel of experts then synthesized key information design strategies from these texts and presented them in tabular and narrative form in the review. Based on this information, the task force is able to identify many elements, although not all are focused specifically on the elderly, that may make patient information easier to read and understood (Raynor et al., 2007). Following is a list of key design elements mentioned by at least four of the six texts (Raynor et al., 2007):

- Use words that are short and familiar, preferably no more than two syllables.
- Use as little jargon as possible and if it must be used, include a glossary.
- Write using the active as opposed to passive voice.
- Keep sentences short, with an average of 15 to 20 words.
- Use plenty of white space.
- Use bullet points to break up and organize information.
- Use boldface text when you want to emphasize a point. Avoid capital letters, italics, and underlining.
- Use a writing style that is relaxed and positive.

In addition to these most frequently agreed on design aspects, the systematic review gives the task force recommendations regarding typeface, line length and spacing, and the use of pictures. Therefore, the task force finds this systematic review to be extremely helpful in the search for evidence related to readability.

There was only one individual study published after 2007 that addresses the topic of understanding medications. The focus of this study was to examine ways to write prescription drug warnings so they could be more easily understood (Wolf, Davis, Bass, et al., 2010). The authors of this study found that the patients in the sample who received drug warnings written in simplified language or simplified language in combination with icons were able to understand the drug warnings better than did the patients who received the standard information.

In addition to the systematic review and related medication information study, the task force finds one narrative review with some relevance to the question at hand (Schaefer, 2008). One focus of this review was to identify the most effective interventions aimed at persons with low health literacy. Among the studies reviewed, four addressed written materials. Two of these studies found the intervention had no effect, and two studies, one of which was focused on the elderly population, did find an outcome of increased knowledge (Schaefer, 2008). However, because this review did not follow systematic review methods, the task force is not able to evaluate its quality using the CASP tool.

The task force is not able to locate systematic reviews of primary research focused specifically on the effectiveness of using easy-to-read instructional materials with the elderly. Nonetheless, in spite of this lack of ideal evidence of effectiveness, the task force knows it needs to change the format of the medication instruction sheets to meet national calls for clear writing and plain language to convey health information (IOM, 2004). The task force decides to use the health information design recommendations published in widely referenced sources such as Doak et al. (1996), Office of Disease Prevention and Health Promotion's guide to health literacy and older adults (2007), the Web-based information publication posted by the National Cancer Institute (2003), and the CMS toolkit for making material clear and effective (2010). After analyzing these sources, the task force finds they contain similar recommendations. The task force also finds these design recommendations are very similar to those published in the systematic review by Raynor et al. (2007). Therefore, in spite of the lack of high-level evidence, task force members are comfortable that the information contained in these publications is the best available evidence at this point in time. The task force also takes into consideration the various calls for using plain language (Plain Language.gov, 2010) as another rationale for moving forward with providing easy-to-read medication information material to patients.

As you begin to question nursing practices, you may encounter similar situations in which practice guidelines and/or systematic reviews are not available to inform your practice. Therefore, expert opinion and published practice standards might be the best available evidence to support a practice change.

As a result of this evidence review, the task force decides to make the following recommendations to the evidence-based practice committee. They pair these recommendations with the levels of evidence corresponding with the JBI (2010) evidence rating system. According to this system, level 1 refers to meta-synthesis/meta-analysis or experimental studies; level 2 refers to smaller randomized controlled trials or quasi-experimental studies; level 3 refers to cohort, case-controlled, or observational studies; and level 4 refers to expert opinion or consensus. The specific recommendations of the task force are as follows:

- Ensure that written patient information materials are written at an appropriate level. (level 4)
- Ensure that written patient information materials incorporate design characteristics that are recognized as being easy-to-read. (level 4)
- Always give patients a verbal explanation of the topic of instruction in addition to written information. (level 3)

Apply/Implement

Kristin and her task force take their recommendations to the next evidence-based practice committee. Along with their recommendations, they prepare a slide presentation that outlines the easy-to-read design characteristics they have learned from the literature. The evidence-based practice committee is quite interested in this material and discusses it at length. As a result, the committee decides it is important to redesign the current written medication information materials to make them easy to read.

Before moving forward with implementation, the Committee discusses the best way to put this information into practice. The committee uses the **Promoting Action on Research Implementation in Health Services (PARIHS) framewor**k (see Chapter 5) to guide the evidence implementation activities (Rycroft-Malone, 2004). This model addresses the need to consider three main elements as components of successful evidence implementation, evidence, context, and facilitation. With respect to evidence, the model states that evidence consists of research, clinical experience, patient experience, and local data. The model indicates that evidence will more likely be implemented when research, clinical experience, and patient experience are at high levels (Rycroft-Malone, 2004). In this case, there is not a great deal of research data, but there is a significant amount of consistently strong opinions regarding the formatting of written materials for patients. The patient experiences described in the literature are good and the committee has good local data.

Regarding context, the PARIHS framework refers to the setting in which the evidence will be implemented. The three components of context include culture, leadership, and evaluation (Rycroft-Malone, 2004). The context in this situation is the hospital where Kristin works. The culture in this hospital is quite supportive of changing practice based on evidence and provides multiple opportunities for the staff to try new ways of doing things. The top leadership is quite visible on the patient care areas and promotes autonomy of staff. Finally, hospital employees frequently participate in evaluation of care processes in the hospital and are kept informed regarding the outcome of their evaluation activities. Therefore, the committee has reason to believe this practice change will be supported in the current context.

The final component of the model is facilitation. Aspects of facilitation include appropriate roles, skills and knowledge (Rycroft-Malone, 2004). In this case, the committee decides the best way to facilitate this practice change is to establish a multi-disciplinary task force that includes current evidence-based practice task force members as well as the adult health clinical nurse specialist, a pharmacist, a physician, and a patient educator (Box 21■3). The clinical nurse specialist is assigned to chair the task force. The committee is confident that the implementation process for this practice change will proceed smoothly based on the high ratings for each component of the PARIHS model.

Assess/Evaluate

As part of the planning process for using easy-to-read medication information materials, the implementation task force needs to identify the best measures to assess the

BOX 21■3 **Interdisciplinary Implementation Task Force**

It takes a team of health-care providers to implement easy-to-read medication instruction sheets in a hospital setting. Consider involving the following individuals:

- Bedside nurses
- Clinical nurse specialists
- Clinical pharmacists
- Nurse researcher
- Patient educators
- Physicians
- Quality/safety specialists
- Risk managers

integration of the evidence into practice (the process) as well as measures to assess the impact of the change on knowledge and understanding (the outcome). It is important to evaluate the process to make sure that the practice change is actually taking place. Therefore, the task force needs to ensure that new medication sheets are actually available on each unit and that nurses explain the medication sheets when giving them to patients. Nurses can assess the implementation process by making rounds on the units, conducting audits, and giving feedback.

Because there was little research-based information in the literature, the task force decides to carry out a research project to examine the effect of easy-to-read medication instruction sheets on knowledge and understanding among elderly patients. Members prepare a research proposal and obtain approval through the hospital's human subjects committee. While collecting baseline data, they search for appropriate preprinted, easy-to-read materials. If they cannot find preprinted materials, the task force members are prepared to create their own instruction sheets using guidelines from their initial evidence search. After this phase is completed, the task force can then follow the steps outlined in the research protocol to implement the new forms and to evaluate the outcome of the change.

■ Summary

The process of applying evidence in daily nursing care occurs at many levels, ranging from individual nurses to an entire organization. In this chapter's Clinical Story, Kristin took the unit-based problem of lack of understanding of medication instructions to the hospital-wide evidence-based practice committee and found the problem actually applied to all units with elderly patients. Kristin worked with a task force and the hospital's librarian to assess the scope and scale of the situation, ask questions, and acquire evidence. They appraised the evidence and made recommendations based on this evidence. Although they were not able to locate clinical practice guidelines or systematic reviews specifically addressing the question they were exploring, they did locate consistent expert opinions. Therefore, they decided to change the hospital's practices related to printed medication information for the elderly. They also recognized the need for additional research testing the effectiveness of using easy-to-read methods. As a result, they decided to perform a study to test this intervention.

In nursing, you may find that clinical practice guidelines and systematic reviews are not available to answer all of your questions and that more research needs to be performed. In this chapter's Clinical Story, you can see how a team of nurses and other health-care professionals can make contributions to nursing practice and the larger community by exploring, applying, and creating evidence. For practice using the evidence-based practice process, refer to Box 21■4.

BOX 21■4 **Tools for Learning and Practice**

- Generate additional PICO questions related to patient education at discharge.
- Search for evidence using keywords in your PICO questions following the strategy supplied in this chapter's Clinical Story as an example.
- Develop one medication information sheet using the criteria identified in the chapter. Check the readability level using the FOG method and assess the suitability of the information sheet using the SAM format.
- Develop a simple audit tool that incorporates evidence-based recommendations for developing written health information.
- Conduct an audit of medication information sheets/materials, summarize data, and provide feedback to colleagues.
- Identify policies that address development of written patient education materials and evaluate the strength and currency of the supporting evidence. If warranted, recommend changes to policies based on best available evidence.

CHAPTER QUESTIONS

1. This chapter's Clinical Story presented the problem of elderly patients not understanding medication instructions. What steps of the evidence-based process were used to address the identified problem?

2. What were the strengths of the evidence that the medication information task force found?

3. Given the evidence that was implemented in the Clinical Story, construct a simple tool to evaluate whether nurses are using the easy-to-read medication information sheets. If the audit reveals that some nurses are not using the easy-to-read medication information sheets, suggest some strategies to implement their use.

4. To evaluate the impact of the easy-to-read medication information sheets, it is necessary to identify some appropriate outcomes and measure them. What are some outcomes that you think would be applicable to measure the effectiveness of the easy-to-read medication sheets? What are some potential ways to go about doing this?

5. Patient education involves more than the use of printed materials. What is another PICO question that you could ask about teaching patients?

6. Using this alternative PICO question, search for a systematic review or practice guideline. Using an appropriate appraisal instrument, critique the evidence you found. Based on that critique, explain whether you would use this evidence and provide a rationale for your decision.

7. If you found more than one guideline or systematic review, compare them and identify the similarities and differences in the findings.

8. If you were to use the evidence-based recommendations you found in your search, explain how you would implement them using the PARIHS framework.

References

Baker, D. W., Wolf, M., Feinglass, J., et al. (2007). Health literacy and mortality among elderly persons. *Archives of Internal Medicine, 167,* 1503–1509.

Centers for Medicare & Medicaid Services. (2010). Toolkit for making written material clear and effective. Retrieved from http://www.cms.gov/WrittenMaterialsToolkit/01_Overview.asp#TopOfPage

Doak, C. C., Doak, L. G., & Root, J. H. (1996). *Teaching patients with low literacy skills.* Philadelphia: Lippincott.

Fry, E. (1977). Fry's readability graph: Clarifications, validity, and extensions to level 17. *Journal of Reading, 21,* 242–252.

Harris, T. L., & Hodges, R. E. (eds.). (1995). *The literacy dictionary: The vocabulary of reading and writing.* Newark, DE: International Reading Association.

Institute of Medicine of the National Academies. (2004). *Health literacy: A prescription to end confusion.* Washington, DC: National Academies Press.

Joanna Briggs Institute. (2010). Levels of evidence. Retrieved from http://www.joannabriggs.edu.au/pubs/approach.php

Joint Commission on Accreditation of Healthcare Organizations. (2007). *Comprehensive accreditation manual for hospitals: The official handbook.* Oakbrook Terrace, IL: Joint Commission Resources.

Kutner, M., Greenberg E., Jin, Y., et al. (2006). *The health literacy of America's adults: Results from the 2003 National Assessment of Adult Literacy* (NCES 2006-483). Washington DC: U.S. Department of Education, National Center for Education Statistics.

National Cancer Institute. (2003). *Clear and simple: Developing effective print materials for low-literate readers.* Retrieved from http://www.cancer.gov/cancerinformation/clearandsimple

National Collaborating Center for Primary Care. (2009). *Medicines adherence. Involving patients in decisions about prescribed medicines and supporting adherence.* Retrieved from http://www.guideline.gov/content.aspx?id=14342&search=medication+adherence

Nicolson, D., Knapp, P., Raynor, D. K., et al. (2009). Written information about individual medicines for consumers. *Cochrane Database of Systematic Reviews, 2.* Art. No.: CD002104. doi:10.1002/14651858.CD002194.pub3

Office of Disease Prevention and Health Promotion. (2007). Quick guide to health literacy and older adults. Retrieved from http://www.health.gov/communication/literacy/olderadults/default.htm

Plain Language.gov. (2010). What is plain language? Retrieved from http://www.plainlanguage.gov/whatisPL/index.cfm

Public Health Research Unit. (2007). Critical appraisal skills program. Retrieved from http://www.phru.nhs.uk/pages/phd/resources.htm

Ratzan, S. C., & Parker, R. M. (2000). Introduction. In *National Library of Medicine current bibliographies in medicine: Health literacy.* Retrieved from http://www.nlm.nih.gov/archive//20061214/pubs/cbm/hliteracy.html

Raynor, D. K., Blenkinsopp, A., Knapp, P., et al. (2007). A systematic review of quantitative and qualitative research on the role and effectiveness of written information available to patients about individual medicines. *Health Technology Assessment, 11*(5).

Rycroft-Malone, J. (2004). The PARIHS framework—a framework for guiding the implementation of evidence-based practice. *Journal of Nursing Care Quality, 19,* 297–304.

Schaefer, C. T. (2008). Integrated review of health literacy interventions. *Orthopaedic Nursing, 27,* 312–317.

Vernon, J. A., Trujillo, A., Rosenbaum, S., et al. (2007). *Low health literacy: Implications for national health policy.* Retrieved from http://npsf.org/askme3/pdfs/Case_Report_10_07.pdf

Wallace, L. S., Rogers, E. S., Turner, L. W., et al. (2006). Suitability of written supplemental materials available on the Internet for nonprescription medications. *American Journal of Health-System Pharmacy, 63,* 71–78.

Weiss, B. D. (1998). *20 common problems in primary care.* New York: McGraw Hill.

Wolf, M. S., Davis, T. C., Bass, P. F., et al. (2010). Improving prescription drug warnings to promote patient comprehension. *Archives of Internal Medicine, 170,* 50–56.

CHAPTER 22

Community Health Nursing

Dolores Huffman

LEARNING OBJECTIVES

■ Given the ill-structured description of a community-based clinical case, apply all phases of the evidence-based practice process to guide decisions related to an area of community health.

■ Analyze the challenges to making evidence-based decisions in a complex and community-based health-care environment.

■ Generate next-step strategies to put better evidence into practice.

KEY TERMS

Qualifications
Research
School health provider
School health services

School nurse
School nurse guidelines
School nurse role
Systematic reviews

Clinical Story

Leanna is the head school nurse in an urban public school system that serves a racially and ethnically diverse population. Most of the district's population is medically underserved. The school nurse's office in the district meets the needs of both students and families by providing day-to-day care, education, and consultations. In addition, through partnerships with the medical and business communities, a robust referral system allows students and families to access services that might otherwise be difficult to procure. In all locations across the district, the school nurse's office is seen as a valuable asset by the community.

Unfortunately, Leanna has just been informed by the superintendent that the school board is considering terminating the school nurse positions. The board is considering replacing the nurses with unlicensed assistive personnel (UAP) and parent volunteers, with one nurse supervisor for the entire school district. This potential action is meant as a cost-cutting measure and is legal in this partic-ular state because registered nurse licensure is not required for the school nurse position. At the board's request, Leanna has 2 weeks to prepare data to justify keeping the current system in place.   ■

Introduction

School nurses are an extension of the public health system and play a vital role in assisting children to successfully adapt to the school environment. On a daily basis, 50 million school-age children with an array of health problems, chronic illnesses, and disabilities attend approximately 97,000 public schools in the United States and are in contact with school nurses (National Association of School Nurses [NASN], 2010a). The responsibilities of school nurses are varied and challenging because a significant amount of health care is provided in the schools (NASN, 2010b). Every day school nurses handle emergencies, complete health screenings, identify out-breaks of communicable disease, administer medication, verify immunization records, and plan health-care strategy. In addition, the school nurse provides psychological support for the students, families, teachers, and administration while addressing the specific health-care needs of school children living with various disabilities and chronic illness. The NASN (1999) defines school nursing as "a specialized practice of professional nursing that advances the well-being, academic success, and lifelong achievement of students. To that end, school nurses facilitate positive student responses to normal development; promote health and safety; intervene with actual and potential health problems; provide case management services; and actively collaborate with others to build student and family capacity for adaptation, self-management, self-advocacy, and learning" (p. 1)

Healthy People (HP) 2020, the federal initiative to improve America's health, recognizes the multifaceted and demanding role of the school nurse. HP 2020 has specifically identified objectives related to the suggested proportion of school nurses to students at all grade levels (U.S. Department of Health and Human Services [USDHHS], 2010). Specifically, the HP objective for Educational and Community Based Program No. 5 says to "increase the proportion of the nation's elementary, middle, and senior high schools that have a full-time registered nurse-to-student ration of at least 1:750" (p. 9). In addition, the NASN Position Statement (2002) and the American Academy of Pediatrics (AAP, 2008) posit that students and staff are entitled to quality health services and that these services can be ensured when school nurses earn appropriate education, licensure, and certification. The AAP recommends that every school have a full-time school nurse, thereby ensuring a strong connection with each student's medical treatment (AAP Council on School Health, 2008). It is the position of the NASN (2002) "that every school-aged child deserves and needs a school nurse who is baccalaureate degree prepared from an accredited college or university and holds licensure as a registered nurse (RN) by their employing state" (p. 1). According to both the NASN and the AAP, these requirements are the minimal preparation needed at the entry level of school nursing practice.

In this chapter's clinical story, as Leanna thinks about her response to the school board, she realizes she needs the best available evidence to make a convincing argument to support her belief that every school-age child in her community deserves and benefits from a baccalaureate prepared school nurse. She knows the school health issue is complex, and her community has unique health needs. It has been hit hard by the economic downturn and is experiencing high rates of unemployment. In addition, if her district succeeds in eliminating school nurses, the decision will set a precedent for eliminating the school nurse position and replacing that nurse with UAP, which could affect other schools. Leanna is aware that her arguments are vital not only to her school nurse colleagues but also to the children, families, teachers, staff, and administrators within her employing school district.

This chapter applies the evidence-based practice process to a community problem. In an attempt to keep this complicated problem controllable, the chapter focuses on the effectiveness of the school nurse in maintaining and promoting school health.

What Are the Key Issues?

Leanna needs credible resources that will support a solution to this grave community dilemma. She begins by asking a series of questions, both general and specific:

1. What is the role of the school nurse in meeting the health needs of school-age children in the United States?
2. How should she factor in the uniqueness of her local community when making this cogent argument to the school board?
3. What are the experiences of communities that do not currently employ RNs as school nurses?
4. What are the sources of support for her argument?
5. Are there established standards for school nurses' academic and professional qualifications—locally, by state, and nationally?

6. If there are established standards, what sources of evidence informed them?
7. Are there national, state, and/or local data to support the employment of school nurses?
8. Are there systematic reviews that focus specifically on the effectiveness of school nurses related to school health?
9. Are there primary studies that have investigated the effectiveness of school nurses?
10. Is there expert opinion about the need for school nurses in our kindergarten through twelfth grade educational system?
11. Are there any places in the United States that have achieved the Healthy People objective of one nurse to every 750 students?

The evidence-based practice process starts with a willingness to answer these questions by considering data that both support and contradict your position. Leanna approaches these questions by first searching the Internet for professional organizations devoted to school nursing and school health. Leanna is a member of her state School Nurses Association (SNA), an affiliate of the NASN, so she starts her search on their Web sites. While reading their position, she finds the AAP supports the NASN position: schools should employ only RNs with at least a baccalaureate degree as school nurses. However, her state SNA *prefers* a baccalaureate but does not *require* even an RN for those who provide school health services. In her state, the exception is that school districts must employ an RN to supervise UAP providing school health services.

In addition, Leanna discovers the ANA supports the employment of RNs in schools, based on the premise that those with RN competencies are better equipped to maintain the health of the school children (ANA, 2007). As she seeks data, Leanna knows she may benefit from a listing of national nursing organizations and specific state SNAs. She also wants to consult federal mandates regarding school health from the U.S. Department of Education, Centers for Disease Control and Prevention, and Healthy People 2020. She will also consider her state's department of education, which is directly responsible for school health services. She realizes that international sources and studies may be judged irrelevant to her school system because other nations differ in school policy and organizational structure. Because of this, she decides not to pursue global sources in this undertaking.

A next important step in developing a position is verifying the *scope* and *scale* of the problem. Leanna has identified many questions associated with this problem, and its complexity seems overwhelming. However, she knows she must be realistic. The scope means identifying the breadth of the problem. Scale is finding out, in this case, if the elimination of the school nurse position is just an isolated experience occurring only in her school system. In the school nurse dilemma, national data will outline the scope of the problem: Leanna can consult the Centers for Disease Control and Prevention (CDC) School Health Policies and Programs Study (SHPPS), which is conducted every 6 years. In addition, the primary purpose of the biannual National Youth Risk Behavior Survey is to identify health-risk behaviors among youth ninth through twelfth grade and ascertain changes in risk behaviors over time every 6 years. The 2009 Risk Behavior Survey shows that in her specific state, health-risk behaviors have increased in key areas: alcohol and drug use, obesity, sexual behaviors that contribute to unintended pregnancy and sexually transmitted infections, tobacco use, violence and suicide.

To further define the scope of the problem Leanna searches the NASN, federal mandates regarding laws that affect school health practices, the American School Health Association (ASHA), the National Association of Elementary and Secondary Principles (NAESP), and the Robert Wood Johnson Foundation (RWJF). The NASN (2010a) reports that 16% of the 52 million students in the U.S. school systems have some type of health problem and need a more comprehensive health-care delivery system in the schools. The No Child Left Behind Act of 2001, Individuals with Disabilities Education Act (originally authored in 1975), and the Vocational Rehabilitation Act (1973) are federal mandates that require children with disabilities to receive health-related services in school. However, none of these federal laws legislates that health-related services must be delivered by nurses, an important distinction for Leanna. The ASHA (2010) considers schools vital in assisting the physical, emotional, social, and environmental factors related to student health and indicates that student well-being can affect the learning process, although it does not address the qualifications for those providing school health services. The NAESP, in its 2008–2009 platform, "strongly recommends that school districts ensure proper health care, including the dispensing of medication, for all children by providing every school with a full-time school nurse" (p. 39). Furthermore, the NAESP (2008–2009) "believes that school health services provided by a qualified school nurse are essential to the education of children. The school nurse is trained to recognize the complexity of physical, social, and psychological factors that interact in the total growth of children. Also, the school nurse is trained to work with parents, school personnel, and community agencies to assess student health needs and initiate appropriate action to meet those needs" (p. 39).

The RWJF identifies too much variance in school health services—over half of the nation's schools lack an RN—and notes that this variance contributes to the vast health disparities among our school-age children. In addition, the RWJF reports a wide range of medical health problems as well as an increase in social issues, such as poverty and homelessness, affecting school children. The RWJF also reports that 13% of school children are taking prescription drugs during school, an increase of 9% a decade earlier (RWJF, 2010).

The *scale* of the problem includes whether the elimination of school nurse positions is an isolated occurrence or a trend across the United States. The 2006 SHPPS results indicate that 81.5% of schools in the United States offer health services. However, only 35.7% of schools had a full-time school nurse (RN or licensed practical nurse [LPN] present in the school for at least 30 hours per week); 50.6% of schools employed a part-time school nurse (one present fewer than 30 hours a week); and 45.1% of all schools reported a nurse-to-student ratio of 1:750 or better (Kann, Brener, and Wechsler, 2007). These data suggest the scale of the problem transcends this local community. Ultimately, Leanna views this problem of eliminating school nurse positions as being both large in scope and scale. After reviewing some of the data acquired from her initial search, she begins to think about how to best approach this problem. Her next step is to develop a PICO question that will assist her in searching for the best available evidence.

Ask/Assess

Both the nursing process and evidence-based practice processes start with assessment and asking questions that direct you to the best available evidence. In Leanna's case, the evidence will serve as a basis for her justification to the school board. Leanna starts her assessment by seeing if needed data concerning this problem are already available through her state department of education and or the state SNA, an affiliate of the NASN. The state department of education Web site provides definitions and laws relevant to health services provided in schools. She notes that it presents the state's nurse practice act as a source of information, but the act fails to address school nursing specifically. She discovers that state law allows for UAP to provide health services, and there must be an RN with a baccalaureate degree in nursing as a school district supervisor, although not necessarily on-site. The state law specifically states that licensed personnel are preferred but not required to provide school health services.

On the SNA Web site, Leanna locates a district map and identifies the area representatives who are responsible for overseeing school nursing and school health services in public schools for all the counties in the state. She contacts these representatives and asks the following questions:

- How many schools represent their district?
- How many school nurses are employed in the district?
- How many school districts use the model of UAP who provides health services with an RN supervisor?
- Have these schools ever employed school nurses, and if yes, when and why did their policy change?
- What is the ratio of school nurses to children?

These *local data* are particularly important because they reveal trends across the state and allow Leanna to compare her state to the nation. She can obtain data from neighboring school districts that encounter the same or similar challenges as hers. According to the state SNA documents, out of 42 school systems in her district, only three school systems employ UAP with one supervising RN. Statewide there are 19 school systems using this model out of a total of 342 state school systems.

Based on this information, Leanna believes she has enough initial data to provide the basis for her response to the school board. To guide her in finding the best available evidence, she formulates the following two PICO questions:

1. What is the effectiveness of the school nurse in providing school health services to students, staff, faculty, and administrators?
2. What is the effectiveness of UAP in providing school health services to students, staff, faculty, and administrators?

See Table 22■1 for more guidelines for developing PICO questions.

Table 22■1   **Narrowing the Focus and Generating Questions**

Broad	What are the best practices for providing school health services?
Narrow	What are the best practices for providing school health services in the United States?
Narrow	What are the best practices for providing school health services for urban school districts with a diverse student population?
Searchable PICO	What is the effectiveness of the school nurse in providing school health services versus the use of Unlicensed Assistive Personnel to students, staff, faculty and administrators?

Population: students, staff, faculty and administrators.

Intervention: school nurses.

Comparison: unlicensed assistive personnel (UAP).

Outcome: school health services.

Acquire/Diagnose

After assessing the local data and the apparent problem, you can proceed to the next step of the evidence-based practice process and determine how you will *acquire the best available evidence*. Depending on your experience with searching, this step may be challenging and in some circumstances it may be prudent to request the assistance of your local school, public, or academic librarians. However, prior to meeting with the librarian, you will need to take some steps to expedite this process. You may want to provide the librarian with your question(s) and a list of key words. Look at the key words used in related articles; frequently, you can locate these key words on the first page of the article. For example, you may have been using the term "school nurse" but notice that other authors use "school health providers" as a keyword. In addition, you may want to access the U.S. National Library of Medicine, Medical Subject Headings Web site (U.S. National Library of Medicine, n.d.). This site provides an online MeSH browser to assist you in identifying descriptors/keywords. For example, when you enter "school health services," the site will display a list of related descriptors such as "health services school," "school health," and "school-based health." This is a good method for adding to and verifying your list of keywords. Be sure to use words from your PICO question, and thinking of synonyms and alternate spellings will assist you in your search.

For the first PICO question (effectiveness of school nurses), Leanna searches for clinical practice guidelines that are based on systematic reviews of randomized clinical trials and tested health services outcomes in schools with RNs and in schools using UAP. If there is no guideline, she can search for systematic reviews or primary research using bibliographic databases such as CINAHL or Medline. After developing a list of keywords, Leanna works with a local community college academic librarian and uses the search strategy and keywords listed in Table 22■2.

In an effort to find ideal sources first, Leanna and the academic librarian first search the online National Guideline Clearinghouse (NGG) (http://www.guidelines.gov).

Table 22■2 **Keywords and Search Strategy for Bibliographic Databases**

PICO	Synonyms	Search Strategy
What is the effectiveness of the school nurse in providing school health services versus the use of UAP to students, staff, faculty and administrators?		
I = school nurse	Nursing, School	Link with OR
C = UAP	UAP Nurse's Aides Nursing Assistants Certified Nurses Assistants Certified Nurses Aides	Link with OR
O = school health services	Health services school School health School-based health services Services, school health	Link with OR
I + C + O		Link with AND

UAP = unlicensed assistive personnel

Using a Boolean search strategy, Leanna uses the term "school nurs*" to start her search. This strategy reveals 15 recommended guidelines; however, on close review, the guidelines focus more on management of chronic illnesses found in school-age children. No results yield guidelines focusing on the overall "effectiveness" of the school nurse. When she searches "school nurs*" and "school health" together, the results reveal two guidelines, but they are also not specific to her question.

Leanna and the librarian discuss expanding the search to find any pertinent synthesized evidence or primary research published within the past 5 years, using bibliographic databases such as CINAHL and Medline. They use the same key words plus the word "research" and limit the search for publications between 2005 and the present. That strategy results in 10 articles. However, on close review, two articles refer to school nursing in the United Kingdom, three are integrative reviews, and four do not specifically address the effectiveness of the school nurse.

One study by Baisch, Lundeen, and Murphy (2011), "Evidence-Based Research on the Value of School Nurses in an Urban School System," warrants further scrutiny. To widen her search, Leanna closely reviews the reference lists in the integrative review articles, seeking hitherto undiscovered but relevant research. This hand searching is an additional strategy that sometimes reveals pertinent literature. Then she searches using "Unlicensed Assistive Personnel" or "UAP" plus "school health services," and identifies one additional study. Unfortunately, the study examined an educational program for UAP and did not specifically address their effectiveness in providing school health services.

Finally, a search of the Cochrane Library and Joanna Briggs Institute Library of Systematic Reviews did not reveal any relevant systematic reviews pertinent to her question. Because Leanna has found only one research article for possible use, she decides to broaden her strategy to find studies relevant to nursing outcomes in other areas of nurse practice. She uses the following Boolean strategy: "quality nursing care" OR "nursing outcomes" OR "failure to rescue" AND "ped* nurs*" OR "nurs*" AND "research." Leanna selects Search All Text to find more results. Her search result identifies two research articles, but she discards both studies because they do not apply to her circumstances and locality.

Not discouraged by the absence of synthesized and limited primary research, Leanna decides the one study applies to her situation, and it warrants further appraisal in her quest for the best available evidence. In addition, she identifies the three national organizations or associations whose position or opinion statements regard qualifications and the need for school health services by school nurses. These statements are possible evidence for justifying the retention of school nurses in her district. The position papers and statements would constitute expert opinion narrative—not the strength of evidence she was hoping for but still evidence that warrants critical appraisal.

Appraise/Plan

You must critically appraise each research study to determine if it is done well and is it basically good enough to use in your argument. Leanna wants only solid research as she makes the case that the school board should retain the school nurse positions. The study she has found must be of high quality and apply to her question. There are various tools available for critical appraisal of primary research. Standardized appraisal tools are important in evaluating research to answer the basic questions:

- What were the results of the study and what do they mean to my problem?
- Are the results valid?
- Can the findings of the study be applied locally to this situation?

The answers to these three questions are not a simple yes or no; many times the answer is somewhere in the middle and ambiguous. Therefore, it is important for you to use a standardized appraisal tool that matches the type of evidence that you are considering. For example, in the study by Baisch et al. (2011), the authors identify their research design as mixed method, but it is not the traditional mix of quantitative and qualitative methods. This study used two quantitative approaches: descriptive (survey) and quasi-experimental. Because of this, it requires two distinct critical-appraisal tools, both applicable to quantitative research. First, Leanna appraises the study's cross-sectional descriptive approach; she uses the Joanna Briggs Institute Critical Appraisal Checklist for Descriptive/Case Series Studies (Fig. 22■1). Here is her evaluation of the descriptive design in the study by Baisch et al. (2011):

- *Authors selected an appropriate sample* for this descriptive study and reflected an urban school environment; 81% of schools meeting the inclusion criteria responded.
- *Inclusion criteria* were clear; the study used only schools funded by Title I, and all employ only baccalaureate-prepared RNs to provide school health services.

JBI Critical Appraisal Checklist for Descriptive/Case Series Studies			
	Yes	No	Unclear
1. Was study based on a random or pseudo-random sample?	☐	☐	☐
2. Were the criteria for inclusion in the sample clearly defined?	☐	☐	☐
3. Were confounding factors identified and strategies to deal with them stated?	☐	☐	☐
4. Were outcomes assessed using objective criteria?	☐	☐	☐
5. If comparisons are being made, were there sufficient descriptions of the groups?	☐	☐	☐
6. Was follow-up carried out over a sufficient time period?	☐	☐	☐
7. Were the outcomes of people who withdrew described and included in the analysis?	☐	☐	☐
8. Were outcomes measured in a reliable way?	☐	☐	☐
9. Was appropriate statistical analysis used?	☐	☐	☐

Overall appraisal: ☐ Include ☐ Exclude ☐ Seek further info.

Comments (including reasons for exclusion):

FIGURE 22▪1 JBI Critical Appraisal Checklist for Descriptive / Case Series Studies. (Courtesy of the Joanna Briggs Institute, Adelaide, Australia.)

- *Confounding factors* were identified and strategies to deal with them were stated.
- Outcomes were assessed using *objective criteria.*
- *Description of comparison groups* was adequate (described by position within schools: principals/assistant principals, clerical staff and teachers).
- *Follow-up* was carried out over a sufficient *period of time* (10-week data collection period; surveys were collected directly after a meeting).
- *Outcomes of those who withdrew* were described—this criterion does not apply because the survey was anonymous, making it impossible to identify nonresponders.
- Outcomes were measured in a *reliable but not necessarily valid* way; although the researchers acknowledge the satisfaction survey was used with nurses in other settings, it was validated for use with school nurses.
- *Appropriate statistical analysis* was used and appropriate for the level of measurement reflected in the survey.

   In this appraisal process, Leanna's biggest challenge is her doubt that she understands the appropriateness of the statistical procedure in relationship to the data. To overcome that doubt, she calls on nursing faculty from her undergraduate program and consults them. She feels better after discussing the problem with more experienced nurses, and they confirm she is on the right track.

Next, Leanna appraises study's second method: the quasi-experimental matched control design. For this method, Leanna selects the Joanna Briggs Institute's Critical Appraisal Checklist for Comparable Cohort/Case Control Studies (Fig. 22■2). She identifies the following strengths of the study by Baisch et al. (2011):

- The *sample* is clearly representative of the population for this district: health records of elementary students in schools with and without a school nurse.
- *Data collection*: All elementary student records were reviewed at the same point.
- *Bias* has been minimized in the selection of cases because the study used all health records for elementary students.
- Outcomes are clearly assessed using *objective criteria*.
- *Follow-up* was carried out over a sufficient period of time.
- *Outcomes of people who withdrew* were not pertinent to this study: it included all health records of students and reported no exclusions.
- Outcomes were clearly measured in a *reliable* way: the researchers reported completeness of health records and immunization rates between program and matched schools—data obtained from official school records.
- Appropriate *statistical analysis* was used in analyzing health record data.

JBI Critical Appraisal Checklist for Comparable Cohort/ Case Control			
	Yes	No	Unclear
1. Is sample representative of patients in the population as a whole?	☐	☐	☐
2. Are the patients at a similar point in the course of their condition/illness?	☐	☐	☐
3. Has bias been minimized in relation to selection of cases and controls?	☐	☐	☐
4. Are confounding factors identified and strategies to deal with them stated?	☐	☐	☐
5. Are outcomes assessed using objective criteria?	☐	☐	☐
6. Was follow-up carried out over a sufficient time period?	☐	☐	☐
7. Were the outcomes of people who withdrew described and included for analysis?	☐	☐	☐
8. Were outcomes measured in a reliable way?	☐	☐	☐
9. Was appropriate statistical analysis used?	☐	☐	☐

Overall appraisal: ☐ Include ☐ Exclude ☐ Seek further info.

Comments (Including reasons for exclusion):

FIGURE 22■2 JBI Critical Appraisal Checklist for Comparable Cohort / Case Control (Courtesy of the Joanna Briggs Institute, Adelaide, Australia.)

Beyond published research and systematic reviews, policymakers also base their decisions on expert opinion. As Craig and Smyth (2007) point out, "Indeed, in instances where there is no good-quality research evidence to underpin practices, expert opinion becomes the source of evidence on which clinical recommendations/ guidelines are based" (p. 216). For Leanna's question, three professional organizations explicitly support having a school nurse located in every school to provide school health services. The three organizations were the NASN, AAP, and NAESP. Leanna is curious about the origin of the NASN recommendation, as it was not evident on the organization's Web site. She makes a mental note of this issue and decides she will contact the organizations personally to obtain an explanation for the basis for their recommendations. Leanna contacts the nurse researcher at NASN and discusses the association's recommendation regarding the use of registered nurses with baccalaureate degrees as providers of school health services; she wants to know how that specific position originated. The researcher says she believes the decision was based on consensus opinion but could not offer any particulars about the discussions or concerns of the panel working on the "Position Statement on Education, Licensure, and Certification of School Nurses" (NASN, 2002). In addition, Leanna requests information concerning her knowledge of gray literature sources related to her question.

From her previous search, Leanna has selected three expert opinion sources to critically appraise. Although expert opinion is not the level of evidence Leanna originally hoped to find, she acknowledges this is still important available evidence to justify her position to the school board. She chooses the position statements of NASN and the APP, and the NAESP 2008–2009 platform document. The NASN (2002) statement asserts that "it is the position of the National Association of School Nurses that every school-aged child deserves a school nurse who is a graduate of a baccalaureate degree program from an accredited college or university and licensed by that state as a registered nurse. These requirements are the minimal preparation for the skills needed at the entry level of school nursing practice" (p. 1).

To assess these position statements, Leanna uses NOTARI, the Joanna Briggs Institute Critical Appraisal Checklist for Narrative, Opinion, and Textual Papers (Fig. 22■3). Leanna identifies the following strengths of the expert opinion by the NASN:

- Although the statement is signed by the authors, it is unclear if other persons were involved in this opinion.
- The source of opinion does have standing as an expert in the community. The NASN is the recognized professional organization for school nurses; it currently has 50 affiliate state school nurses' organizations.
- The interest of the school nurse in providing health services to students is clearly the focus of the opinion, as seen in the goal of the organization to "provide children and youth with access to the primary school health-care resource, the school nurse."
- The opinion's basis in logic/experience is clearly argued. The authors describe the issue with relevant factors that impact children and support the need for a more comprehensive delivery of health-care services in schools.

JBI NOTARI Critical Appraisal Checklist for Narrative, Opinion, and Textual Papers			
	Yes	No	Unclear
1. Is the source of the opinion clearly identified?	☐	☐	☐
2. Does the source of the opinion have standing in the field of expertise?	☐	☐	☐
3. Are the interests of patients the central focus of the opinion?	☐	☐	☐
4. Is the opinion's basis in logic/experience clearly argued?	☐	☐	☐
5. Is there reference to the extant literature/evidence and any incongruence with it logically defended?	☐	☐	☐
6. Is the opinion supported by peers?	☐	☐	☐

Overall appraisal: ☐ Include ☐ Exclude ☐ Seek further info.

Comments (including reasons for exclusion):

FIGURE 22■3 JBI NOTARI, Critical Appraisal Checklist for Narrative, Opinion, and Textual Papers. (Courtesy of the Joanna Briggs Institute, Adelaide, Australia.)

- The argument is developed analytically: authors identify a detailed rationale about why they take their position.
- An extensive reference list is provided, incorporating many other associated professional organizations' statements.
- The position statement indicates the support of the American Academy of Pediatrics.

Overall appraisal: Include this study when developing justification for retaining school nurses as the provider of school health services.

Leanna appraises her second expert opinion, the American Academy of Pediatrics' position statement on the role of the school nurse in providing school health services. Again using NOTARI, the Joanna Briggs Institute Critical Appraisal Checklist for Narrative, Opinion, and Textual Papers (see Fig. 22■3), Leanna identifies the following strengths of the expert opinion by the APP's Council on School Health:

- An extensive list of members of the council on school health is provided.
- The source of opinion does have standing as an expert in the community. The APP is a recognized professional organization of 60,000 pediatricians; in addition, the association has a council specifically focusing on school health and the role of the school nurse.
- The interest of the students/children is clearly the focus identified in the background discussion supporting their position.
- The opinion's basis in logic/experience is clearly argued through a detailed discussion of the crucial role of the school nurse in providing school health services.

- The argument is developed analytically, identifying a detailed rationale for the AAP's position and focusing on the importance of a working relationship between school nurse and pediatrician to promote the health of children.
- The AAP authors provide an extensive list of research references that serves as a basis for its position.
- The position statement indicates the support of the National Association of School Nurses.

Overall appraisal: Include this study when developing justification for retaining school nurses as the provider of school health services.

As her third expert opinion, Leanna identifies the 2008 platform of the National Association of Elementary School Principals (NAESP). NOTARI, the Joanna Briggs Institute Critical Appraisal Checklist for Narrative, Opinion, and Textual Papers (see Fig. 22■3), will serve as the appraisal guide. Appraising this expert opinion, Leanna identifies the following strengths and weaknesses:

- The source of the opinion is clearly identified as the Delegate Assembly; however, the opinion does not list names of the members.
- The source of opinion does have standing as an expert in the community. The NAESP is a recognized professional organization that has both state and international affiliates; it sponsors conferences and offers considerable opportunities for professional development for members.
- The interest of the students/children and the need for school nurses are clearly two of the many focuses of their platform document.
- The opinion's basis in logic/experience is clearly presented; the oganization discusses meeting the health needs of children by providing every elementary school with a full-time school nurse.
- The argument is developed analytically, identifying the many health problems to which elementary children may be exposed.
- An extensive reference list is *not* provided in the platform document.
- There was *no* specific evidence that the opinion was supported by peers or other similar professional groups.

Overall appraisal: Include this study when developing justification for retaining school nurses as the provider of school health services.

After careful appraisal and recommendations of her sources, Leanna selects the levels of evidence and the strength of each recommendation. Levels of evidence are usually related to how much confidence you can have in the appraised sources. To rank the sources, Leanna uses the following A to D scale:

- Grade A = strong support that merits application; evidence from a systematic review or from a precise, randomized controlled trial
- Grade B = moderate support that merits consideration; evidence from single well-defined studies
- Grade C = moderate support that merits consideration; evidence from case series or expert consensus
- Grade D = evidence that does not support the adoption of the practice

Apply/Implement

Although Leanna would have preferred finding stronger evidence regarding the effectiveness of school nurses in providing school health services, she is feeling confident she has the best available evidence at this point in time. She is pleased the appraised documents are unmistakably consistent regarding the necessity for school nurses to assume direct responsibility for school health services. Reflecting on her college courses, she now understands why her professors stressed that nursing needs research evidence as a catalyst for change. However, she also acknowledges the complexity of her current situation.

As a guiding implementation framework for evidence-based decisions, she selects the PARIHS model (Promoting Action on Research Implementation in Health Service) (Kitson, Harvey, and McCormack, 1998; Kitsen, Rycroft-Malone, Harvey, et al., 2008). This model asserts that successful implementation of the evidence is based on the type of evidence, the context in which the evidence is implemented, and the facilitation of the process. As a facilitator for changing minds and policies in this chapter's clinical story, Leanna realizes she cannot reach that goal merely by presenting the evidence. She also needs to examine the context of the situation (school, school board, and community). Ultimately, she will need to include her colleagues and vested stakeholders related to retaining school nurse positions in every school.

Leanna arranges a meeting with all the school nurses in her district and informs them of evidence findings. In the course of their meeting, they identify key stakeholders who need to be involved. The group identifies parents, administrators, teachers, staff, local pediatricians, and community clinic health-care personnel, and Leanna arranges another meeting to discuss the situation and evidence with them.

In addition, Leanna turns to her state SNA to assist her through this process by identifying the strength of the context and illustrating how to use the best evidence to change thinking and policy. As Mallory (2010) points out, "Although implementing evidence based practice changes in the practice setting is usually seen as a major responsibility of the practice environment, nursing societies are ideally positioned to provide expert knowledge about the best evidence for practice and readily available resources for facilitating practice changes" (p. 283).

In this situation, leaders from the state SNA can best serve and support Leanna by helping her gain a clearer perspective on the organizational culture that surrounds the school district and school board. She turns to them for their expertise and assistance in convincing the school board to implement the evidence. Here are some strategies:

- Assess if the professional societies related to school health services and school nurses have established toolkits to address this issue, including identified leaders who have expertise in this area (Eagle, Garson, Beller, et al., 2010).
- Identify a core group and/or change champions to support the policy of retaining school nurses as the providers of school health services (Eaton, 2009).
- Provide the school board with quality-evaluation evidence that school nurses positively influence immunization rates, absenteeism, the accuracy of student health records, and efficient management of student health concerns.

- Provide the school board with quality data that show the relationship /impact between nurses as the health service providers and the child's school performance and satisfaction of parents and staff (Maughan, 2003; Read, Small, Donaher, et al., 2009; Winland and Shannon, 2004).

Assess/Evaluate

Part of the evidence-based process is evaluating the effectiveness of a combined strategy to change policy. Leanna assesses all components of her strategy to persuade the school board to uphold the recommendations of professional associations and organizations that every school should have an RN. She knows the outcome of the school board's decision will have a profound effect on the community. In an effort to enhance the recognition of the school nurses, she is going to study for school nurse certification and encourage her colleagues to follow her example.

The health-care services provided for the students are the main concern for the school nurses. However, the process of implementing those services is an important assessment. Leanna will continue to work with her state SNA to enhance the practice of school nursing and to implement established evidence-based practices relevant to her role (Box 22■1).

■ Summary

As Leanna continues functioning as head nurse in her school district, she realizes that the field of school nursing needs both more primary research and systematic

---

BOX 22■1 **Tools for Learning and Practice**

- Generate your own list of keywords and then access the National Library of Medicine Web site (http://www.nlm.nih.gov/nlmhome.html) and click on MeSH. Type in one of your keywords then click on Find Exact Words to see what other terms are identified. Compare your list to those identified.
- Search the Internet for the term "gray literature." What is the relevance of gray literature to evidence-based practice?
- Search the Internet for the relevance of hand searching to evidence-based practice.
- Search for additional organizations with opinions concerning school nurses providing health-care services.
- Search the Internet for the 2006 SHPPS summary report. Identify states that require specific student-to-nurse and school-to-nurse ratios meeting Healthy People guidelines.
- Search the Internet to find states that require newly hired school nurses to have specific educational, licensure, and certification status.

reviews. She feels fortunate to have congruent expert opinion evidence to support her position, as it enhances her confidence in attempting to sway the school board. The *asking of the question* was paramount in preceding to *acquiring data*—that is, her search for the best available evidence. Her *appraisal of the evidence* was challenging, and she learned to rely not only on expert opinion but the expertise of others such as the librarian, nursing faculty, and professional organizational leaders. In the *application* of the evidence, she realizes this process is best done in collaboration with others. As she *evaluates* retrospectively, Leanna knows she has learned a great deal through this endeavor. Most important, she now sees the evidence-based process along with the nursing process as co-contributors to her role as a school nurse.

CHAPTER QUESTIONS

1. In this example chapter's clinical story of justifying the effectiveness of the school nurse, how would you compare and contrast the steps of the evidence-based process and the nursing process?

2. In this example, Leanna uses three professional organizations' position statements or platforms as expert-opinion evidence. What are your thoughts regarding the selection of these organizations to justify her position? Were they appropriate? Should she only have used only the two professions (NSNA and APP) whose priorities directly relate to health needs of children as sources of evidence? Was it suitable to use the NAESP's platform as a source of evidence?

3. Knowing that there are many other factors that can affect this situation, what other PICO questions could you Leanna have asked?

4. Reflecting on some of the implementation strategies offered, what other strategies would you suggest? What evidence do you have to support your proposed strategies?

5. What challenges did Leanna encounter in applying the PARIHS framework to this situation? What are the nature and type of evidence? What are the qualities of the context? How is the process facilitated?

6. Develop a plan for how Leanna and her colleagues could achieve stakeholder support to back up their position. Would you identify additional stakeholders?

7. Pearson, Field, and Jordan (2007) argue that in the absence of rigorously derived research, it is not defensible to discount expert opinion as nonevidence. Do you agree or disagree with this statement?

8. What do you think will be the school board's response to Leanna's arguments? What additional questions do you think the board might have for Leanna? What do you think board members will identify as strengths in her arguments? What weaknesses might be apparent to the board?

References

American Academy of Pediatrics. (2008). The role of the school nurse in providing school health services. *Pediatrics, 21,* 1052–1056. doi:10.1542/ppeds.2008-0382

American Academy of Pediatrics (AAP) Council on School Health. Retrieved from www.app.org/sections/schoolhealth.

American Nurses Association. (2007). *Assuring safe, high quality health care in pre-k through 12 educational settings* [Monograph]. Silver Spring, MD: Author.

American School Health Association. (2010). What school administrators can do to enhance student learning by supporting a coordinated approach to health. Retrieved from http://www.ashaweb.org/files/public/Miscellaneous/Administrators_Coordinated_Approach_Support.pdf

Baisch, M. J., Lundeen, S. P., & Murphy, M. K. (2011). Evidence-based research on the value of school nurses in an urban school system. *Journal of School Health, 81,* 74–80.

Craig, J. V., & Smyth, R. L. (eds.). (2007). *The evidence-based practice manual for nurses.* New York: Elsevier.

Eagle, K. A., Garson, A. J., Beller, G. A., et al. (2003). Closing the gap between science and practice. *Health Affairs, 22,* 196–201. doi:10.1377/hlthaff.22.2.196

Eaton, L. H. (2009). Oncology nursing science priorities. In J. Phillips & C. King (eds.), *Advancing oncology nursing science.* Pittsburgh, PA: Oncology Nursing Society.

Kann, L., Brener, N. D., & Wechsler, H. (2007). Overview and summary: School health policies and programs study 2006. *Journal of School Health, 77,* 385–397.

Kitson, A., Harvey, G., & McCormack, B. (1998). Enabling the implementation of evidence based practice: A conceptual framework. *Quality Health Care, 7,* 149–158. doi:10.1136/qhsc.7.3.14.9

Kitson, A., Rycroft-Malone, J., Harvey, G., et al. (2008). Evaluating the successful implementation of evidence into practice using the PARIHS Framework: Theoretical and practical challenges. *Implementation Science, 3.* doi:10.1186/1748-5908-3-1

Mallory, G. A. (2010). Professional nursing societies and evidence-based practice: Strategies to cross the quality chasm. *Nursing Outlook, 58,* 279–286.

Maughan, E. (2003). The impact of school nursing on school performance: A research synthesis. *The Journal of School Nursing, 19,* 163–171.

National Association of Elementary and Secondary School Principals. *NAESP platform, 2008–2009.* (Obtained in PDF format from the NAESP, 1615 Duke St., Alexandria, VA 22314; *NAESP platform 2010–2011* is available at http://www.naesp.org/naesp-platform-2010-2011)

National Association of School Nurses. (1999). Definition of school nursing. Castle Rock, CO: Author. Retrieved from http://www.nasn.org.

National Association of School Nurses. (2002). Position statement on education, licensure, and certification of school nurses. Retrieved from http://www.nasn.org/Default.aspx?tabid=219

National Association of School Nurses. (2010a). Caseload assignments: Position statement. Retrieved from http://www.nasn.org/Portals/0/positions/2010pscaseload.pdf

National Association of School Nurses. (2010b). Public comment submitted March 15, 2010, on the proposed rule for the meaningful use of electronic health records. Retrieved from http://www.nasn.org/portals/0/legislation/2010_03_15_meaningful_use_comment.pdf

Pearson, A., Field, J., & Jordan, Z. (2007). *Evidence-based clinical practice in nursing and health care: Assimilating research, experience, and expertise.* Oxford: Blackwell.

Read, M., Small, P., Donaher, K., et al. (2009). Evaluating parent satisfaction of school nurse services. *Journal of School Nursing, 25,* 205–213.

Robert Wood Johnson Foundation. (2010). Charting nursing's future: Unlocking the potential of school nursing: Keeping children healthy, in school, and ready to learn. Retrieved from http://www.rwjf.org/files/research/cnf14.pdf

U.S. Department of Health and Human Services, Office of Disease Prevention and Health Promotion. Objectives. Retrieved from http://healthypeople.gov/2020/topicsobjectives2020/pdfs/Educational-Programs.pdf

U. S. National Library of Medicine. (n.d.). Suggestions for authors. Retrieved from http://www.nlm.nih.gov/mesh/authors.html

Winland, J., & Shannon, A. (2004). School staff's satisfaction with school health services. *The Journal of School Nursing, 20,* 101–106.

Academic detailing— An expert, usually from an academic organization, who works closely with staff to develop evidence-based interventions.

Accountability— An assumption of responsibility for one's actions and decisions.

Acquire— Using your question to determine how to search for the evidence and find the best information that links the question related to the patient problem with potential solutions.

Acute care setting— An entity that provides services to patients with acute care needs as opposed to chronic rehabilitative or palliative needs, such as a medical-surgical hospital unit.

Ad hoc committees— Committees that spawn from the original group, allowing key stakeholders to work with nurses to support implementation of evidence-based practice innovations.

Advocate— To champion or support the patient to meet her needs and wishes.

Agency for Healthcare Research and Quality (AHRQ)— A U.S. federal-level agency that supports research and policies to help people make more informed decisions and improves the quality of health-care services.

AGREE tool— A standardized appraisal tool for practice guidelines, rigorously developed by an international group of experts.

American Health Policy Association— An association whose mission is to advance quality of care and patients safety nationwide.

American Health Quality Association— An association whose mission is to advance quality of care and patients safety nationwide.

ANCC Magnet Recognition [registered symbol]— A program, offered by the credentialing arm of the American Nurse's Association, that recognizes health-care organizations for quality patient care, nursing excellence and innovations in professional nursing practice. Consumers rely on the designation as the ultimate credential for high-quality nursing.

Animal assisted therapy— The use of animals as a tool to achieve a therapeutic effect.

Apply— Putting evidence into action and practice.

Appraise— To critically evaluate the evidence for its quality and applicability.

Ask— To state a clear question that will lead to the right evidence for your problem.

Assess— To gather data from physical assessment, laboratory data, and from what the patient says in order to make a judgment about a patient's condition. In the 5 As of evidence-based practice, assess means to evaluate outcomes using the same methods that could be used to assess a patient's condition.

Attitude of inquiry— Being curious, somewhat skeptical, and willing to pursue the evidence.

Audit and feedback— The process of making clinical observations of behaviors against specific criteria and feeding back the findings of the audit to the stakeholders.

Authority to change practice— Ability to have control over or influence practice.

Autonomy— Independence or free will to make choices.

Available resources— In the context of evidence-based practice, the resources available to implement evidence including the right people (human resource), technology, equipment, and money.

Barriers— Any organizational, person, or resource gap or impediment that will challenge change.

Benchmarking— A standard, based either an average performance among agencies or other means of setting a standard. The purpose is to establish a level of quality that can then be used to judge the quality care.

Beneficence— A moral obligation to help another.

Best available research evidence— Best available represents two principles, available and best. *Available* implies the evidence that is accessible but only after an exhaustive and transparent search of multiple databases of published and unpublished literature. *Best* means that the investigator has rigorously appraised the evidence and determined it to be the highest, although often less than ideal, evidence.

Best practice— Generally accepted, informally standardized techniques, methods, or processes that seem to accomplish given tasks. Some best practices reflect the best available evidence, whereas others represent consensus opinion.

Beveridge model— A single-payer system in which health care is provided and financed by the government through a system of tax payments.

Bias— When a study is conducted in a way that might lead to an erroneous conclusion.

Bibliographic database— Searchable index of published literature that contains abstracts, a synopsis of articles, and (sometimes) the full text of articles. It is organized by taxonomy of keywords. Examples include the Cumulative Index of Nursing and Allied Health Literature (CIHAHL) and MEDLINE.

Bismark model— A model that uses an insurance system jointly financed by employers and employees. Bismark-type health insurance plans are mandated to cover all citizens, and they do not make a profit. Although this is a multipayer system, tight regulations give government as much cost control clout as in the singlepayer system.

Boolean operators— Logical connectors including OR, AND, and NOT combined with keywords and phrases to structure a search in a bibliographic database.

"Borderless" evidence/knowledge— External, global evidence that crosses the boundaries of countries or disciplines.

Case-controlled study— Study in which researchers select cases (those with a particular condition) and the control group (those without the condition) and compare the two groups' outcomes.

Centers for Disease Control and Prevention (CDC)— A U.S. federal agency providing expertise, information, and tools to protect the public's health—through health promotion; prevention of disease, injury, and disability; and preparedness for new health threats.

Centers for Medicare & Medicaid Services (CMS)— A U.S. federal agency that administers the Medicare program, providing health-care security and choice for aged and disabled people. Jointly with the state governments, CMS administers the Medicaid program and the State Children's Health Insurance Program (SCHIP).

Centre for Reviews and Dissemination (CRD)— An online source of internationally developed systematic reviews. The CRD is made available from the National Institute for Health Research (NIHR) and the University of York.

Chief nursing officer (CNO) or chief nursing executive (CNE)— The most senior nursing leader in the organization who is administratively responsible for all aspects of the nursing care, including budget, patient care services, and so on. Sometimes the CNO or CNE carries the title of vice president.

Clinical decision making— When health-care providers choose among alternatives to affect a health outcome of individuals or groups.

Clinical expertise— Practical know-how that comes from professional experience. It is often integrated automatically when making decisions; it is tacit and intuitive but is strongest when exposed for critique and analysis.

Clinical nurse specialist (CNS)— An advanced practice nurse with graduate preparation (master's or doctoral degree); a clinical expert in a specialized area of nursing practice and in the delivery of evidence-based nursing interventions. The CNS provides direct and indirect care to patients and families as well as influences nursing personnel and organizations.

Clinical practice guidelines— When well constructed, they are a form of synthesized evidence designed to provide comprehensive recommendations about the diagnosis, management, or treatment of a particular condition or clinical question. The best guidelines are built upon systematic reviews.

Cochrane Collaboration— An international network of people founded in 1993. Multiple disciplines write systematic reviews and publish them in the Cochrane Library. The collaboration provides access to the reviews and other resources to help health-care providers, policy makers, patients, and their advocates make well-informed decisions about health care.

Cochrane Library— One of the most comprehensive collections of systematic reviews, controlled trials, and evidence-based health-care sources. It is composed of six databases: the Cochrane Database of Systematic Reviews (CDSR), Cochrane Central Register of Controlled Trials (CENTRAL), Cochrane Methodology Register (CMR), Database of Abstracts of Reviews and Effects (DARE), Health Technology Assessment (HTA) Database, and NHS Economic Evaluation Database (EED).

Cohort study— A study with a control group and a cohort group in which the cohorts share a characteristic (e.g., having a condition or having an occupation) and the control group is alike in all respects except the unique cohort characteristic.

Comparison— In a PICO question, the *C* stands for comparison. When comparing one intervention against another, one may include a comparison intervention in the question. The comparison may be another nursing intervention or taking no action at all.

Complex problems— Tend to be unique, are associated with a great deal of uncertainty, and are less predictable than other problems.

Complicated problems— Usually made up of a series of simple problems.

Conceptual framework— An abstract, theoretical approach that describes, explains, or predicts a set of variables and relationships to explain a phenomenon.

Conceptual research utilization— One thinks differently after understanding research but does not change his or her behavior.

Conduct and Utilization of Research in Nursing (CURN) Project— One of two large national projects aimed at improving how nurses evaluate and use research.

Context— The practice environment, including the subelements of organizational culture, leadership, and evaluation practices; the surroundings of the phenomenon or person.

Context of care— The environment or setting in which the proposed change is to be implemented.

Core measures— A set of care processes that helps institutions improve quality of patient care by focusing on outcomes.

Cost sharing— Employers require individuals to pay a portion of their health-care premium.

Credibility— In appraisal of qualitative research, it refers to how well the researcher made every effort to report an honest representation of the true voices of the participants.

Critical appraisal— Judging the quality of information in terms of its validity and degree of bias (quantitative research) and credibility and dependability (qualitative research). This is a critical step in the evidence-based practice process.

Critical Appraisal Skills Program (CASP)— Provides a set of tools appropriate for critical appraisal of both quantitative and qualitative methodologies.

Cumulative Index to Nursing and Allied Health Literature (CINAHL)— Bibliographic database that contains over 2 million abstracts from nearly 3000 English-language journals and full-text English-language journal articles from over 600 journals published since 1981.

Data— Observations, narrative, or measurements produced through the conduct of either qualitative or quantitative research.

Deductible— The amount of out-of-pocket expenses before the insurance company will cover remaining costs.

Dependability— In qualitative research, it refers to whether the results are logical, transparent, and clearly documented.

Descriptive framework or model— A framework or model that describes the nature of the elements of a phenomenon or process without making claims about the nature or direction of relationships among phenomena or concepts.

Easy to read— See Readability. Sometimes "easy to read" is used instead of readability, meaning that a piece is written so it can be read by people with lower literacy skills.

Effectiveness— The extent to which an intervention, when used appropriately, achieves the intended effect. Clinical effectiveness is about the relationship between an intervention and clinical or health outcomes.

Embase— Bibliographic database that contains over 20 million abstracts and full-text articles from over 7000 peer-reviewed global journals published since 1974. Viewed as one of the most global sources of abstracts and full-text articles, Embase may have limited availability in U.S. nursing schools and hospital libraries.

Embedded evidence— When policies, protocols, and pathways transparently use evidence.

Empirical quality outcome— A measurement of patient-centered and organizational health outcomes that is the result of an organizational commitment of excellent nursing care.

Empowerment— Increasing the spiritual, political, social, or economic strength of individuals and communities.

Enculturation— The process by which a person learns the requirements of the surrounding culture, and acquires values and behaviors appropriate or necessary in that culture.

Environment— Immediate surroundings or sociopolitical or economical context of the person.

Epistemology— Foundations of knowledge or ways of knowing.

Evidence-based health care— Clinical decision making that considers the best available evidence, the context in which the care is delivered, client preference, and the professional judgment of the health professional.

Evidence-based medicine movement— An approach to clinical decision making in medicine that uses research evidence instead of pathophysiological rationales, intuition, previous clinical experience, and expert opinion to determine appropriate interventions for patient care.

Evidence-based practice (EBP)— The conscientious, explicit, and judicious use of current best evidence in making decisions about the care of individual patients. It means integrating individual clinical expertise and patient preferences with the best available external clinical evidence from systematic research in a context of limited resources.

Evidence-based practice movement— A global initiative aimed at using an evidence-based approach to clinical decision making.

Evidence-based practice process— Problem solving that includes the following steps: identifying a problem, asking specific questions, acquiring evidence, appraising the evidence for its quality, applying the evidence, and assessing the outcomes of the intervention.

Evidence generation— Process of conducting primary research.

Evidence hierarchies— Systems used to rank evidence statements according to certain criteria.

Evidence/knowledge transfer— The act of transferring knowledge to individual health professionals, health facilities, health systems, and consumers by means of journals, other publications, electronic media, education, training, and decision support systems so that practitioners and patients can understand and use it in decision making.

Evidence synthesis— A pooling of available research findings through the process of systematic review.

Evidence utilization— The use of evidence to bring about practice or system change at point of care.

Experience— Knowledge and skill acquired through being involved in or exposed to practice over a period of time.

Expert consensus opinion— Occurs when experts in an area of science discuss and come to an agreement about the best approach to a problem. The best expert consensus opinion would involve a systematic and rigorous method to determine a conclusion that is then exposed to public opinion or external critique.

Expertise— See Clinical expertise.

Expert opinion— Presentation of pertinent data by one with special skill or knowledge representing a mastery of a particular subject. Evidence that draws on the expert knowledge of individuals or group; it is not research-based evidence.

Explanatory framework or model— A framework or model that specifies cause-and-effect relationships and mechanisms.

External evidence— Evidence from rigorous research, external to a local setting.

Facilitation— The process of enabling or making easier the implementation of evidence into practice.

Facilitators— Those who enable others to bring about an outcome or change in behavior through skillful negotiation, coaching, teaching, etc.

Forces of Magnetism— A term associated with the Magnet recognition program, it refers to the attributes or outcomes that exemplify excellence in nursing. Organizations must fully operationalize these 14 attributes in order to be considered for recognition. The new model of the program consolidates these 14 attributes into 5 components: transformational leadership, structural empowerment, exemplary professional practice, new knowledge, innovation and improvements and empirical quality results.

Google Scholar— Internet search engine in which results include only information that is freely available from the Internet; therefore, the results do not include abstracts or articles found only within subscription-based bibliographic databases. Use caution and understand that results will not be comprehensive and often do not freely link to the full-text journal articles.

Grading of Recommendations Assessment, Development, and Evaluation (GRADE) Working Group— The GRADE Working Group is an international group of evidence-based medicine experts who aim to provide a standard system that guideline developers can use to grade the quality of the evidence and the strength of recommendations and clinicians can understand without deep backgrounds in critical appraisal.

Hand searching— Looking through the references cited or a bibliography.

Health— How a person experiences wellness and illness along a continuum.

Health Care Commission— An agency that regulates care provided by the NHS, local authorities, private companies, and voluntary organizations. Aiming to make sure better care is provided for everyone—in hospitals, care centers, and people's own homes. It seeks to protect the interests of people whose rights are restricted under the Mental Health Act.

Health literacy— The degree to which individuals have the capacity to obtain, process, and understand basic health information and services needed to make appropriate health decisions.

Heuristic— A "rule of thumb" or structure for problem solving.

High-alert medications— Those medications that can cause significant harm if administered incorrectly.

Homogeneity— The degree that different studies measure the effects of interventions in the same way with limited variability to enable them to be combined in a meta-analysis.

Hospital-acquired conditions (HACs)— Conditions that are (a) high cost or high volume or both, (b) result in the assignment of a case to a diagnostic-related group (DRG) that has a higher payment when present as a secondary diagnosis, and (c) could reasonably have been prevented through the application of evidence-based guidelines.

Implementation science— The scientific study of methods to promote the systematic uptake of clinical research findings and other evidence-based practices into routine practice, and hence to improve the quality and effectiveness of health care. It includes the study of influences on health-care professional and organizational behavior.

Incidence— The occurrence rate of new conditions.

Indian Health Services (IHS)— An operating division within the U.S. Department of Health and Human Services that provides medical and public health services to member of federally recognized Native American tribes and Alaskan tribes.

Innovation— The creation or improvement of interventions, products, technologies, or ideas.

Institute for Healthcare Improvement (IHI)— An independent, not-for-profit organization based in Cambridge, Massachusetts, IHI focuses on motivating and building the will for change; identifying and testing new models of care in partnership with both patients and health-care professionals; and ensuring the broadest possible adoption of best practices and effective innovations.

Institute of Medicine (IOM)— A nongovernmental organization within the National Academies of Science. It is highly regarded for its reports, as it recruits the highest level of experts to study and advise the decision makers on scientific matters including health.

Instrumental research utilization— Application of research in some concrete way.

Intervention— The nursing treatment or action that is the *I* part of a PICO question.

Iowa model— Developed at the University of Iowa Hospital, the purpose of this evidence-based practice model is to guide practitioners through a series of decision points as they move through the evidence implementation process.

Iterative— Dynamic, back-and-forth way of considering information.

Joanna Briggs Institute (JBI)— Founded in 1996 by Alan Pearson PhD, RN. It is a multidisciplinary international collaboration of centers and groups that engages in all aspects of evidence-based practice including evidence synthesis, evidence transfer, and implementation. The institute provides many different resources for health-care providers.

Joanna Briggs Institute (JBI) Library of Systematic Reviews— A subscription-based library of rigorous, peer-reviewed systematic reviews. Protocols, another term for systematic review proposals, can also be found in the library.

Joanna Briggs Institute (JBI) model— Describes the role of evidence generation, synthesis, transfer, and utilization in improving global health with an emphasis on tools and strategies to make each phase operational for local providers.

Joint Commission (JC)— An independent, not-for-profit organization that accredits and certifies more than 18,000 health-care organizations and programs in the United States.

Joint Commission Patient Safety Goals (NPSGs)— Established to help accredited organizations address specific areas of concern regarding patient safety.

Joint Commission Performance Standard— A health-care leadership standard used to judge the eligibility of health-care agencies (such as hospitals) to become accredited.

Journal clubs— Clinician or student groups that meet to discuss research, systematic reviews, and evidence-based practice protocols to generate an awareness of evidence-based practice.

Keyword— A significant or descriptive word used as a reference point for finding other words or information.

Knowledge translation (KT)— The transmission of knowledge from research and other sources into everyday practice.

Levels of evidence— A system to rank confidence in research designs to control extraneous variables (questions of effectiveness) or offer credibility (questions of meaning).

Levels of recommendations— A system to rank recommendations based on the quality of the evidence, the magnitude of the effect, and the balance of harm and effectiveness. Some systems such as GRADE (the Grading of Recommendations, Assessment, Development, and Evaluation) incorporate both quality of the evidence and the strength of the recommendations.

Literature review— Often the first step in writing a paper or developing a research proposal. Its purpose is to summarize information from various authors and sources. Literature reviews help in the understanding of background issues and determining the scope of an area of literature. However, because they lack the rigor of other types of reviews, you should not directly inform your clinical decisions using casual literature reviews.

Lobbyists— Persons who attempt to influence legislation on behalf of special interests.

Local context— The environment in which the evidence is used and that affects the uptake of the evidence. The local context can be as narrow as a unit or as broad as a country.

Local evidence— See Local data.

Local data— Internal evidence that is obtained systematically from local sources and may include audit data, performance evaluations, feedback from a wide range of stakeholders, knowledge about the culture of an organization, and patient stories and narratives.

Local evidence— See Local data.

Magnet model— Now in its second generation, the model illustrates a framework for nursing practice and research that serves as a road map for organizations pursuing Magnet recognition. It describes five components encompassed by the global issues in nursing and health care and encompasses the previous 14 forces of magnetism conceived in the first-generation model.

Magnitude— Refers to the "so-what" factor, or how big an effect the intervention makes on the outcome.

Meaning— The subjective interpretation that an individual places on something.

Meaningfulness— The extent to which someone experiences an intervention, activity, or phenomena.

Medicaid— Funded by both the federal government and the states. It is administered at the state level. It covers low-income children and their families.

Medical Literature Analysis and Retrieval System (MEDLINE)— The National Library of Medicine's bibliographic database, available by subscription through most nursing school libraries. It contains over 18 million abstracts and full-text journal articles from over 5400 global journals published since 1947.

Medicare— A U.S., federally funded program that insures persons 65 years and older and some individuals with disabilities. Part A pays for hospital care, Part B, for physician services, and Part D, for prescription benefits.

MeSH subject headings— Medical subject headings (MeSH) were designed as a controlled vocabulary for medicine by the U.S. National Library of Medicine. Arranged in alphabetical and hierarchical structure, MeSH subject headings allow for more organized and accurate searching.

Meta-aggregation— A process of combining findings of individual qualitative studies (cases) to create summary statements that authentically describe the meaning of themes.

Meta-analysis— A statistical method that allows for the combination of the results of many studies to aggregate the conclusions into data that is stronger than that of just one study.

Meta-synthesis— A process of combining findings of individual qualitative studies (cases) to create summary statements that authentically describe the meaning of themes.

Meta-paradigm— Meta-paradigm is the broadest perspective of a discipline. The nursing meta-paradigm describes the concepts that are essential to the nursing domain. The four concepts in the nursing meta-paradigm are person, health, environment, and nursing.

Model— Representations of a real phenomenon that are narrower than theories or frameworks. They usually represent a specific situation, and are made of more precise assumptions.

Moral decision making— A step-by-step guide to decision making that includes the following steps: recognizing the moral issue, identifying the participants/ stakeholders, distinguishing the values involved, weighing the benefits and burdens, looking for analogous situations, discussing with appropriate people, ascertaining organizational rules and legal codes, and examining one's own comfort with the decision.

Multipayer system— System in which more than one party is responsible for payment of health care.

Narrative data— Narrative data are data elicited through stories and verbal communications, often gathered through qualitative research methods.

Narrow confidence intervals— A statistical term that means how precisely the statistic estimates the true population value and to what degree of probability you can be sure of the estimate.

Nasogastric/orogastric (NG/OG) tube— A tube inserted either through the nostrils or mouth into the esophagus and advanced to the stomach.

National Association of Elementary and Secondary Principles (NAESP)— An organization whose mission is to advocate for every child to receive the world's best elementary and secondary education.

National Association of School Nurses (NASN)— A nonprofit specialty nursing organization that represents school nurses and is dedicated to improving the health and educational success of children.

National Guideline Clearinghouse— An online collection of clinical practice guidelines hosted by the Agency for Healthcare Quality and Research.

National Health Insurance model— Contains elements of both the Beveridge and Bismark models. It uses providers from the private sector, but reimbursement comes from a government-run insurance company that is funded by all residents.

National Health Service (NHS)— Manages the publicly funded health-care system in the United Kingdom. It was designed by William Beveridge.

National Hospital Quality Measures— Efforts by the Centers for Medicare & Medicaid Services and the Joint Commission to establish common national hospital performance measures and to share a single set of common documentation.

National Institute for Health and Clinical Excellence (NICE)— In the United Kingdom, an independent organization responsible for providing national guidance on promoting good health and preventing and treating ill health. NICE develops and defines the standards of health care that people can expect to receive. These standards indicate when a clinical treatment (or set of clinical procedures) is considered highly effective, cost effective, and safe as well as being viewed as a positive experience by patients.

National Quality Forum (NQF)— A U.S. nongovernmental organization that operates under a three-part mission to improve the quality of American health care by building consensus on national priorities and goals for performance improvement and working in partnership to achieve them; endorsing national consensus standards for measuring and publicly reporting on performance; and promoting the attainment of national goals through education and outreach programs.

National Service Framework (NSF)— Strategies that set clear quality requirements for care. These are based on the best available evidence of what treatments and services work most effectively for patients.

Nature of evidence— Fundamental characteristics of evidence and knowledge such as its purpose, type, quality, and usefulness.

Never events— Extremely serious, preventable, patient safety incidents that should not occur if the relevant evidence-based practice measures are in place.

Nonmaleficence— A moral obligation to not harm.

Nursing— The protection, promotion, and optimization of health and abilities; prevention of illness and injury; alleviation of suffering through the diagnosis and treatment of human response; and advocacy in the care of individuals, families, communities and populations.

Nursing actions— How nurses intervene to protect, promote, and optimize health and abilities. Nurses act to prevent illness and injury; alleviate suffering; and advocate for individuals, families, communities, and populations to produce beneficial outcomes.

Nursing process— The nursing process serves as an organizational framework for practicing nursing. It includes assessment, nursing diagnosis, planning, implementation, and evaluation.

Nursing-sensitive indicators— Reflect the structure, process, and outcomes of nursing care. Patient outcomes that are determined to be nursing sensitive are those that change based on the quantity or quality of nursing care (e.g., pressure ulcers, falls, and intravenous infiltrations).

Nursing-sensitive patient outcomes (NSPOs)— Confirm nurses' contributions to patient care in areas such as quality of life, symptom management, safety, functional status, and utilization of nursing resources.

Nursing standard— An authoritative statement by which the nursing profession describes the responsibilities for which its practitioners are accountable; the outcomes for which registered nurses are responsible; and by which the quality of practice, service, or education can be evaluated.

Nursing theory— Aims to describe, predict, and explain the phenomena important to nursing.

Nursing traditions— Nurses performing as they do for no other reason than habit.

Observational study— A study that draws inferences about the possible effect of a treatment on subjects, in which the assignment of subjects into a treated group versus a control group is outside of the control of the investigator.

Occupational hazard— A working condition that places a person at increased risk for harm as a result of his or her job.

Occupational Safety and Health Act (OSHA) of 1970 — An act that mandates that, in addition to compliance with hazard-specific standards, all employers have a general duty to provide their employees with a hazard-free workplace.

Opinion leaders— Well-respected colleagues who can influence others in the setting.

Organizational culture— The psychology, attitudes, experiences, beliefs, and values of an organization. It depends on the type of leadership, available resources, enculturation of value for evidence-based practice, expectation of nurses, and the individual nurse.

Ottawa Model of Research Use (OMRU)— A model focused on three phases that prescribe how to assess, monitor, and evaluate the evidence implementation process. It focuses on the innovation, the adopters, the practice environment, implementation strategies, and the outcomes.

Outcome— The specific effect(s) of an intervention or what matters to the nurse, patient and/or the health-care system. It is what the nurse would use to evaluate whether the intervention had a beneficial or harmful effect on the patient, nurse, or organization.

Out-of-pocket model— In nations that are too poor to have any formalized health care, rich citizens pay out of pocket for health care, whereas the poor citizens cannot afford care and usually stay sick or die.

PARIHS (Promoting Action on Research Implementation in Health Services) framework— A framework describing the factors that contribute to successful implementation of evidence. It can be described as SI = f(E, C, F), where SI is successful implementation of evidence, f = function of, E is evidence, C is context, and F is facilitation.

Patient education— The process by which health professionals and others impart information to patients for the purpose of empowering them to make decisions that will improve their health status.

Patient preference— The right of an individual to be involved in the planning of his or her own care and ultimately having the final say about which interventions he or she chooses to accept or not accept. A patient's values, desires, and contributions to clinical decision making in the evidence-based practice process.

Patient Protection and Affordable Care Act (PPACA)— A recently enacted, large bill in the United States with many provisions that may change over time. Although the law is currently being challenged in the courts, and it is difficult to predict what will be the final outcome, it includes provisions to enhance effective health practices in the United States.

Patient-mediated strategies— Strategies to actively engage patients to improve their knowledge, experience, service use, health behavior, and health status.

Pay-for-performance— Reimbursement based on outcomes.

Peer-reviewed journals— Journals containing scholarly articles are approved through a peer-review process of multiple reviewers who hold advanced degrees within the discipline, teach within the field, are experts in the profession, and are very knowledgeable about the topic.

Person— Individuals, families, communities, and the integrated aspects of the biophysical, psychological, sociological, and spiritual person/family/community.

Persuasive research utilization— Using research to influence others.

Phenomenon of interest— The part of a patient's experience that you want to understand.

PICO question— A question about the effectiveness of interventions in which *P* represents population, *I* equals intervention, *C* stands for comparison intervention, and *O* is outcome.

PICo question— A question in which *P* represents population, *I* stands for phenomena of interest, and *Co* stands for context.

Pluralistic approach— In evidence-based practice, accepting evidence from quantitative and qualitative research as well as discourse as legitimate sources of evidence.

Population— The group of people that are of concern in the question. This group may be related by a disease, a health condition, risk profile, the environment in which they exist, age, or any combination of these factors.

Potential adopters— Practitioners, policy makers, patients, and other stakeholders who may accept or play a role in change guided by evidence.

Practice environment— Setting and social factors in which a change will occur; includes governing rules and cultural and social factors such as local politics, power structures, resource availability, leadership approaches, and peer groups.

Pre-appraised, digested evidence— Evidence sources where someone else has already done the hard work of searching, appraising, and summarizing the evidence.

Pre-appraised evidence— Evidence that has already been appraised and ranked for its quality and/or strength.

Predictive framework or model— Forecast of how phenomena will behave and how they relate to each other and tend to generate propositions and hypotheses.

Pressure ulcer— Localized injury to the skin and/or underlying tissue, usually over a bony prominence, as a result of pressure or pressure in combination with shear.

Printed information sheets— Printed patient information sheets prior to discharge that describe medications.

Prevalence— The ratio (for a given time period) of the number of occurrences of a disease or event to the number of units at risk in the population.

Primary source or primary study— An article or report in which researchers publish data they collected first hand.

Problem solving— Defining problem and cause, generating alternative solutions, selecting alternative solutions, carrying out solutions, and evaluating effects.

Professional standards— Appropriate standards of care based on the Nursing Scope and Standards of Practice developed by professional organizations.

Prompts— Cues in the clinical setting to enhance attention to an intervention.

Public Health Resource Unit (PHRU)— A division of the United Kingdom's National Health Service that provides Critical Appraisal Skills Program (CASP) tools.

Public policy— Whatever governments choose to do, or choose not to do.

PubMed Central— A free Internet resource made available by the U.S. National Institutes of Health (NIH) and managed by the National Center for Biotechnology Information (NCBI) at the National Library of Medicine. It provides access to Medline's 18 million abstracts and limited full-text articles from participating journals, publisher Web sites, and other Internet sites.

PubMed Central's Clinical Queries— A place to search for free, full-text systematic reviews within the National Library of Medicine's database, PubMed.

Qualifications— A quality/accomplishment that fits a person for some function.

Qualitative research— Methods of inquiry that include an array of methodologies that attempt to explore the meaning and experience of phenomena.

Questions of appropriateness— Clinical questions that address how appropriate a given activity or intervention is related to the context in which the care is given.

Questions of effectiveness— Clinical questions that relate to the efficacy of interventions on patient outcomes.

Questions of feasibility— Clinical questions that relate to the extent a particular activity would be practical or practicable.

Questions of meaningfulness— Clinical questions that address how people experience a particular phenomenon.

Randomized controlled trial (RCT)— An experimental research design in which the investigator randomly assigns participants in a trial to either a treatment or control (no treatment) group.

Randomized controlled trial (RCT) with concealed randomization— RCT in which participants are assigned to a treatment or control group and the researcher manipulates whether or not the group receives the treatment or control.

RAPid— A program from the Joanna Briggs Institute (JBI) used to perform rapid appraisals of primary research.

Rapid critical appraisal— A method allowing clinicians to quickly appraise evidence to determine its validity and applicability to practice, and a user-friendly critical appraisal approach.

Readability— How easy it is to read and understand written material.

Regression equation— A statistical technique that is used to predict the behavior of a dependent variable.

Reminders— An embedded memory aid.

Research— A diligent and systematic inquiry or investigation into a subject to discover or revise facts, theories, applications, etc.

Research knowledge— Knowledge gained through investigation.

Research process— A formal, systematic process of identifying and developing an area of inquiry and a research question, and using a methodology to generate data to answer the question.

Research utilization— A complex process in which knowledge, in this case in the form of research, is transformed from the findings of one or more studies into possible nursing interventions, the ultimate goal of which is use in practice.

Respect for patients' values— To give particular attention or regard to what patients deem important.

Review of the literature (ROL)— Encompasses a strategic search for current knowledge on a given subject. A person searches all literature on a specific topic to find out what has been published on the subject. Depending on the focus, the search may include multiple databases within multiple disciplines. The results of the search may include informational articles, research findings, and theoretical papers.

Rigor— In the context of research, the degree that the researchers ensure high-quality methods are used that lead to valid or credible results or findings.

School health nurse— A professional nurse who provides health services in schools.

School health provider— A broader term for people who provide health services in schools.

School health services— Services provided to children and sometimes families through the school.

Scale— Relates to how much of the scope of the issue you wish to address.

Scope— Relates to the breadth of the question. You might define scope in terms of setting, population, age, group, or other category.

Search strategy— The plan to find evidence in various databases that includes the keywords, how to link keywords together and filter sources by their type, year of publication, language, etc.

Secondary sources— Report on the work of others, not on the author's own original research findings.

Shared decision making— A decision-making process jointly shared by patients and their health-care provider; it is a key part of evidence-based practice because it brings together clinical expertise and patient preference.

Shared governance— A structural configuration of councils and committees that provides formal mechanisms that ensures nurses' responsibility, right, and power to make decisions and to control nursing practice.

Single-payer system— A system in which only a single entity pays the bill.

Skill set— A set of basic techniques that you need to carry out a task.

Social contract— The explicit or implicit obligations nurses meet in their relationship with patients and their families.

Social policy— Policies that address things such as welfare, crime, education, and health care.

Standards of nursing practice— Authoritative statement by which the nursing profession describes the responsibilities for which its practitioners are accountable; the outcomes for which registered nurses are responsible; and by which the quality of practice, service, or education can be evaluated.

Standardized subject headings— Specific subject terms developed by the Library of Congress to organize large subjects logically into categories.

State Children's Health Insurance Program (SCHIP)— Funded by both the federal government and the states to provide health care to children whose families earn too much income to qualify for Medicaid but do not have enough money to pay for private insurance.

Strength (of evidence)— Relates to the quality or believability of the evidence.

Structural supports— Supports that help nurses achieve expected performance levels and externalize the internal cultural value for evidence-based nursing practice.

Synopses— Short, abridged summaries of a longer source of evidence.

Syntheses— Systematic reviews of quantitative or qualitative evidence that follow explicit methods of search, appraisal, and analysis of the evidence.

Systematic reviews— A rigorous secondary research method that incorporates a comprehensive search, critical appraisal, and synthesis of either quantitative or qualitative research; it addresses a focused clinical question using methods designed to reduce the likelihood of bias.

Tacit knowledge— Implicit or unspoken knowledge largely associated with expertise, experience, and tradition.

Theory-guided practice— The use of theory to describe, predict, and explain the phenomena important to nursing for the purpose of improving practice.

Tradition— An inherited pattern of thought or action that leads to a specific, long-standing practice.

Transferability— The degree to which the results of the study can be applied to other contexts.

Transparent— When an evidence source is transparent, the authors provide a great deal of details about purpose and methods so that someone else might reproduce the study or systematic review.

TRICARE— A program that provides health coverage to all military retirees, their spouses, survivors, and other qualified dependents.

Truncation— A symbol, typically an asterisk (*) in bibliographic databases, that can be applied to the end of a keyword to retrieve all the words beginning with that word.

Unit practice councils— A formal venue to allow nurses to voice their concerns and be involved in making practice changes. They allow for the exploration of practice issues and create opportunities for supporting evidence-based practice.

U.S. Department of Health and Human Services (HHS)— The federal agency with primary responsibility of protecting the health of Americans and providing essential human services, especially for the most needy.

Veterans Health Administration (VHA)— A federally funded and administered program for veterans. Health care is delivered in government-run health-care facilities.

Western Interstate Commission on Higher Education (WICHE) Project— Like the Conduct and Utilization of Research in Nursing (CURN) Project, a national project aimed at increasing nurses' utilization of research.

Wildcards— A symbol, typically a question mark in bibliographic databases, that can be inserted within a word to retrieve all the words with alternate spellings of the same word.

Workplace violence— Violence or the threat of violence against workers.

World Health Organization (WHO)— WHO is the directing and coordinating authority for health within the United Nations system. It is responsible for providing leadership on global health matters, shaping the health research agenda, setting norms and standards, articulating evidence-based policy options, providing technical support to countries, and monitoring and assessing health trends.

Worldview— Frame of reference and how we fit our experiences into our representation of the world.